Updates in Clinical Dermatology

Series Editors

John Berth-Jones, University Hospitals Coventry & Warwickshire, NHS Trust, Coventry, UK

Chee Leok Goh, National Skin Centre, Singapore, Singapore

Howard I. Maibach, Department of Dermatology
University of California San Francisco Department of Dermatology
ALAMEDA, CA, USA

Shari R. Lipner, Dermatology, Weill Cornell Medicine
New York, NY, USA

Updates in Clinical Dermatology aims to promote the rapid and efficient transfer of medical research into clinical practice. It is published in four volumes per year. Covering new developments and innovations in all fields of clinical dermatology, it provides the clinician with a review and summary of recent research and its implications for clinical practice. Each volume is focused on a clinically relevant topic and explains how research results impact diagnostics, treatment options and procedures as well as patient management. The reader-friendly volumes are highly structured with core messages, summaries, tables, diagrams and illustrations and are written by internationally well-known experts in the field. A volume editor supervises the authors in his/her field of expertise in order to ensure that each volume provides cutting-edge information most relevant and useful for clinical dermatologists. Contributions to the series are peer reviewed by an editorial board.

Hazel H. Oon • Chee Leok Goh

Editors

COVID-19 in Dermatology

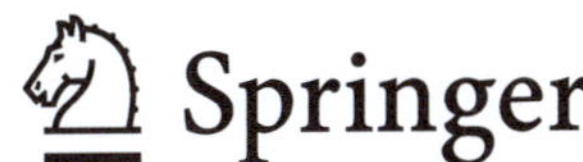

Editors
Hazel H. Oon 🆔
National Skin Centre
Singapore, Singapore

Chee Leok Goh
National Skin Centre
Singapore, Singapore

ISSN 2523-8884 ISSN 2523-8892   (electronic)
Updates in Clinical Dermatology
ISBN 978-3-031-45588-9 ISBN 978-3-031-45586-5   (eBook)
https://doi.org/10.1007/978-3-031-45586-5

© The Editor(s) (if applicable) and The Author(s), under exclusive license to Springer Nature Switzerland AG 2023
This work is subject to copyright. All rights are solely and exclusively licensed by the Publisher, whether the whole or part of the material is concerned, specifically the rights of translation, reprinting, reuse of illustrations, recitation, broadcasting, reproduction on microfilms or in any other physical way, and transmission or information storage and retrieval, electronic adaptation, computer software, or by similar or dissimilar methodology now known or hereafter developed. The use of general descriptive names, registered names, trademarks, service marks, etc. in this publication does not imply, even in the absence of a specific statement, that such names are exempt from the relevant protective laws and regulations and therefore free for general use.
The publisher, the authors, and the editors are safe to assume that the advice and information in this book are believed to be true and accurate at the date of publication. Neither the publisher nor the authors or the editors give a warranty, expressed or implied, with respect to the material contained herein or for any errors or omissions that may have been made. The publisher remains neutral with regard to jurisdictional claims in published maps and institutional affiliations.

This Springer imprint is published by the registered company Springer Nature Switzerland AG
The registered company address is: Gewerbestrasse 11, 6330 Cham, Switzerland

Paper in this product is recyclable.

SARS-CoV-2, the etiologic agent of COVID-19, caught the world by surprise. The pandemic as declared by the World Health Organization (WHO) lasted slightly more than 3 years and was declared not a global public health emergency on 5 May 2023. But the virus lingers on, and the disease has become endemic. Although the respiratory system is the primary target, the infection is systemic in nature and the skin is not excluded from its direct or indirect effects.

This book is timely and aptly collates skin manifestations, explores the possible biological mechanisms, sets up of a skin registry and delves into therapeutic approaches. The use of face masks, an effective non-pharmaceutical intervention, has led to unintended consequences on the skin. The long hours of use of tight-fitted N95 respirator masks by healthcare workers left injuries to the skin, and even prolonged use of surgical masks resulted in rashes and other skin conditions. Similarly, mRNA vaccine has its own unintended effect on the skin.

I applaud and congratulate the editors and all contributors to this book that undoubtedly will serve as a valuable educational material.

National Centre for Infectious Diseases   Yee Sin Leo
and National Healthcare Group
Singapore, Singapore

Preface

Since the first cases of an acute respiratory illness were reported in China in 2019, the pathogen SARS-coV-2 (severe acute respiratory syndrome coronavirus 2) and its disease COVID-19 have disrupted the world and changed the course of medical history. Dermatologists, residents and allied health professionals were sent out to care for patients with COVID-19, clinics were under lockdown and supplies of critical drugs such as biologics and meladinine were delayed. The prolonged impact of disease has taken its toll on patients, their carers, medical staff, research and medical education. Throughout this period, the dermatology community has stepped forward by quickly characterising COVID-19 rashes, their various morphologies and pathogenesis, drafted guidelines and implemented measures on how best to deliver care with new means such as teledermatology, and whether immunosuppressive medication should be halted or continued during infection. Medical education in dermatology has changed with more asynchronous and online learning. Yet with the move to more technology-based means and social distancing, how can we retain the personal touch and prevent burnout and depersonalisation amongst our patients, healthcare workers, residents and medical students?

Shortly after the first landmark studies of COVID-19 vaccine trial data were made known, global mass vaccination programmes were underway. Vaccine technology has expanded beyond messenger RNA (mRNA) to include non-replicating viral vectors, inactivated virus and protein subunits. Cutaneous manifestations of vaccine reactions, including non-mRNA and their morphological patterns, indications and contraindications, vaccine global access, equity, allocation of booster doses, emerging COVID variants and subvariants, waning vaccine and treatment efficacy are the issues that begged to be explored. New oral therapies are available for treatment of COVID-19 but they bring with them drug-drug interactions and potential side effects.

This book represents a compilation of the concerted efforts of dermatologists across the globe to join hands against COVID-19. We bring you content from experts in each individual chapter. They have, each of them, first-hand experience on their topic and have synthesised the literature to bring you up to date on this fast-paced, changing landscape of COVID-19 in dermatology. We hope that together we can future-proof our practices to better meet the demands and challenges of this elusive disease.

Singapore, Singapore
Singapore, Singapore

Hazel H. Oon
Chee Leok Goh

Contents

The Science of COVID-19

Shi Yu Derek Lim, Pei Hua Lee, Laurent Renia,
Jean-Marc Chavatte, Raymond Tzer-Pin Lin,
Lisa F. P. Ng, and Hazel H. Oon

Introduction

The severe acute respiratory syndrome coronavirus-2 (SARS-CoV-2), responsible for coronavirus disease 2019 (COVID-19), was first identified in January 2020, after the initial outbreak of a mysterious respiratory illness in Wuhan, Hubei province, China (Wu et al. 2020).

The virus rapidly spread worldwide. As of writing, over 750 million cases and 6.8 million deaths have been reported globally, with only Turkmenistan having no reported cases thus far (World Health Organization 2023). However, as underreporting of cases exists, these figures probably underestimate the global disease burden of COVID-19.

S. Y. D. Lim (✉) · H. H. Oon
National Skin Centre, Singapore, Singapore
e-mail: dereklimsy@nsc.com.sg;
derm@hazeloon.com

P. H. Lee
National Centre for Infectious Diseases,
Singapore, Singapore

Department of Infectious Diseases, Tan Tock Seng
Hospital, Singapore, Singapore
e-mail: peihua_lee@ttsh.com.sg

L. Renia
Lee Kong Chian School of Medicine, Nanyang
Technological University, Singapore, Singapore

A*STAR Infectious Diseases Labs (A*STAR ID
Labs), Agency for Science, Technology and Research
(A*STAR), Singapore, Singapore
e-mail: renia_laurent@idlabs.a-star.edu.sg;
lcsrenia@ntu.edu.sg

J.-M. Chavatte
National Public Health Laboratory, National Centre
for Infectious Diseases, Singapore, Singapore
e-mail: Jean-Marc_CHAVATTE@moh.gov.sg

R. T.-P. Lin
National Public Health Laboratory, National Centre
for Infectious Diseases, Singapore, Singapore

Department of Microbiology and Immunology, Yong
Loo Lin School of Medicine, National University of
Singapore, Singapore, Singapore
e-mail: Raymond_Lin@ncid.sg;
micltprv@nus.edu.sg

L. F. P. Ng
A*STAR Infectious Diseases Labs (A*STAR ID
Labs), Agency for Science, Technology and Research
(A*STAR), Singapore, Singapore

National Institute of Health Research, Health
Protection Research Unit in Emerging and Zoonotic
Infections, University of Liverpool, Liverpool, UK

Institute of Infection, Veterinary and Ecological
Sciences, University of Liverpool, Liverpool, UK
e-mail: Lisa_Ng@idlabs.a-star.edu.sg

© The Author(s), under exclusive license to Springer Nature Switzerland AG 2023
H. H. Oon, C. L. Goh (eds.), *COVID-19 in Dermatology*, Updates in Clinical Dermatology,
https://doi.org/10.1007/978-3-031-45586-5_1

Virology

SARS-CoV-2 has a single-stranded, positive-sense RNA genome, enclosed by a double-layered lipid envelope and containing the spike (S), envelope (E), membrane (M), and nucleocapsid (N) structural proteins. The S glycoprotein enables the virus to penetrate the host cells by binding to ACE2 cellular receptors (Triggle et al. 2021), E protein aids virulence (Nieto-Torres et al. 2014), M glycoprotein assembles viral particles (Fu et al. 2021), and the N protein assembles and packages viral RNA (Zhu et al. 2020). Other than genes expressing the structural proteins, the genome also includes open reading frames, which encode for 16 nonstructural proteins (Chan et al. 2020). Figure 1.1 depicts a diagrammatic representation of the virus.

Upon entry into the host cell cytoplasm, SARS-CoV-2 releases its RNA genome, which is translated into replicase polyproteins, which are then further cleaved into nonstructural proteins. These drive replication and transcription with endoplasmic reticulum–derived double-membrane vesicles. Subgenomic RNA is translated to structural and accessory proteins, which are inserted into the endoplasmic reticulum–Golgi intermediate compartments. Incorporation of the positive-sense RNA genome leads to the formation of new virions, which are released from the plasma membrane (Harrison et al. 2020). Figure 1.2 depicts the virus replication

Fig. 1.1 Diagrammatic representation of SARS-CoV-2

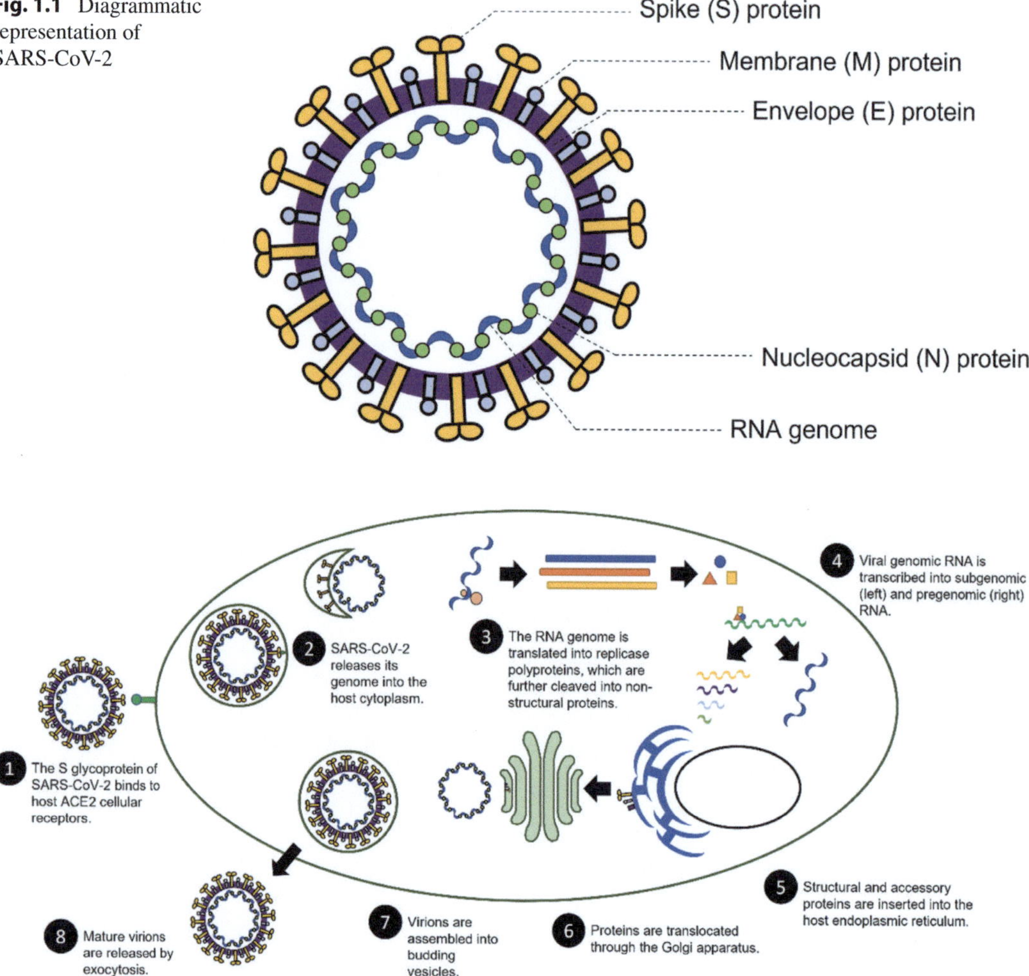

Fig. 1.2 Virus replication cycle of SARS-CoV-2

cycle of SARS-CoV-2. By inhibiting interferon production and signaling, SARS-CoV-2 proteins can evade host immunity (Rashid et al. 2022).

Genomic sequencing has revealed a high degree of genetic similarity to bat-derived betacoronaviruses, and thus, bats are believed to be the natural reservoir for the virus, with a yet-unconfirmed intermediate animal host (Lu et al. 2020).

Transmission

The primary mode of transmission of SARS-CoV-2 is via respiratory droplets and short-range airborne particles (Tabatabaeizadeh 2021). Indirect contact of mucous membranes with viral particles may also result in infection. Most transmission takes place from 1 day prior to 3 days after onset of symptoms (Del Aguila-Mejia et al. 2022). A meta-analysis found the average incubation period to be 6.57 days, with a decrease in the duration with each new variant of concern, reducing to 3.42 days with the Omicron variant (Wu et al. 2022).

Pathogenesis

SARS-CoV-2 is believed to target and first enter multiciliated cells in the upper respiratory tract or sustentacular cells lining the olfactory epithelium and ultimately disseminate to the lower respiratory tract, where it primarily infects alveolar type 2 cells, leading to alveolar damage and impairment of gas exchange. Infection triggers a host immune response with the initiation of a signaling cascade, promoting the production of type I

and III interferons. Subsequent downstream cytokine production activates adaptive responses to clear the virus (Lamers and Haagmans 2022). However, the inflammatory cascade may also contribute to the development of hypoxemia and subsequently acute respiratory distress syndrome (ARDS).

Treatment

Three main categories of therapies for COVID-19 have emerged, based on current understanding of the virology of SARS-CoV-2 and disease pathophysiology (Murakami et al. 2023). These are briefly outlined in Table 1.1.

Vaccines

The rapid development, manufacture, and administration of COVID-19 vaccines has occurred at an unprecedented pace. To date, globally combined, there are 40 different vaccines authorized for use. COVID-19 vaccines can be divided into five main categories: viral vector vaccines, nucleic acid vaccines, inactivated vaccines, live-attenuated vaccines and protein vaccines. The mechanism and examples of each type are outlined in Table 1.2.

Since 2020, COVID-19 vaccines have been rapidly developed and have been shown to be highly effective in preventing severe illness, hospitalization, and death caused by the virus, although efficacy of individual vaccines varies. Data highlight the need for booster-dose vaccines, especially against newer variants (Chenchula et al. 2022; Piechotta and Harder

Table 1.1 COVID-19 treatments, mechanisms, and examples

Treatment category	Mechanism	Examples
Anti-inflammatory agents	Therapies target and reduce hyperinflammation, which causes severe COVID-19, ARDS and death	Baricitinib, tocilizumab
Antiviral agents	Therapies target viral replication, thus reducing disease duration and severity	Molnupiravir, nirmatrelvir-ritonavir, remdesevir, ensitrelvir
Antibody-based therapies	Neutralizing antibodies target the spike protein, preventing viral entry into host cells	Convalescent plasma, bamlanivimab/etesevimab, bebtelovimab, casirivimab/imdevimab, sotrovimab, tixagevimab/cilgavimab

Table 1.2 COVID-19 vaccine types, mechanisms, and examples

Vaccine type	Mechanism	Examples
Nucleic acid	Nucleoside-modified mRNA encoding the SARS-CoV-2 spike glycoprotein is encapsulated in lipid nanoparticles for delivery to human cells. Translation of mRNA into the spike glycoprotein by the host cellular machinery leads to the production of the spike protein, capture and antigen presentation by dendritic cells, resulting in the priming of cellular and humoral immune responses	Elasomeran and davesomeran (Moderna), tozinameran and famtozinameran (Pfizer and BioNTech)
Viral vector	An unrelated virus with limited pathogenicity transmits SARS-CoV-2 genetic material encoding viral antigen proteins into cells. Release of secreted antigens leads to antigen presentation, resulting in a cellular and humoral immune response	Jcovden (Janssen and Johnson & Johnson), Covishield/Vaxzevria (University of Oxford and AstraZeneca), Sputnik V (Gamaleya)
Inactivated	Inactivated, killed SARS-CoV-2 virus particles that are not able to replicate trigger humoral and cellular immune responses	BBIBP-CorV (Sinopharm), CoronaVac (Sinovac Biotech) Covaxin (Bharat Biotech)
Live attenuated	A weakened, live SARS-CoV-2 virus mimics natural infection, stimulating cellular and humoral immunity, and the production of antibodies	COVI-VAC (Codagenix and Serum Institute of India)
Protein	Protein subunits from the SARS-CoV-2 virus (e.g., the S protein) trigger humoral and cellular immunity	Nuvaxovid (Novavax)

2022). At present, the US Centers for Disease Control and Prevention recommends one bivalent mRNA booster dose, given at least 2 months completing primary series vaccination (US Centers for Disease Control and Prevention 2023). Chapter 19 further elaborates on the vaccination recommendations for immunosuppressed patients. The optimal dosing interval and regimen are still being refined.

Lab Testing and Interpretation

Real-time reverse-transcriptase polymerase chain reaction using specimens obtained from the respiratory tract is considered as the most sensitive test for detection of SARS-CoV-2. Rapid point-of-care antigen tests have been developed, with the advantages of shorter turn-around times, though having varying levels of sensitivity, overall ranging from 40 to 80%, depending on several factors, including the quality of the test, the timing of the test, and the viral load of the person being tested (Dinnes et al. 2021; Peto and Team UC-LFO 2021; US Centers for Disease Control and Prevention 2022).

Immunoassays have been developed to detect antibodies (IgG, IgM, and IgA) against SARS-CoV-2S and N proteins. These can assess the presence and stage of infection, as well as to monitor the immune responses to vaccination. Inactivated and live-attenuated vaccines, as well as natural infection, result in the formation of anti-S and anti-N antibodies. On the other hand, only anti-S antibodies will be detected in patients who have received viral vector, nucleic acid, and protein vaccines based on the S antigen, in the absence of prior infection.

In addition, the presence of functional neutralizing antibodies may be quantified by assessing for disruption of the biochemical interaction between the receptor-binding domain of the S protein and human ACE2 receptor (Tan et al. 2020).

Mutations and Implications on Clinical Practice

Genetic mutations may result in changes in viral characteristics, which may potentially result in changes in transmissibility, disease severity, immune response, and diagnostic or therapeutic failure, which result in increased transmission and threat to public health. These are termed variants of interest (VOIs).

Variants of concern (VOCs) are defined as VOIs with actual clinical or epidemiological evidence of increased transmissibility or adverse epidemiological impact, change in presentation of illness and increased virulence, or decreased effectiveness of measures to diagnose, treat, and contain the disease. Diagnostic tests, vaccines, or treatments may have to be modified to increase detection, prevention, and treatment of circulating VOCs.

The incidence of mutations in the S gene, coding for the spike glycoprotein, is high and holds the most relevance for clinical practice. Mutations are predominantly concentrated around the N-terminal domain, receptor-binding domain, and furin cleavage site. These allow the virus to evade neutralizing antibodies and result in reduced effectiveness of vaccines and monoclonal antibodies (McLean et al. 2022). In addition, N protein mutations also allow the virus to evade detection by rapid antigen tests, leading to falsely negative results (Jian et al. 2022).

The most notable VOCs that have emerged since the dawn of the pandemic are:

1. the Alpha variant (B.1.1.7 lineage), first identified in the United Kingdom in late 2020 and quickly spread to many other countries. Multiple mutations in the spike protein result in increased transmissibility compared to the original strain of the virus (Liu et al. 2022).
2. the Beta variant (B.1.351), first identified in South Africa in late 2020. It has mutations in the spike protein that reduce its susceptibility to some of the monoclonal antibody treatments (Singer et al. 2021).
3. the Gamma variant (P.1), first identified in Brazil in late 2020. Like the Beta variant, it has mutations in the spike protein that may make it less susceptible to some treatments and vaccines (Sabino et al. 2021; Charmet et al. 2021).
4. the Delta variant (B.1.617.2), first identified in India in late 2020 and subsequently emerged as the dominant strain in many countries, including the United Kingdom and the United States. It has multiple mutations in the spike protein and is believed to be more transmissible and potentially more virulent than earlier strains of the virus (Tatsi et al. 2021).
5. the Omicron (B.1.1.529 descendant lineages) variant, first identified in South Africa in November 2021 and has since been detected internationally. The Omicron variant has a large number of mutations, including more than 30 mutations in the spike protein of the virus. Reduced disease severity but increased transmissibility are features of this VOC (Pulliam et al. 2022; Kim et al. 2021).

Conclusion

The outbreak of COVID-19 emphasizes unique challenges in public health and clinical medicine. At the same time, the unprecedented pace of vaccine rollout, therapeutics, and test development highlights the power of international, pharmaceutical, and scientific collaboration.

Funding This study is supported by the Singapore National Medical Research Council Centre Grant II Seed funding and National Skin Centre Medical Department Fund.

References

Chan JF, Kok KH, Zhu Z, Chu H, To KK, Yuan S, et al. Genomic characterization of the 2019 novel human-pathogenic coronavirus isolated from a patient with atypical pneumonia after visiting Wuhan. Emerg Microb Infect. 2020;9(1):221–36.

Charmet T, Schaeffer L, Grant R, Galmiche S, Cheny O, Von Platen C, et al. Impact of original, B.1.1.7, and B.1.351/P.1 SARS-CoV-2 lineages on vaccine effectiveness of two doses of COVID-19 mRNA vaccines: results from a nationwide case-control study in France. Lancet Reg Health Eur. 2021;8:100171.

Chenchula S, Karunakaran P, Sharma S, Chavan M. Current evidence on efficacy of COVID-19 booster dose vaccination against the omicron variant: a systematic review. J Med Virol. 2022;94(7):2969–76.

Del Aguila-Mejia J, Wallmann R, Calvo-Montes J, Rodriguez-Lozano J, Valle-Madrazo T, Aginagalde-

Llorente A. Secondary attack rate, transmission and incubation periods, and serial interval of SARS-CoV-2 omicron variant, Spain. Emerg Infect Dis. 2022;28(6):1224–8.

Dinnes J, Deeks JJ, Berhane S, Taylor M, Adriano A, Davenport C, et al. Rapid, point-of-care antigen and molecular-based tests for diagnosis of SARS-CoV-2 infection. Cochrane Database Syst Rev. 2021;3(3):CD013705.

Fu YZ, Wang SY, Zheng ZQ, Yi H, Li WW, Xu ZS, et al. SARS-CoV-2 membrane glycoprotein M antagonizes the MAVS-mediated innate antiviral response. Cell Mol Immunol. 2021;18(3):613–20.

Harrison AG, Lin T, Wang P. Mechanisms of SARS-CoV-2 transmission and pathogenesis. Trends Immunol. 2020;41(12):1100–15.

Jian MJ, Chung HY, Chang CK, Lin JC, Yeh KM, Chen CW, et al. SARS-CoV-2 variants with T135I nucleocapsid mutations may affect antigen test performance. Int J Infect Dis. 2022;114:112–4.

Kim S, Nguyen TT, Taitt AS, Jhun H, Park HY, Kim SH, et al. SARS-CoV-2 omicron mutation is faster than the chase: multiple mutations on spike/ACE2 interaction residues. Immune Netw. 2021;21(6):e38.

Lamers MM, Haagmans BL. SARS-CoV-2 pathogenesis. Nat Rev Microbiol. 2022;20(5):270–84.

Liu Y, Liu J, Plante KS, Plante JA, Xie X, Zhang X, et al. The N501Y spike substitution enhances SARS-CoV-2 infection and transmission. Nature. 2022;602(7896):294–9.

Lu R, Zhao X, Li J, Niu P, Yang B, Wu H, et al. Genomic characterisation and epidemiology of 2019 novel coronavirus: implications for virus origins and receptor binding. Lancet. 2020;395(10224):565–74.

McLean G, Kamil J, Lee B, Moore P, Schulz TF, Muik A, et al. The impact of evolving SARS-CoV-2 mutations and variants on COVID-19 vaccines. MBio. 2022;13(2):e0297921.

Murakami N, Hayden R, Hills T, Al-Samkari H, Casey J, Del Sorbo L, et al. Therapeutic advances in COVID-19. Nat Rev Nephrol. 2023;19(1):38–52.

Nieto-Torres JL, DeDiego ML, Verdia-Baguena C, Jimenez-Guardeno JM, Regla-Nava JA, Fernandez-Delgado R, et al. Severe acute respiratory syndrome coronavirus envelope protein ion channel activity promotes virus fitness and pathogenesis. PLoS Pathog. 2014;10(5):e1004077.

Peto T, Team UC-LFO. COVID-19: rapid antigen detection for SARS-CoV-2 by lateral flow assay: a national systematic evaluation of sensitivity and specificity for mass-testing. EClinicalMedicine. 2021;36:100924.

Piechotta V, Harder T. Waning of COVID-19 vaccine effectiveness: individual and public health risk. Lancet. 2022;399(10328):887–9.

Pulliam JRC, van Schalkwyk C, Govender N, von Gottberg A, Cohen C, Groome MJ, et al. Increased risk of SARS-CoV-2 reinfection associated with emergence of omicron in South Africa. Science. 2022;376(6593):eabn4947.

Rashid F, Xie Z, Suleman M, Shah A, Khan S, Luo S. Roles and functions of SARS-CoV-2 proteins in host immune evasion. Front Immunol. 2022;13:940756.

Sabino EC, Buss LF, Carvalho MPS, Prete CA Jr, Crispim MAE, Fraiji NA, et al. Resurgence of COVID-19 in Manaus, Brazil, despite high seroprevalence. Lancet. 2021;397(10273):452–5.

Singer SR, Angulo FJ, Swerdlow DL, McLaughlin JM, Hazan I, Ginish N, et al. Effectiveness of BNT162b2 mRNA COVID-19 vaccine against SARS-CoV-2 variant Beta (B.1.351) among persons identified through contact tracing in Israel: a prospective cohort study. EClinicalMedicine. 2021;42:101190.

Tabatabaeizadeh SA. Airborne transmission of COVID-19 and the role of face mask to prevent it: a systematic review and meta-analysis. Eur J Med Res. 2021;26(1):1.

Tan CW, Chia WN, Qin X, Liu P, Chen MI, Tiu C, et al. A SARS-CoV-2 surrogate virus neutralization test based on antibody-mediated blockage of ACE2-spike protein-protein interaction. Nat Biotechnol. 2020;38(9):1073–8.

Tatsi EB, Filippatos F, Michos A. SARS-CoV-2 variants and effectiveness of vaccines: a review of current evidence. Epidemiol Infect. 2021;149:e237.

Triggle CR, Bansal D, Ding H, Islam MM, Farag E, Hadi HA, et al. A comprehensive review of viral characteristics, transmission, pathophysiology, immune response, and management of SARS-CoV-2 and COVID-19 as a basis for controlling the pandemic. Front Immunol. 2021;12:631139.

US Centers for Disease Control and Prevention. Guidance for Antigen Testing for SARS-CoV-2 for Healthcare Providers Testing Individuals in the Community. 2022. https://www.cdc.gov/coronavirus/2019-ncov/lab/resources/antigen-tests-guidelines.html. Accessed 4 Apr 2022.

US Centers for Disease Control and Prevention. Interim Clinical Considerations for Use of COVID-19 Vaccines Currently Approved or Authorized in the United States. 2023. https://www.cdc.gov/vaccines/covid-19/clinical-considerations/interim-considerations-us.html. Accessed 11 Feb 2023.

World Health Organization. WHO Coronavirus (COVID-19) Dashboard. https://covid19.who.int/. Accessed 11 Feb 2023.

Wu F, Zhao S, Yu B, Chen YM, Wang W, Song ZG, et al. A new coronavirus associated with human respiratory disease in China. Nature. 2020;579(7798):265–9.

Wu Y, Kang L, Guo Z, Liu J, Liu M, Liang W. Incubation period of COVID-19 caused by unique SARS-CoV-2 strains: a systematic review and meta-analysis. JAMA Netw Open. 2022;5(8):e2228008.

Zhu G, Zhu C, Zhu Y, Sun F. Minireview of progress in the structural study of SARS-CoV-2 proteins. Curr Res Microb Sci. 2020;1:53–61.

Cutaneous Manifestations of COVID-19

Charlene Li Ping Wee, Ding Yuan Wang, and Joel Hua Liang Lim

Introduction

Coronavirus Disease 2019 (COVID-19) is a multisystemic disease, which manifests predominantly with fever and respiratory symptoms. Since its emergence, varying cutaneous manifestations of COVID-19 have been observed. The reported incidence of these manifestations varies from 4.9 to 20.4% (Sanchez-Flores et al. 2021). The main clinical patterns of COVID-19-associated cutaneous manifestations may be classified into the following morphologies: urticarial, maculopapular or morbilliform, papulovesicular, pseudo-chilblains or pernio-like, livedoid or vaso-occlusive, and purpuric (Genovese et al. 2021). Additionally, patients may also present with aggravation of preexisting chronic dermatoses. In this chapter, we will describe the various cutaneous findings associated with COVID-19 (summarized in Table 2.1).

Table 2.1 Summary of the various cutaneous manifestations of COVID-19

	Clinical features	Management
Maculopapular or morbilliform exanthem	Confluent erythematous patches and plaques that starts on the trunk with centrifugal spread; usually pruritic	Supportive management, topical corticosteroids; may consider oral corticosteroids for severe cases
Urticarial rash	Erythematous, migratory pruritic wheals primarily on the trunk that resolves within 1 day; may be associated with angioedema	Oral antihistamines and corticosteroids
Papulovesicular rash	Scattered papules and vesicles on the trunk, and less frequently on the limbs; usually not pruritic	Supportive management

(continued)

C. L. P. Wee (✉) · D. Y. Wang · J. H. L. Lim
National Skin Centre, Singapore, Singapore
e-mail: weecharlene@nsc.com.sg;
dywang@nsc.com.sg; joellimhl@nsc.com.sg

© The Author(s), under exclusive license to Springer Nature Switzerland AG 2023
H. H. Oon, C. L. Goh (eds.), *COVID-19 in Dermatology*, Updates in Clinical Dermatology,
https://doi.org/10.1007/978-3-031-45586-5_2

Table 2.1 (continued)

	Clinical features	Management
Pseudo-chilblains or pernio-like lesions	Blanchable erythematous to violaceous macules and patches with swelling or blistering on the extremities; may be mildly pruritic or tender; varies with positional change	Supportive management, avoidance of cold, topical corticosteroids; may consider topical or oral vasodilatory agents such as calcium channel blockers, and aspirin
Livedoid or vaso-occlusive lesions	*Livedo reticularis*: lace-like dusky patches forming rings with pale centers on the limbs, sparing the trunk; usually mild	Supportive management
	Livedo racemosa or retiform purpura: non-blanching discontinuous erythematous rings, branching macules or plaques, or ulcers	
Purpuric lesions	Erythematous, non-blanchable macules or plaques or hemorrhagic blisters; may occur in a generalized or localized distribution affecting the acral, intertriginous sites or buttocks	Topical or oral corticosteroids

Cutaneous Manifestations of COVID-19

To date, the pathophysiology by which SARS-CoV-2 affects various organs, including the skin, is not yet fully elucidated. The mechanism is multifactorial, involving the innate immune and humoral responses, coagulation pathways, activation of monocytes and macrophages, and release of cytokines. The risk for an organ to be affected is determined by the presence of functional angiotensin-converting enzyme 2 and transmembrane protease serine 2 viral receptors expressed on cells. These proteins are present in the cutaneous capillary endothelial cells and basal layer of the epidermis (Genovese et al. 2021).

While protean in its presentation, the variable cutaneous manifestations of SARS-CoV-2 infection predict the clinical outcome as they mirror the host's ability in eradicating the virus (Tan et al. 2021). For instance, in younger immunocompetent persons, the type 1 interferon-1 (IFN-1) response elicited is greater, resulting in successful cessation of viral replication and milder disease. In turn, the IFN-1 surge induces cutaneous microangiopathy and hence pseudo-chilblains or pernio-like lesions. On the other polar extreme, immunocompromised and elderly individuals have a blunted IFN-1 response, allowing a cytokine storm to rage, culminating in higher mortality. This florid hypercytokinemia causes prothrombosis with livedoid and ulcerative dermatoses, a catastrophic sequalae reproducibly reported in other end organs.

Maculopapular or Morbilliform Exanthem

The most commonly encountered cutaneous manifestation of COVID-19 is a confluent erythematous maculopapular or morbilliform exanthem, which is usually pruritic and predominantly occurs on the trunk and limbs (Freeman et al. 2020) (Fig. 2.1). The rash tends to be symmetrical, starts on the trunk with centrifugal spread, and resolves after approximately 1 week. Typically, the palms, soles, and mucous membranes are not involved. In most cases, the eruption coincides with the onset of other systemic symptoms including fever, cough, dyspnea, asthenia, headache, or gastrointestinal symptoms (Català et al. 2020).

Other reported subtypes of exanthems associated with COVID-19 include purpuric, erythema

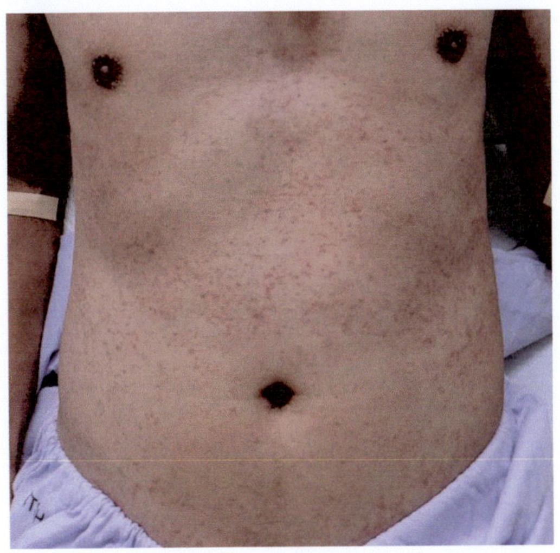

Fig. 2.1 Scattered erythematous macules and papules on the trunk

multiforme-like, pityriasis rosea-like, erythema elevatum diutinum-like, and perifollicular patterns (Català et al. 2020). Hospitalization due to pneumonia was observed more frequently in patients with morbilliform and erythema multiforme-like patterns, suggesting that these may be associated with more severe disease (Català et al. 2020). The induction of a cytokine storm and the direct cytopathic effect of SARS-CoV-2 are thought to drive the development of maculopapular rashes (Fernández-Lázaro and Garrosa 2021).

It is prudent for clinicians to exclude other viral or drug exanthems, which may present similarly. Management of the maculopapular or morbilliform rash is supportive with the use of topical corticosteroids. In more severe cases, oral corticosteroids may be administered (Genovese et al. 2021).

Urticarial Rash

Development of erythematous, migratory pruritic wheals primarily on the trunk may appear simultaneously with fever and systemic symptoms and resolve within a day without scarring. The eruption usually lasts 1 week (Galván Casas et al. 2020). Associated angioedema has been observed (Najafzadeh et al. 2020).

The binding of SARS-CoV-2 to angiotensin-converting enzyme-2 protein disrupts normal protein activity. This induces the formation of reactive oxygen species, vasodilatory molecules, and complement activation. It is proposed that complement activation and sequential degranulation of mast cells result in the formation of urticarial lesions (Abuelgasim et al. 2021). Symptoms may be alleviated with oral antihistamines and corticosteroids (Shanshal 2022a).

Papulovesicular Rash

Patients may develop scattered papules and vesicles on the trunk, and less frequently on the limbs, akin to that of varicella infection (Fig. 2.2). However, unlike true varicella, lesions are usually scattered, pruritus is mild or absent, and the scalp is not involved. The vesicles are also monomorphic, as opposed to the polymorphic nature of varicella (Fernández-Lázaro and Garrosa 2021). The eruption usually occurs 3 days after the onset of systemic symptoms and resolves by 8 days without varioliform scarring (Marzano et al. 2020). It affects middle-aged patients more commonly and is associated with moderate severity of infection (Galván Casas et al. 2020).

Given the resemblance to varicella or disseminated herpetic infection, sampling of blister fluid or fresh erosions for the presence of such viruses is prudent. Moreover, it has been shown that various herpesviridae are reactivated during the clinical course of patients with SARS-CoV-2 infection, which makes exclusion of the former even more pertinent. Should the patient be critically ill, empiric antiviral therapy can be considered. If herpesviruses are excluded, treatment is supportive as lesions are self-limiting.

Pseudo-Chilblains or Pernio-Like Lesions

Pseudo-chilblains present as erythematous to violaceous macules and papules with swelling or blistering on the extremities (Fig. 2.3). The incidence is more abundant in countries in the

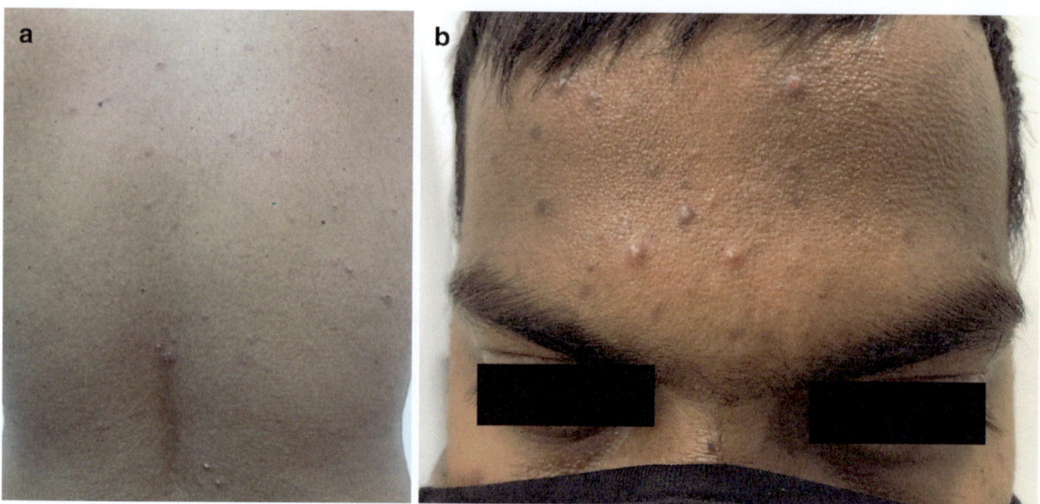

Fig. 2.2 (**a**) Erythematous papules, vesicles, and crusted erosions on the back. (**b**) Erythematous papules and vesicles on the forehead

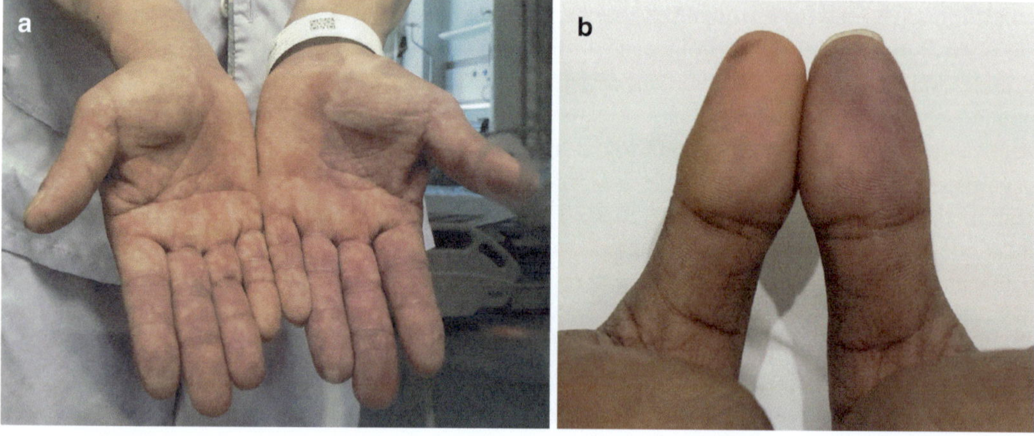

Fig. 2.3 (**a**) Violaceous macules and patches on the hands. (**b**) Reticular purpuric plaque on the left thumb

Northern Hemisphere where colder temperatures are encountered, as compared to equatorial nations with a more tropical climate. Lesions affect the toes and feet more frequently than the fingers and hands and are associated with mild pruritus or tenderness (Wollina et al. 2020). Rarely, pseudo-chilblains may affect other acral sites such as the auricular region (Proietti et al. 2020). Importantly, this has to be distinguished from true perniosis (chilblains), which has differing clinical and prognostic implications. Chilblain eruptions are characterized by acral, tender, and fixed livid lesions, which do not change with position, whereas pseudo-chilblains are typified by transient, blanchable violaceous erythema that is alleviated on limb elevation. The former may herald underlying autoimmune disease or hematological disorders.

Proposed pathogenic mechanisms include increased release of interferons and a subsequent cytokine-mediated inflammatory response, virus-induced endothelial damage, and obliterative microangiopathy and coagulation abnormalities (Genovese et al. 2021). Other postulations include the deposition of immune complexes in blood vessels causing tissue injury and direct vascular damage with secondary ischemia (Sanchez-Flores et al. 2021). Pseudo-chilblains have been reported to affect younger patients, occur later in the course of COVID-19, and are associated with better disease prognosis (Galván Casas et al. 2020).

The lesions are usually self-limiting and resolve after 2 weeks. Patients should be advised to avoid cold temperatures and wear warm clothing, gloves, and socks. Treatment options include topical corticosteroids, topical or oral vasodilatory agents such as calcium channel blockers, and aspirin (Sanchez-Flores et al. 2021).

Last but not least, there have been publications dispelling the association of COVID-19 and pernio-like lesions. However, as chilblains tend to occur in patients with more robust IFN-1 activation, the low rate of SARS-CoV-2 confirmation among these patients may be due to rapid clearance of the virus. SARS-CoV-2 vaccination has also been associated with the development of pernio, suggesting that these lesions represent an immunologic reaction to SARS-CoV-2 (Sun and Freeman 2022).

Livedoid or Vaso-Occlusive Lesions

Livedoid or vaso-occlusive lesions are relatively uncommon in COVID-19. These typically occur in older patients with more severe disease (Galván Casas et al. 2020). The clinical presentation is varied and ranges from livedo reticularis, livedo racemosa, retiform purpura to cutaneous necrosis.

Livedo reticularis-like eruptions are usually mild, transient, and not typically associated with thromboembolic complications. These manifest as lace-like dusky patches forming rings with pale centers on the limbs, sparing the trunk. On the contrary, patients with livedo racemosa-like lesions or retiform purpura may have associated severe coagulopathy (Genovese et al. 2021). Patients may develop non-blanching discontinuous erythematous rings, branching macules or plaques, or ulcers on the skin. These are associated with other thrombotic events such as deep

vein thrombosis, ischemic stroke, and disseminated intravascular coagulation (Seque et al. 2022).

It is suggested that inflammation of the endothelia triggered by COVID-19 results in the alteration of vascular homeostasis and the development of livedoid lesions (Khalil et al. 2020). Purpuric lesions exhibit a pauci-inflammatory thrombogenic vasculopathy, with deposition of C5b-9 and C4d and colocalization of COVID-19 spike glycoproteins in the skin (Magro et al. 2020). Treatment is supportive.

Purpuric Lesions

Patients may develop erythematous, non-blanchable macules or plaques (Fig. 2.4) or hemorrhagic blisters in a generalized or localized distribution affecting the acral or intertriginous sites. This is rare and occurs more commonly in elderly patients with severe disease (Galván Casas et al. 2020). Interestingly, these lesions have been more commonly reported on the gluteal regions and dubbed "COVID-buttocks" (Waqas et al. 2021); this has been ascribed to constant decubitus pressure owing to recumbency when the patient is hospitalized for severe disease and contributed by fecal soilage.

Severe microvascular injury with thrombotic vasculopathy mediated by complement activation or a cytokine storm is key in the development of purpuric lesions (Fernández-Lázaro and Garrosa 2021). Topical corticosteroids can be used to treat

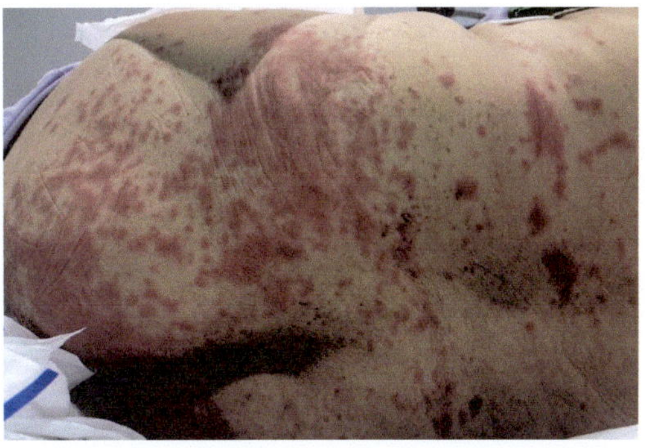

Fig. 2.4 Purpuric plaques on the lower back and gluteal region

purpuric lesions. In widespread or ulcerative lesions, systemic corticosteroids can be considered (Genovese et al. 2021).

Others

Cutaneous manifestations of COVID-19 can mimic severe cutaneous adverse drug reactions, including acute generalized exanthematous pustulosis (Mashayekhi et al. 2021), toxic epidermal necrolysis (Narang et al. 2021), and symmetrical drug-related intertriginous and flexural exanthema (Mahé et al. 2020).

Rare cases of reactivation of herpes simplex virus infections, eruptive cherry angiomas, Grover's disease-like lesions, Melkersson–Rosenthal syndrome, erythema nodosum, Gianotti–Crosti syndrome, erythema annulare centrifugum, and granuloma annulare have been observed (Seque et al. 2022; Daneshgaran et al. 2020).

Apart from affecting the skin, cases of telogen effluvium (Mieczkowska et al. 2021), anagen effluvium (Shanshal 2022b), and alopecia areata (Seque et al. 2022) have been reported.

There have only been a few case reports describing COVID-related nail changes, such as Beau's lines, Mees' lines, and onychomadesis. However, as these nail changes have known associations with other systemic illnesses, they have not been considered to be pathognomonic of COVID-19 infection (Hadeler et al. 2021).

Novel nail findings purported to be unique to COVID-19 infection include (Hadeler et al. 2021; Preda-Naumescu et al. 2021):

(a) the red half-moon sign—a convex, half-moon-shaped, red band appearing just distal to the lunula (Fig. 2.5) (Méndez-Flores et al. 2020).
(b) transverse orange discoloration—orange discoloration of the distal nail, sharply demarcated from the proximal healthy-appearing nail; similar findings have been described in Kawasaki's disease while Lindsay's nails are a close mimic.
(c) diffuse red-white nailbed discoloration—heterogeneous red-white discoloration of nails, with round onycholytic areas distally, surrounded by erythema, in selected digit(s).

At present, there appears to be no association between nail changes and poorer outcomes in COVID patients.

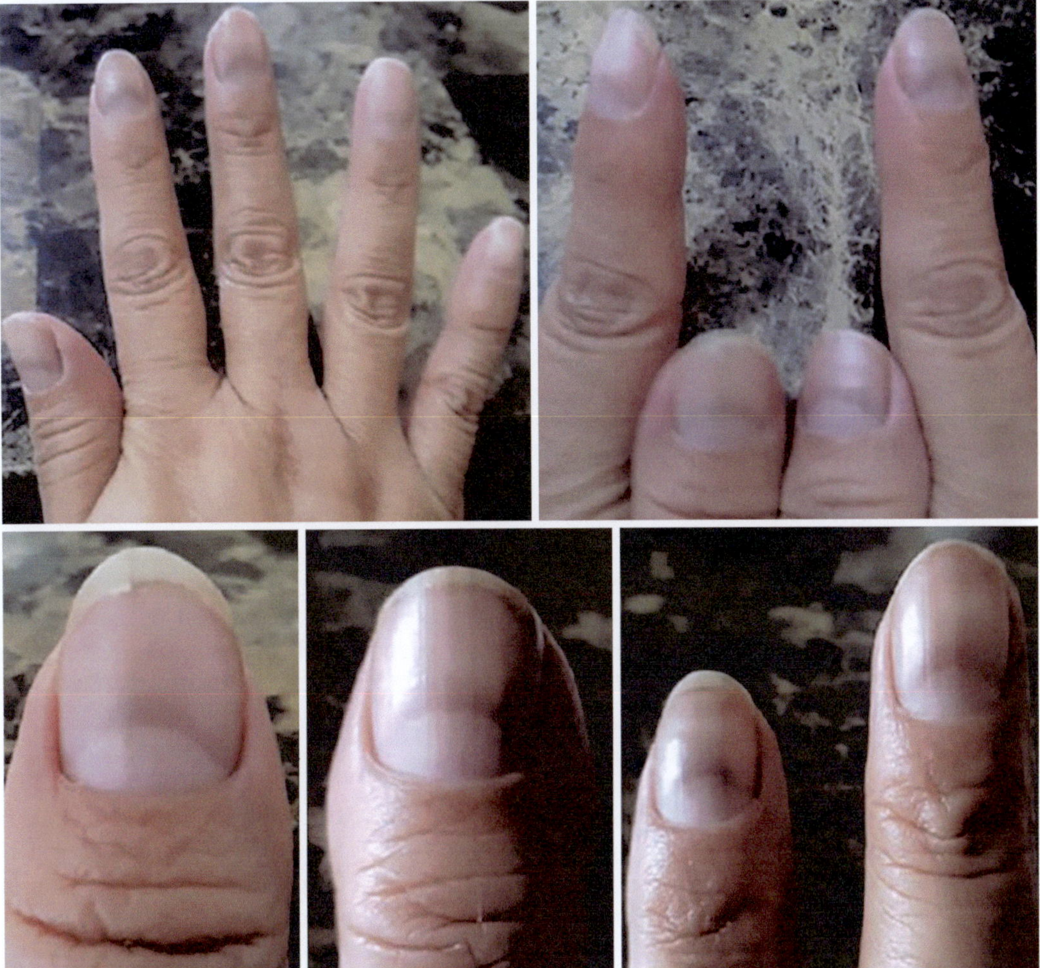

Fig. 2.5 The red half-moon sign. (Permission to use this image was granted by the International Journal of Dermatology on Jan 27, 2023. Fig. 1, page 1414 (Méndez-Flores et al. 2020))

COVID-19 in the Pediatric Population

In children with COVID-19, pseudo-chilblains, maculopapular, urticarial, and vesicular lesions are most frequently encountered. COVID-19 may trigger acute hemorrhagic edema of infancy, resulting in target-like purpuric plaques and swelling of the skin. Despite the dramatic clinical findings, patients generally remain well (Chesser et al. 2017).

Children who develop multisystem inflammatory syndrome can present with a polymorphous eruption involving the trunk and flexures, acral erythema, swelling of the extremities, desquamation, and mucositis (Sanchez-Flores et al. 2021). These cases should be managed in the intensive care unit.

Cutaneous Manifestations in Long-COVID Patients

Some patients develop a multiorgan symptomatic complex that persists even after the acute phase of the disease and are termed "long-COVID patients." In these patients, persistent dermatological manifestations include papulosquamous eruptions, pseudo-chilblains, alopecia, and necrotic skin lesions (Fernández-Lázaro and Garrosa 2021).

COVID-19 and Chronic Skin Diseases

COVID-19 has been associated with exacerbations of prior skin dermatoses, although it is difficult to establish causality definitively.

Atopic Dermatitis

Atopic dermatitis is a common inflammatory skin condition that arises due to the disruption of the epidermal barrier, immune dysregulation, and alteration of the microbiome in the skin. Patients with atopic dermatitis may experience an exacerbation of their skin condition during infection with COVID-19 (Miodońska et al. 2021). Studies have shown that patients with COVID-19 demonstrate higher levels of interleukin-4 and -13, which are key cytokines involved in the pathogenesis of atopic dermatitis (Fan et al. 2022).

Psoriasis

Patients with a history of psoriasis may present with flares of their dermatosis during their illness. Manifestations vary from worsening of chronic plaque psoriasis, pustular eruption, and erythrodermic psoriasis (Aram et al. 2021). While the mechanism for such flares is not known yet, it is proposed that patients with COVID-19 are in a state of hyperinflammation, and this may result in exacerbation of inflammatory conditions such as psoriasis. This is corroborated by increases in the biomarkers of inflammation including C-reactive protein and ferritin levels (Ozaras et al. 2020).

Cutaneous Autoimmune Diseases

This encompasses a wide range of dermatoses mediated by autoimmunity, including autoimmune blistering dermatoses and connective tissue diseases.

Viral infections are known to stimulate the development and aggravation of autoimmune conditions. Similarly, infection with SARS-CoV-2 may induce an exaggerated immune response through antigen mimicry, epitope spreading, cytokine imbalance, and the overwhelming of clearance mechanisms by amplified tissue destruction that increases the availability of self-antigens (Aram et al. 2021).

For the autoimmune blistering disorders, cases of new-onset or aggravation of bullous pemphigoid (Olson et al. 2021), pemphigus foliaceus (Mohaghegh et al. 2022), and pemphigus vulgaris (Zou and Daveluy 2022) have been described. Cytokines associated with COVID-19, such as interleukin-1B, -17, and tumor necrosis factor-α have also been implicated in bullous pemphigoid (Olson et al. 2021).

Lastly, COVID-19 has been reported in association with sclerotic disorders including morphea (Pigliacelli et al. 2022) and systemic sclerosis (Mariano et al. 2020), and other connective tissue diseases such as systemic lupus erythematosus (Zamani et al. 2021).

Conclusion

The cutaneous manifestations of COVID-19 are polymorphic, and to date, the exact pathophysiologic mechanisms and associated disease outcomes of the various clinical patterns remain poorly understood. Nonetheless, it is crucial for the clinician to be aware of such dermatological features as early recognition of these signs can guide the clinician toward a prompt diagnosis of COVID-19 and may even serve as a guide on the latter's clinical prognosis. Further studies will be useful to allow us to better understand the longer-term sequelae of COVID-19 on the skin.

Acknowledgments The authors would like to thank Drs. Benjamin Ho, Derek Lim, and Hong Liang Tey for contributing clinical photographs to this chapter.

References

Abuelgasim E, Dona ACM, Sondh RS, Harky A. Management of urticaria in COVID-19 patients: a systematic review. Dermatol Ther. 2021;34(1):e14328.

Aram K, Patil A, Goldust M, Rajabi F. COVID-19 and exacerbation of dermatological diseases: a review of the available literature. Dermatol Ther. 2021;34(6):e15113.

Català A, Galván-Casas C, Carretero-Hernández G, et al. Maculopapular eruptions associated to COVID-19: a subanalysis of the COVID-Piel study. Dermatol Ther. 2020;33(6):e14170.

Chesser H, Chambliss JM, Zwemer E. Acute hemorrhagic edema of infancy after coronavirus infection with recurrent rash. Case Rep Pediatr. 2017;2017:5637503.

Daneshgaran G, Dubin DP, Gould DJ. Cutaneous manifestations of COVID-19: an evidence-based review. Am J Clin Dermatol. 2020;21(5):627–39.

Fan R, Leasure AC, Damsky W, Cohen JM. Association between atopic dermatitis and COVID-19 infection: a case-control study in the all of us research program. JAAD Int. 2022;6:77–81.

Fernández-Lázaro D, Garrosa M. Identification, mechanism, and treatment of skin lesions in COVID-19: a review. Viruses. 2021;13(10):1916.

Freeman EE, McMahon DE, Lipoff JB, et al. The spectrum of COVID-19-associated dermatologic manifestations: an international registry of 716 patients from 31 countries. J Am Acad Dermatol. 2020;83(4):1118–29.

Galván Casas C, Català A, Carretero Hernández G, et al. Classification of the cutaneous manifestations of COVID-19: a rapid prospective nationwide consensus study in Spain with 375 cases. Br J Dermatol. 2020;183:71.

Genovese G, Moltrasio C, Berti E, Marzano AV. Skin manifestations associated with COVID-19: current knowledge and future perspectives. Dermatology. 2021;237(1):1–12.

Hadeler E, Morrison BW, Tosti A. A review of nail findings associated with COVID-19 infection. J Eur Acad Dermatol Venereol. 2021;35(11):e699–709.

Khalil S, Hinds BR, Manalo IF, Vargas IM, Mallela S, Jacobs R. Livedo reticularis as a presenting sign of severe acute respiratory syndrome coronavirus 2 infection. JAAD Case Rep. 2020;6(9):871–4.

Magro C, Mulvey JJ, Berlin D, et al. Complement associated microvascular injury and thrombosis in the pathogenesis of severe COVID-19 infection: a report of five cases. Transl Res. 2020;220:1–13.

Mahé A, Birckel E, Krieger S, Merklen C, Bottlaender L. A distinctive skin rash associated with coronavirus disease 2019? J Eur Acad Dermatol Venereol. 2020;34(6):e246–7.

Mariano RZ, Rio APTD, Reis F. Covid-19 overlapping with systemic sclerosis. Rev Soc Bras Med Trop. 2020;53:e20200450.

Marzano AV, Genovese G, Fabbrocini G, et al. Varicella-like exanthem as a specific COVID-19–associated skin manifestation: multicenter case series of 22 patients. J Am Acad Dermatol. 2020;83(1):280–5.

Mashayekhi F, Seirafianpour F, Pour Mohammad A, Goodarzi A. Severe and life-threatening COVID-19-related mucocutaneous eruptions: a systematic review. Int J Clin Pract. 2021;75(12):e14720.

Méndez-Flores S, Zaladonis A, Valdes-Rodriguez R. COVID-19 and nail manifestation: be on the look-out for the red half-moon nail sign. Int J Dermatol. 2020;59(11):1414.

Mieczkowska K, Deutsch A, Borok J, et al. Telogen effluvium: a sequela of COVID-19. Int J Dermatol. 2021;60(1):122–4.

Miodońska M, Bogacz A, Mróz M, Mućka S, Bożek A. The effect of SARS-CoV-2 virus infection on the course of atopic dermatitis in patients. Medicina (Kaunas). 2021;57(6):521.

Mohaghegh F, Hatami P, Refaghat A, et al. New-onset pemphigus foliaceus following SARS-CoV-2 infection and unmasking multiple sclerosis: a case report. Clin Case Rep. 2022;10(6):e05910.

Najafzadeh M, Shahzad F, Ghaderi N, Ansari K, Jacob B, Wright A. Urticaria (angioedema) and COVID-19 infection. J Eur Acad Dermatol Venereol. 2020;34(10):e568–70.

Narang I, Panthagani AP, Lewis M, Chohan B, Ferguson A, Nambi R. COVID-19-induced toxic epidermal necrolysis. Clin Exp Dermatol. 2021;46(5):927–9.

Olson N, Eckhardt D, Delano A. New-onset bullous pemphigoid in a COVID-19 patient. Case Rep Dermatol Med. 2021;2021:5575111.

Ozaras R, Berk A, Ucar DH, Duman H, Kaya F, Mutlu H. Covid-19 and exacerbation of psoriasis. Dermatol Ther. 2020;33(4):e13632.

Pigliacelli F, Pacifico A, Mariano M, D'Arino A, Cristaudo A, Iacovelli P. Morphea induced by SARS-CoV-2 infection: a case report. Int J Dermatol. 2022;61(3):377–8.

Preda-Naumescu A, Penney K, Pearlman RL, Brodell RT, Daniel CR, Nahar VK. Nail manifestations in COVID-19: insight into a systemic viral disease. Skin Appendage Disord. 2021;183(6):1–6.

Proietti I, Tolino E, Bernardini N, et al. Auricle perniosis as a manifestation of Covid-19 infection. Dermatol Ther. 2020;33(6):e14089.

Sanchez-Flores X, Huynh T, Huang JT. Covid-19 skin manifestations: an update. Curr Opin Pediatr. 2021;33(4):380–6.

Seque CA, Enokihara MMSES, Porro AM, Tomimori J. Skin manifestations associated with COVID-19. An Bras Dermatol. 2022;97(1):75–88.

Shanshal M. Low-dose systemic steroids, an emerging therapeutic option for COVID-19 related urticaria. J Dermatolog Treat. 2022a;33(2):1140–1.

Shanshal M. COVID-19 related anagen effluvium. J Dermatolog Treat. 2022b;33(2):1114–5.

Sun Q, Freeman EE. Chilblains and COVID-19-an update on the complexities of interpreting antibody test results, the role of interferon α, and COVID-19 vaccines. JAMA Dermatol. 2022;158(2):217–8.

Tan SW, Tam YC, Oh CC. Skin manifestations of COVID-19: a worldwide review. JAAD Int. 2021;2:119–33.

Waqas B, Salgado F, Harp J. Retiform purpura on the buttocks in 6 critically ill COVID-19 patients. Cutis. 2021;108(5):E13–4.

Wollina U, Karadağ AS, Rowland-Payne C, Chiriac A, Lotti T. Cutaneous signs in COVID-19 patients: a review. Dermatol Ther. 2020;33(5):e13549.

Zamani B, Moeini Taba S-M, Shayestehpour M. Systemic lupus erythematosus manifestation following COVID-19: a case report. J Med Case Rep. 2021;15(1):29.

Zou H, Daveluy S. Pemphigus vulgaris after COVID-19 infection and vaccination. J Am Acad Dermatol. 2022;87(3):709–10.

Cutaneous Reactions to COVID-19 mRNA Vaccines

Alexis G. Strahan and Esther E. Freeman

Abbreviations

AA	Alopecia areata
DLL	Delayed large local
PR	Pityriasis rosea
TE	Telogen effluvium
V-REPP	Vaccine-related eruption of papules and plaques
VZV	Varicella Zoster virus

Introduction

In late 2019, a novel coronavirus, termed SARS-CoV-2, was identified and subsequently spread rapidly across the globe. The World Health Organization designated the disease process COVID-19; as of December 2022, there have been nearly 650 million cases of COVID-19 and 6.6 million deaths worldwide (World Health Organization 2023). In response to a novel disease process, mRNA vaccine technology was utilized to target the rapid spread and reduce morbidity and mortality. mRNA vaccine technology, first established in the 1990s, had been under investigation for other infectious processes including influenza and Zika viruses (Pardi et al. 2018). In response to the impact of COVID-19, the Food and Drug Administration issued Emergency Use Authorizations for Pfizer/BioNTech (BNT162b2) and Moderna (mRNA-1273) COVID-19 vaccines, which proved to be effective at mitigating the morbidity and mortality associated with COVID-19 (U.S. Food and Drug Administration 2020).

As of December 2022, nearly 13 billion doses of vaccines have been administered. Initial reporting of cutaneous findings in phase 3 trials of Pfizer/BioNTech (BNT162b2) and Moderna (mRNA-1273) included mention of local injection site reactions (83%, 84.2%) and rare instances of urticarial, macular, papular, exfoliative, and dermal filler–related cutaneous reactions (Baden et al. 2021; Polack et al. 2020). Compared to clinical trial data, rollout of vaccines worldwide introduced a spectrum of cutaneous reactions. Pooled incidence of cutaneous adverse reactions to all vaccine types in real-world data, not encompassing local site reactions, is estimated to be 5% (ranging from <0.01 to 19%) with that number decreasing to 3% for

A. G. Strahan
Department of Dermatology, Massachusetts General Hospital, Boston, MA, USA

Mercer University School of Medicine,
Savannah, GA, USA
e-mail: astrahan@mgh.harvard.edu

E. E. Freeman (✉)
Department of Dermatology, Massachusetts General Hospital, Boston, MA, USA

Medical Practice Evaluation Foundation,
Massachusetts General Hospital, Boston, MA, USA
e-mail: efreeman@mgh.harvard.edu

© The Author(s), under exclusive license to Springer Nature Switzerland AG 2023
H. H. Oon, C. L. Goh (eds.), *COVID-19 in Dermatology*, Updates in Clinical Dermatology,
https://doi.org/10.1007/978-3-031-45586-5_3

mRNA specific vaccines (Bellinato et al. 2022). The incidence was similar in those receiving first and second dose vaccination. The time to onset of cutaneous reactions on average was 7 days, with a shorter interval seen with subsequent doses (McMahon et al. 2021). The American Academy of Dermatology and International League of Dermatological Societies collaborated to create a registry to capture vaccine-associated cutaneous reactions from healthcare providers across the world. Frequently reported findings ranged from local site reactions and delayed large local reactions to chronic urticaria and reactivation of varicella zoster virus (McMahon et al. 2021).

As variants continue to emerge, COVID-19 vaccination and booster doses remain an important component of control of viral spread and reduction of morbidity and mortality. Dermatologists are posed with the unique position to recognize and counsel patients on cutaneous findings post-mRNA vaccination. Accurate understanding and counseling on the overall benign and self-limiting nature of most cutaneous reactions are crucial to maintain trust in the safety of vaccines. In this article, we will examine the most frequently reported cutaneous reactions to mRNA vaccines, relevant clinical and histologic findings, and treatment options (Table 3.1).

Table 3.1 Summary: cutaneous reaction types, clinical findings, and treatment for COVID-19 mRNA vaccine-associated reactions

	Clinical findings	Treatment
Local injection site reactions	Erythematous, edematous, or indurated papules or plaques at the site of injection	Self-resolving Symptomatic treatment-cool compress, oral analgesics
Delayed large local reactions	Edematous, erythematous, or indurated patch or plaque of variable size at the site of vaccination-often associated with pain, warmth, and itching	Self-resolving Symptomatic treatment-topical corticosteroids, oral antihistamines, cool compress, or analgesics (World Health Organization 2023)
Morbilliform rashes/diffuse erythematous eruption	Erythematous macules and papules reminiscent of the classic measles eruption, most often affecting the trunk and extremities	Self-resolving Symptomatic treatment-topical or systemic corticosteroids or antihistamines
Urticaria	Transient, edematous, well-circumscribed papules and plaques (wheals) extending beyond the site of injection—characterized by timing: *Acute*—greater than 4 h after vaccination & persists for less than 6 weeks *Chronic*—persistence of urticaria greater than 6 weeks	Oral antihistamine therapy (second generation >first generation) (Pardi et al. 2018), H2 antihistamines, corticosteroids (U.S. Food and Drug Administration 2020), Omalizumab (Baden et al. 2021; Polack et al. 2020)
Dermal filler reaction	Erythematous, edematous, or inflamed papules or nodules at the prior dermal filler sites (Bellinato et al. 2022)	Self-resolving Lisinopril 5–10 mg for 3–5 days (McMahon et al. 2021), hyaluronidase, or corticosteroids (Sharif et al. 2021)
Pernio/chilblains	Pink to violaceous macules, papules, or nodules of acral areas—most commonly on the fingers and toes	Minimize exposure to cold, insulated gloves and footwear Topical corticosteroids, oral nifedipine (Avallone et al. 2022a; Gidudu et al. 2008; Center for Disease Control and Prevention 2022)
Varicella zoster virus reactivation	Grouped vesicles on an erythematous base in a unilateral, dermatomal distribution	Anti-viral agents—acyclovir or valacyclovir

Table 3.1 (continued)

	Clinical findings	Treatment
Vaccine-related eruption of papules and plaques (V-REPP)	*Mild-VREPP:* papulosquamous changes, consisting of pink oval or annular papules occasionally coalescing into plaques with or without mild scale *Moderate V-REPP:* oval, pink edematous papules and plaques with occasional trailing scale or crust *Robust V-REPP:* discrete, edematous papules with occasionally crusting or vesiculation	Mild: Symptomatic treatment Moderate/severe: Medium potency topical corticosteroids, oral antihistamine therapy (Blumenthal et al. 2021)
Erythema Multiforme	Targetoid papules consisting of two or three classic zones: a dusky central zone, a deep red inflammatory zone with associated ring of pale edematous skin, and an outer rim of erythema	Removal of trigger Topical or oral corticosteroids, oral antihistamines (Català et al. 2022; Kempf et al. 2021; Kroumpouzos et al. 2022)
Autoimmune bullous disease	Varied-flaccid or tense blistering of the skin and mucous membranes and painful erosions with easy bleeding and crusting	Immunosuppressant and anti-inflammatory agents in accordance with disease-specific guidelines (includes topical corticosteroids, oral corticosteroids, azathioprine, mycophenolate (Ohsawa et al. 2021; Jedlowski and Jedlowski 2021), rituximab, dupilumab, and intravenous immune globulin therapy)
Hair loss Alopecia Areata Telogen effluvium	Smooth, discrete patches of complete hair loss occurring over the scalp and other hair-bearing areas Decreased density of hair (typically up to 50% loss)	AA: Intralesional corticosteroids, topical clobetasol, or oral JAK inhibitors such as baricitinib (McMahon et al. 2022; CDC 2022) TE: Identification of trigger, psychological support

mRNA Vaccine-Associated Cutaneous Reactions

Local Injection Site Reaction

Local injection site reactions are the most commonly reported cutaneous finding after COVID-19 vaccination, both in vaccine trials and real-world reports occurring in up to 84% and 34% respectively, most often occurring in younger populations (Baden et al. 2021; Sharif et al. 2021; Avallone et al. 2022a). Local site reactions are often described as erythematous, edematous, or indurated papules or plaques at the site of injection appearing within 1–3 days of vaccination (Gidudu et al. 2008). In lighter skin tones, the area may appear pink to red and in darker skin tones more violaceous (McMahon et al. 2021; Gidudu et al. 2008). Local injection site reactions may be associated with lymphadenopathy near the vaccinations site (Center for Disease Control and Prevention 2022).

No treatment is necessary for local injection site reactions as they are self-limited, most resolving within 1 week of vaccination. If symptomatic relief is desired, over-the-counter analgesics or cool compress to the area may relieve discomfort.

Delayed Large Local Reaction

Delayed large local (DLL) reaction, also referred to as "COVID Arm," is a type of local injection site reaction occurring 4 or more days, with a median of 7–8 days, after vaccination (McMahon et al. 2021; Blumenthal et al. 2021). A DLL reaction is described as an edematous, erythematous,

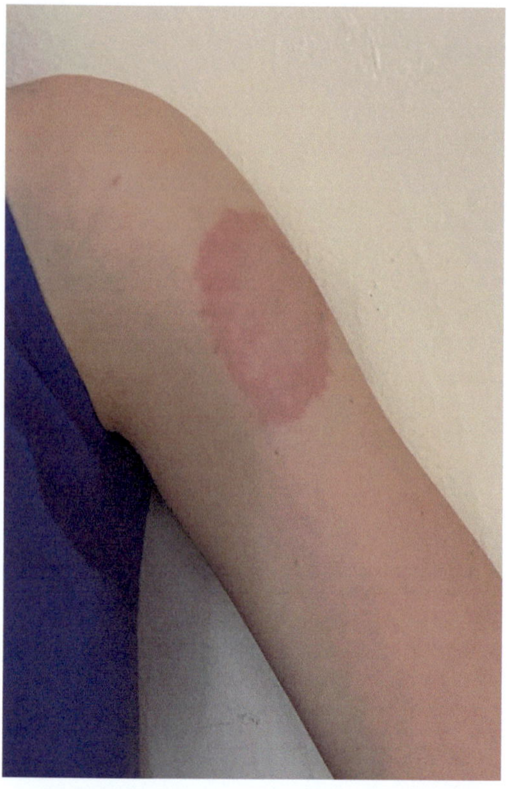

Fig. 3.1 Delayed large local (DLL) reaction, consisting of an erythematous patch on the upper arm. (Reprinted from Journal of the American Academy of Dermatology; Vol 85; McMahon et al.; Cutaneous reactions reported after Moderna and Pfizer COVID-19 vaccination: A registry-based study of 414 cases; Pages 46–55; Copyright (2021), with permission from Elsevier)

or indurated patch or plaque of variable size at the site of vaccination (Fig. 3.1) (McMahon et al. 2021; Blumenthal et al. 2021; Català et al. 2022). The lesion may appear annular or targetoid and is often associated with pain, warmth, and itching.

Histologic findings can include focal epidermal changes, prominent spongiosis, and associated superficial perivascular or perifollicular lymphocytic infiltrates. Rare eosinophils and mast cells may also be seen (Blumenthal et al. 2021; Kempf et al. 2021). Proposed mechanisms for delayed large local reactions in response to mRNA vaccination include a T-cell-mediated, delayed hypersensitivity response to an mRNA component or vaccine element (Kroumpouzos et al. 2022).

Although less than local injection site reaction, delayed large local reactions were reported in mRNA vaccine trials in up to 0.8% of participants (Baden et al. 2021; Polack et al. 2020). Of cutaneous reactions associated with vaccination, delayed large local reactions DLL reactions are reported more often in females and are often associated with more systemic symptoms than other vaccine-associated cutaneous findings (Català et al. 2022). Some studies have shown a dose–response relationship where DLL reactions occur earlier, on day 2–3, with a second vaccine dose but have been found to be milder in severity (McMahon et al. 2021).

DLL reactions are self-limited and typically resolve within 3–4 days without intervention (McMahon et al. 2021). If symptomatic treatment is desired, various interventions such as topical corticosteroids, oral antihistamines, ice-packs, and pain-relieving medications have shown improvement in real-world reports (Blumenthal et al. 2021). A DLL reaction is not a contraindication to future vaccination. DLL reactions should not be confused with cellulitis and do not require antibiotics.

Morbilliform Rashes/Diffuse Erythematous Eruptions

Morbilliform eruptions are described as erythematous macules and papules reminiscent of the classic measles eruption, most often affecting the trunk and extremities. Diffuse erythematous eruptions have been described in 2% of all reports of cutaneous vaccine-associated reactions (Avallone et al. 2022a), Histologic findings can include perivascular lymphocytic infiltrate, basal call vacuolization, and spongiosis (Ohsawa et al. 2021; Jedlowski and Jedlowski 2021; McMahon et al. 2022).

Mechanisms underlying the spectrum of morbilliform and diffuse erythematous rashes are still under investigation. Similarities to eruptions seen during SARS-CoV-2 active infection favor immune-mediated mechanisms, one suggestion including a type of immune-mediated response modulated by a prior SARS-CoV-2 infection cross-reacting with antigens encoded by vaccination (Ohsawa et al. 2021).

Most morbilliform and diffuse erythematous rashes resolve without intervention. Symptomatic treatment options include topical or systemic corticosteroids or oral-antihistamine medication.

Acute and Chronic Urticaria

Urticaria is described as transient, edematous, well-circumscribed papules and plaques (wheals) extending beyond the site of injection. Urticaria may occur as part of a Type 1 hypersensitivity reaction, occurring within 4 h of vaccination. Immediate-onset urticaria is important to distinguish from urticaria that occurs more than 4 h after vaccination, as urticaria within 4 h may be either a contraindication to future vaccination or require vaccine administration under medical supervision (CDC 2022; Chu et al. 2022) Acute urticaria occurs greater than 4 h after vaccination, is often transient, and persists for less than 6 weeks. Chronic urticaria is defined by persistence of urticaria greater than 6 weeks.

Acute urticaria is often associated with angioedema—an edematous process involving deeper layers, papillary and deep vascular plexus of the skin (Wolff et al. 2006). Dermatographism, or urticarial lesions at the site of external contact with the skin, and significant pruritus may also co-occur (Fig. 3.2). The mechanism of acute urticaria after vaccination is proposed as an IgE-mediated reaction to vaccine additives or excipients. Chronic urticaria is thought to be less IgE-mediated and more often related to anti-FcεR auto-antibodies, mast-cell-derived histamine, eicosanoids, or neuropeptides in the skin (Wolff et al. 2006). Histologic findings may include dermal edema, perivascular lymphocytes, neutrophils, or eosinophils (McMahon et al. 2022).

Acute and chronic urticaria has been reported in nearly 11% of all COVID-19-associated vaccine reactions in mRNA and non-mRNA vehicles (Avallone et al. 2022a). Effective treatment options include oral antihistamine therapy with

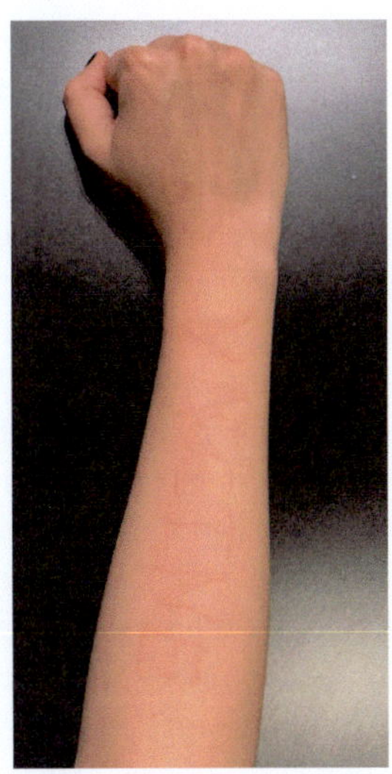

Fig. 3.2 Dermatographism over the forearm. (Reprinted from JAAD Case Reports; Vol 25; Strahan et al.; Chronic spontaneous urticaria after COVID-19 primary vaccine series and boosters; Pages 63–66; Copyright (2022), with permission from Elsevier)

second-generation H1 antihistamines preferred over first-generation H1 antihistamines for adults and children (Zuberbier et al. 2009). H2 antihistamines and corticosteroids are alternative options that have shown promise (Pescosolido et al. 2022). Omalizumab, a monoclonal antibody inhibiting IgE binding to the high-affinity IgE receptor (FcεRI), is approved for chronic spontaneous urticaria and has been used in recalcitrant cases with some success (Picone et al. 2022; Strahan et al. 2022).

Dermal Filler Reactions

Dermal tissue filler is one of the most common cosmetic procedures and most often involves the injection of hyaluronic acid, a biocompatible product to the naturally occurring component of the extracellular matrix of the skin. Dermal filler reactions are described as erythematous, edematous or inflamed papules or nodules at the prior dermal filler sites (Kroumpouzos et al. 2022). Most reported cases noted a reaction 2–5 days after vaccination and had received filler injections 1–2 years prior (Kalantari et al. 2022).

Dermal filler reactions are proposed to be a type of delayed hypersensitivity reaction to filler elements after introduction of an immunologic trigger (Rice et al. 2021). Immunologic triggers post filler have included acute infections, trauma, contaminated or low-quality product or vaccination (Kalantari et al. 2022). Favorable response to angiotensin-converting enzyme (ACE) inhibitor medications has further suggested that mRNA-encoded spike protein may interact with ACE receptors, promoting a proinflammatory response (Munavalli et al. 2022). This idea is reinforced by similar inflammatory filler reactions seen during SARS-CoV-2 acute infection. One study by Decates et al. proposes that patients with human leukocyte antigen subtypes HLA-B*08 and DRB1*03 haplotypes have a four-fold increased odds of dermal filler reactions in general (Decates et al. 2021). Additionally, a larger volume of dermal filler (>1 mL) has been associated with more severe reactions (Safir et al. 2022).

Similar to other mRNA vaccine-associated reactions, dermal filler reactions often resolve without intervention. A promising treatment option in patients with filler reactions includes the use angiotensin-converting enzyme inhibitors such as lisinopril at a dose of 5–10 mg for 3–5 days. Additional successful symptomatic treatment in the literature includes hyaluronidase, to dissolve the filler, or corticosteroids (Kalantari et al. 2022). A filler reaction does not constitute a contraindication for future vaccination or future dermal filler use, and for the general population, providers may consider recommending a 4–8-week interval between filler administration and vaccination (Rice et al. 2021; American Society of Plastic Surgeons 2021).

Pernio/Chilblains

As one of the first and most prominent SARS-CoV-2-related cutaneous findings, pernio and chilblains, otherwise referred to as "COVID toes," have similarly presented after mRNA COVID-19 vaccination. Traditionally, pernio/chilblains are associated with exposure to cold—manifesting more often during winter months—with improvement seen after warming; but pernio can be secondary to systemic processes including autoimmune disorders, paraproteinemia, or malignancies (Takci et al. 2012).

Pernio/chilblains are described as pink to violaceous macules, papules, or nodules of acral areas—most commonly on the fingers and toes. Findings can have associated pain, pruritus, edema, ulceration, or blistering of affected areas. Histologic findings include perivascular lymphocytic infiltrate, without thrombi or vasculitis, in the superficial to deep dermis with dermal edema (Lopez et al. 2021; Kha and Itkin 2021).

The proposed underlying mechanism of pernio after vaccination is largely tied to similar exanthems seen in active SARS-CoV-2 infection. Suggested pathways include small vessel damage secondary to vaccine-induced microangiopathy or accumulation of immune complexes in dermal vasculature of endothelial cells activating an inflammatory cascade (Lopez et al. 2021). Rather than possible direct viral effects, vaccine-induced pernio may represent a strong type 1 interferon host response to vaccine-produced viral components (Sahin et al. 2020; Sun and Freeman 2022).

Pernio/chilblains can be classified acute or chronic. Acute pernio resolves within 3 weeks of onset (Takci et al. 2012). Pernio associated with a systemic process is more likely to be chronic or recurrent (Takci et al. 2012). Treatment options for vaccine-associated pernio/chilblains mirror traditional pernio recommendations—the primary intervention being minimizing exposure to cold with insulated gloves and footwear. Additional studies have supported the use of topical corticosteroids or oral nifedipine (Lopez et al. 2021; Kha and Itkin 2021; Cappel and Wetter 2014).

Varicella Zoster Virus Reactivation

The varicella-zoster virus (VZV), known to cause varicella (chickenpox) in primary infection, can lay dormant in sensory ganglia and upon reactivation causes herpes zoster (shingles). VZV reactivation has been reported in numerous case studies and in 35 patients from an international registry, though if there is a true increase in incidence after COVID vaccination is not yet known (Fathy et al. 2022; Rodríguez-Jiménez et al. 2021; Lee et al. 2021; Furer et al. 2021). A systematic review of VZV after COVID-19 vaccination noted an average latency time of 6 days after vaccination to reactivation symptoms (Martinez-Reviejo et al. 2022; Katsikas Triantafyllidis et al. 2021). VZV reactivation lesion morphology is described as grouped vesicles on an erythematous base in a unilateral, dermatomal distribution. The exanthem is most often associated with a prodrome of neuritis in the affected region that persists throughout the infection and may persist for weeks following resolution. Diagnosis is made on clinical features and may be confirmed via PCR testing or direct fluorescent antibody (DFA) testing of most recently erupted lesions (Dahl et al. 1997). The mechanism of ZVZ reactivation after vaccination is largely thought to occur due to immunomodulation or immune response to vaccination induces a lower nidus of cell-mediated immune control over the latent pathogen (Català et al. 2022; Corbeddu et al. 2021).

Of all reported cases, 90% were non-serious, defined as not requiring hospitalization (Martinez-Reviejo et al. 2022). Treatment options include the use of antiviral agents such as acyclovir or valacyclovir.

V-REPP (Vaccine-Related Eruption of Papules and Plaques)

Vaccine-related eruptions of papules and plaques (V-REPP) are a spectrum of cutaneous reactions encompassing mild papulosquamous (mild-VREPP), erythematous pityriasis rosea-like (moderate V-REPP), to edematous, crusted papulovesicular eruptions (robust V-REPP) (McMahon et al. 2022). V-REPP is characterized by histopathologic findings that exist on a spectrum of the extent of interface and spongiotic changes: mild V-REPP is associated with interface change, moderate V-REPP has both interface and spongiotic elements, while severe V-REPP is associated with substantial spongiosis (Fig. 3.3) (McMahon et al. 2022).

More specifically, mild V-REPP is characterized by papulosquamous changes, consisting of pink oval or annular papules occasionally coalescing into plaques with or without mild scale, and is most commonly found on the trunk and extremities. Histologically, mild V-REPP shows minimal spongiosis with prominent interface changes and occasional eosinophils. Median onset of mild V-REPP was 16 days post-vaccination (McMahon et al. 2022).

Moderate V-REPP, or pityriasis rosea-like eruption, is characterized by oval, pink edematous papules and plaques with occasional trailing scale or crust. PR-like eruptions are infrequently reported vaccine-associated cutaneous findings, reported in 2% of all cutaneous reactions in both mRNA and non-mRNA vehicles (Avallone et al. 2022a). PR-like eruptions are associated with a trigger, often a drug, and can differ in symptomatology from typical pityriasis rosea (PR). In contrast to PR, PR-like eruptions can lack a "herald" patch and consist of more diffuse lesion distribution and associated pruritus (Panda et al. 2014). Moderate V-REPP/PR-like eruptions histologically show spongiotic dermatitis with interface dermatitis and eosinophils (McMahon et al. 2022; Panda et al. 2014; Drago et al. 2016). PR-like eruptions have been noted after other vaccinations, including smallpox, tuberculosis, and influenza, and have been reported after SARS-CoV-2 infection (Drago et al. 2016; Freeman et al. 2022). Median onset was 13 days post-vaccination. In some studies, PR-like eruptions persisted longer than any other vaccine-associated cutaneous reaction—with averages nearing 25 days and some up to 90 days (Català et al. 2022). PR-like eruptions have shown a potential to flare with subsequent vaccine doses but do not constitute a contraindication to future vaccination (McMahon et al. 2022).

Robust V-REPP is characterized by papulovesicular changes, consisting of discrete, edematous papules with occasionally crusting or vesiculation, and is most often found on the trunk and extremities. Histologically robust V-REPP exhibits marked spongiosis, intraepidermal vesi-

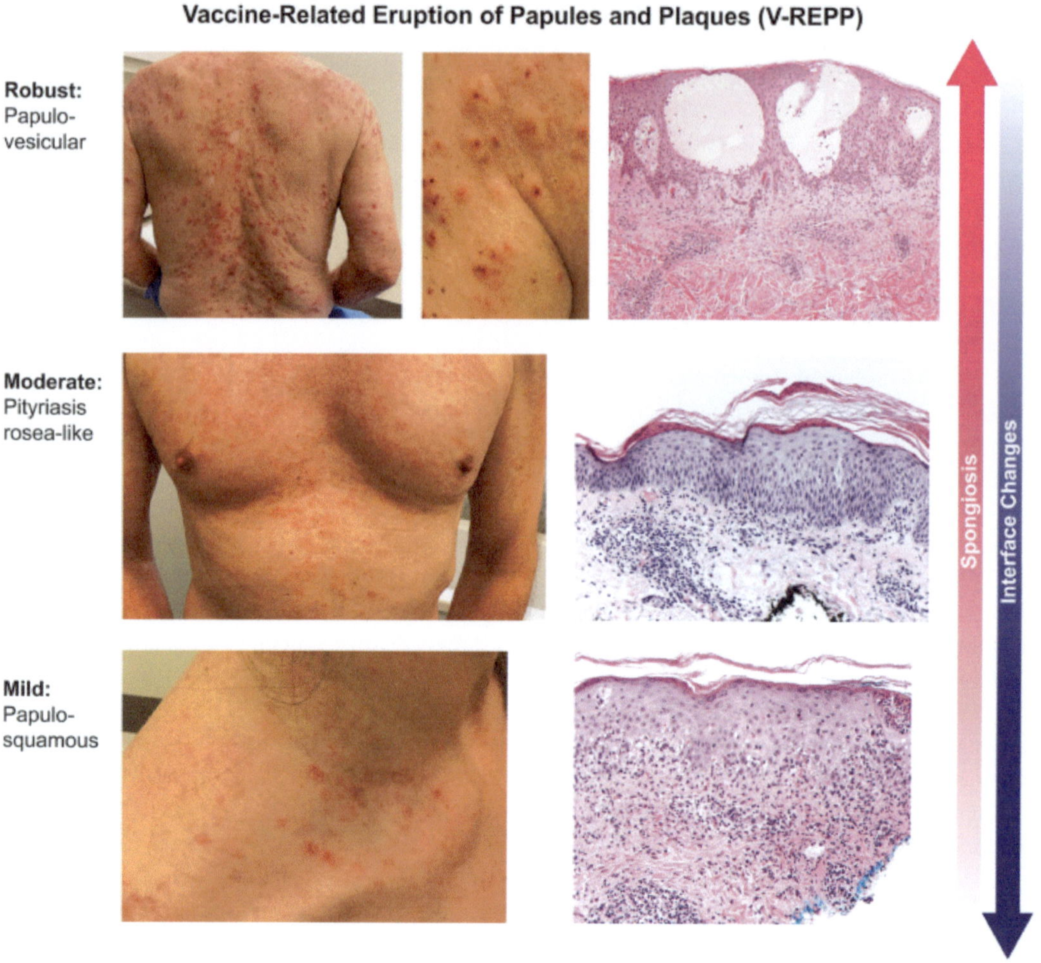

Fig. 3.3 V-REPP by degree of spongiosis and interface changes present on histopathologic examination. (Reprinted from Journal of the American Academy of Dermatology; Vol 86, McMahon et al.; Clinical and pathologic correlation of cutaneous COVID-19 vaccine reactions including V-REPP: A registry-based study; Pages 113–121; Copyright (2022), with permission from Elsevier)

cles, and minimal interface changes. The median time to onset post-vaccination was the shortest of all V-REPP variants at 5.5 days after vaccination and persisted for a maximum of 49 days as reported in an internationally registry (McMahon et al. 2022).

The mechanism of V-REPP remains unknown, but proposed mechanisms include: (1) immuno-modulation following vaccination that allows for reactivation of latent viruses (HHV-6 or HHV-7) for PR-like or moderate V-REPP; (2) cell-mediated response to a viral epitope encoded by the mRNA vaccine inducing molecular mimicry; (3) or delayed hypersensitivity response to vac-cination (Kroumpouzos et al. 2022; McMahon et al. 2022). Treatment of V-REPP-type eruptions is largely supportive. For pruritus, medium potency topical corticosteroids may be used along with oral antihistamine therapy (Chuh et al. 2016).

Erythema Multiforme

Erythema multiforme (EM) is an acute, type IV sensitivity reaction associated with infectious agents, most commonly herpes simplex virus, and medications. Erythema multiforme and

EM-like reactions have been reported in 0.6% of all reported vaccine-associated reactions, with 85% occurring specifically after vaccination with mRNA-based vaccines (Avallone et al. 2022a). Lesion morphology is described as targetoid papules that may consist of two or three classic zones including a dusky central zone, a deep red inflammatory zone with associated ring of pale edematous skin, and an outer rim of erythema (Wolff et al. 2006; Huff 1985). Lesions commonly occur in a symmetrical distribution on the acral extremities and may have associated pruritus or burning.

Histology findings seen in vaccine-associated EM has exhibited vacuolar interface dermatitis with necrotic keratinocytes and a superficial perivascular inflammatory infiltrate with scattered eosinophils, papillary dermal edema, or red blood cell extravasation (Karatas et al. 2022).

The mechanism of EM and EM-like reactions to mRNA vaccines remains under investigation, but it is thought to be of similar etiology to classic EM—vaccine-generated antigens cause a T-cell dominated immune response at the surface of resulting in cell necrosis and dermoepidermal junction separation (Lavery et al. 2021). EM has been reported after vaccination for other infectious processes including smallpox, measles, mumps, and rubella, meningococcus, and influenza (Rosenblatt and Stein 2015).

The treatment of erythema multiforme is largely symptomatic and requires removing the trigger, if identifiable. EM after vaccination may be treated with topical or oral corticosteroids and oral antihistamines as needed for symptomatic relief (Karatas et al. 2022; Lavery et al. 2021; Borg et al. 2022). EM typically persists for less than 2 weeks but can persist for as long as 5 weeks (James et al. 2006).

Autoimmune Bullous Disease

A spectrum of autoimmune bullous diseases has been reported following vaccination against COVID-19 with mRNA-based vaccines. Bullous diseases encompass various blistering processes of the skin and mucosa caused by autoantibodies targeting desmosomal proteins—including pemphigus vulgaris and bullous pemphigoid. Bullous diseases can manifest as flaccid or tense blistering of the skin and mucous membranes and painful erosions with easy bleeding and crusting. Pruritus can be associated with some variants. Of reported cases of bullous disease postvaccination, 81% occurred after vaccination with mRNA versus other vaccines—with 6% acquiring a new-onset and 10% a flare of previously diagnosed bullous disease. Onset occurred up to 6 weeks post-vaccination (Kasperkiewicz and Woodley 2022a). The mechanistic connection remains unknown—some studies suggest molecular mimicry between SARS-CoV-2 spike protein components to endogenous human antigens in predisposed individuals (Huang et al. 2022). Other studies have shown no cross-reactivity between SARS-CoV-2 antibodies and pemphigus and pemphigoid autoantibodies (Kasperkiewicz and Woodley 2022b). One study hypothesized that in those with rapid bullous development after initial vaccination it is possible that subsequent immune activation unmasked preexisting subclinical autoreactivity (Tomayko et al. 2021).

Bullous diseases have been linked to other vaccines including influenza, tetanus, and diphtheria (Kasperkiewicz and Woodley 2022a). For clinicians, it is important to note that reports of bullous disease post vaccination have shown no increased risk to unvaccinated age-matched cohorts and therefore may be a result of coincidence (Birabaharan et al. 2022).

Treatment options comprise immunosuppressant and anti-inflammatory agents used for classic pemphigus and pemphigoid processes including high-potency topical corticosteroids, oral corticosteroids, azathioprine, or mycophenolate (Tomayko et al. 2021; Martora et al. 2022). In a series of 12 patients from an international registry, seven improved over a median of 3 weeks using a combination of topical and systemic corticosteroids, doxycycline, and nicotinamide (Tomayko et al. 2021). Rituximab, dupilumab, and intravenous immune globulin therapy are also included in guidelines for management of these processes.

Hair Loss

Hair loss after vaccination with mRNA-based vaccine has been reported in individuals both with a history of alopecia and those with no history of hair loss (Ganjei et al. 2022; Fusano et al. 2022; Aryanian et al. 2022). Alopecia areata (AA), one type of hair loss reported after mRNA vaccination, is caused by an immune-mediated targeting of hair follicles in the anagen (growth) phase and results in non-scarring hair loss. AA described as smooth, discrete patches of complete hair loss occurring over the scalp and other hair-bearing areas. Similar to other vaccine-induced autoimmune processes, AA is hypothesized to mechanistically result from autoimmune activation secondary to molecular mimicry from vaccine components or adjuvants in genetically susceptible individuals (May Lee et al. 2022). Treatment options may be based on extent of disease and comorbid conditions and include intralesional corticosteroids, topical clobetasol, or oral JAK inhibitors such as baricitinib (Tassone et al. 2022; King et al. 2022).

Telogen effluvium (TE), another non-scarring alopecia, results from an interruption in the hair follicle growth cycle—anagen (growth), catagen (transformation), and telogen (rest)—where an increase in follicles enters telogen phase, and subsequently they are shed in larger quantities. Clinically patients present with decreased density of hair, typically up to 50% loss (Trüeb 2010). Telogen effluvium has been widely reported after active SARS-CoV-2 infection with a prevalence of up to 74% of all cases with reported hair loss (Czech et al. 2022; Hussain et al. 2022). Though fewer reports of post-vaccination TE exist and association remains difficult to ascertain, TE has been reported in those who received mRNA vaccines (Alharbi 2022). Though investigations are ongoing, one hypothesis for TE post-vaccination is that it could be triggered by vaccine-related fear or stress rather than the vaccine itself (Alharbi 2022).

Other Cutaneous Reactions

Other less commonly reported cutaneous reactions to mRNA vaccination include new onset or flare of psoriasis, lichen planus, vitiligo, morphea, and erythromelalgia.

New onset psoriasis and flares of previously diagnosed psoriasis were reported in 0.08% and 0.61% of vaccine-associated cutaneous reaction reports respectively (Sharif et al. 2021). Clinical and histologic findings mirror classic findings and include well-demarcated papules and plaques with overlying scale seen on the trunk, extremities, head, and neck. Histologic findings include epidermal acanthosis, parakeratosis, and diminished thickness of the granular layer (McMahon et al. 2022).

New-onset lichen planus (LP) and lichenoid reactions were reported in 0.07% and 0.05% of vaccine-associated cutaneous reaction reports, respectively (Avallone et al. 2022a). Histologic findings included the characteristic lichenoid interface dermatitis with saw-tooth appearance and hypergranulosis, vacuolar degeneration of basal layer, and dense lymphocytic infiltrate in the superficial dermis (McMahon et al. 2022; Hiltun et al. 2021). Reports of vitiligo post-vaccination are reported in 0.03% of vaccine-associated cutaneous findings. Loss of pigmentation has occurred both at the site of vaccination and distant sites (Singh et al. 2022; Ciccarese et al. 2022). Morphea, an indurated, light to dark brown, atrophic plaque usually at the injection site, has been reported in the literature in few isolated cases after mRNA vaccination (Català et al. 2022; Antoñanzas et al. 2022). Erythromelalgia is a syndrome of intermittently red, hot, painful extremities—most often the lower extremities but can include the upper extremities. Erythromelalgia has been reported in 0.32% of vaccine-associated cutaneous reactions, all in relation to mRNA vaccines (McMahon et al. 2021; McMahon et al. 2022).

Booster Vaccinations

mRNA-based booster vaccinations were introduced in 2021 in response to waning immunity and the emergence of SARS-CoV-2 variants. Cutaneous reactions to booster doses of mRNA vaccines have been seen in both individuals with no prior reactions and those with previous reported reactions alike. In a registry study of 36 patients with reactions to booster vaccination, 26 reported new reactions to booster vaccination. The most commonly reported reactions included local site reactions, delayed large local reactions, urticaria, erythromelalgia, and vesicular reactions (Prasad et al. 2022; Judd et al. 2022). A multicenter Italian study found that of 13 patients, all were isolated reactions to booster vaccination (Avallone et al. 2022b). The same study found that a heterologous booster regiment, i.e., introduction of the mRNA1273 vaccine after the BNT162b2 showed greater reactogenicity (Avallone et al. 2022b). Patients reporting cutaneous reactions to booster vaccination, particularly urticaria, report high rates of vaccine hesitancy or unwillingness to receive future recommended COVID-19 vaccine (Judd et al. 2022). Investigations into the immunologic mechanism of cutaneous reactions to both primary series and newer bivalent mRNA-based vaccines remain imperative to combat vaccine hesitancy and improve vaccination rates.

Characterizing the Severity of Cutaneous Vaccine Reactions

Cutaneous reactions to mRNA vaccination vary significantly. To date, there is no standardized grading scale for assessing the severity of reactions. One study proposed a method of standardizing terminology, which included mapping localized and generalized cutaneous reactions to vaccination to two preexisting scales, the FDA's Toxicity Grading Scale and the National Cancer Institute's Common Terminology Criteria for Adverse Events (CTCAE) respectively (Singh et al. 2023). Although not yet adopted as a standardized tool, these scales may provide dermatologists the terminology needed to assess severity and response to treatment.

Cutaneous Reactions in Context

The reporting of cutaneous reactions is subject to multiple external factors. There was a significant difference in case reporting by patient sex, with percent women ranging from 62 to 82% in large studies (Avallone et al. 2022a; McMahon et al. 2022; Al Salmi et al. 2022). The difference by sex has been hypothesized to be due to an increase in reactogenicity to vaccines in women or due to reporting bias (Klein et al. 2010). Additionally, with disease processes such as varicella zoster, autoimmune bullous diseases, and pityriasis rosea, it is important to consider the background rate of these disease processes in the general population. Assessing causality can prove challenging: in future, larger-scale epidemiologic studies may help distinguish whether there is a true increase in incidence in some of these reactions post-vaccination (Singh et al. 2023).

Conclusion

With nearly 13 billion doses administered globally, vaccines are an integral tool in mitigating the impacts of SARS-CoV-2. The spectrum of cutaneous reactions reported after vaccination with mRNA-based vaccines vary widely but are largely non-severe and self-limiting in nature. Interestingly, many reaction types seen in response to mRNA vaccination mimic those reported in SARS-CoV-2 infection, suggesting a similar host immune response to viral infection and vaccination (McMahon et al. 2022). Despite being labeled as non-severe, many of the above reactions can have significant impact on the quality of life of affected patients. Dermatologists have the opportunity to recognize and counsel on vaccine-associated reactions with the available information and engage in dialogue and investigations into the underlying pathophysiology of many cutaneous reactions. A better understanding of the underlying mechanisms is key to combat hesitancy in affected patients and to further vaccination efforts. With much still left to learn regarding cutaneous reactions, dermatologist play a role in combatting the hesitancy that may result from a cutaneous reaction after vaccination and provide appropriate reassurance that vaccination remains an integral tool in the efforts to decrease SARS-CoV-2 morbidity and mortality.

References

Al Salmi A, Al Khamisani M, Al Shibli A, Al MS. Adverse cutaneous reactions reported post COVID-19 vaccination in Al Buraimi governorate, Sultanate of Oman. Dermatol Ther. 2022;35:e15820.

Alharbi M. Telogen effluvium after COVID-19 vaccination among public in Saudi Arabia. J Family Med Prim Care. 2022;11(10):6056–60.

American Society of Plastic Surgeons. ASPS guidance concerning FDA reported adverse events in patients with dermal fillers receiving the SARS-CoV-2 mRNA Vaccine. 2021. https://www.plasticsurgery.org/for-medical-professionals/covid19-member-resources/covid19-vaccine-dermal-fillers.

Antoñanzas J, Rodríguez-Garijo N, Estenaga Á, Morelló-Vicente A, España A, Aguado L. Generalized morphea following the COVID vaccine: a series of two patients and a bibliographic review. Dermatol Ther. 2022;35(9):e15709.

Aryanian Z, Balighi K, Hatami P, Afshar ZM, Mohandesi NA. The role of SARS-CoV-2 infection and its vaccines in various types of hair loss. Dermatol Ther. 2022;35(6):e15433.

Avallone G, Quaglino P, Cavallo F, Roccuzzo G, Ribero S, Zalaudek I, et al. SARS-CoV-2 vaccine-related cutaneous manifestations: a systematic review. Int J Dermatol. 2022a;61(10):1187–204.

Avallone G, Cavallo F, Astrua C, Caldarola G, Conforti C, De Simone C, et al. Cutaneous adverse reactions following SARS-CoV-2 vaccine booster dose: a real-life multicentre experience. J Eur Acad Dermatol Venereol. 2022b;36(11):e876–e9.

Baden LR, El Sahly HM, Essink B, Kotloff K, Frey S, Novak R, et al. Efficacy and safety of the mRNA-1273 SARS-CoV-2 vaccine. N Engl J Med. 2021;384(5):403–16.

Bellinato F, Fratton Z, Girolomoni G, Gisondi P. Cutaneous adverse reactions to SARS-CoV-2 vaccines: a systematic review and meta-analysis. Vaccines (Basel). 2022;10(9):1475.

Birabaharan M, Kaelber DC, Orme CM, Paravar T, Karris MY. Evaluating risk of bullous pemphigoid after mRNA COVID-19 vaccination. Br J Dermatol. 2022;187(2):271–3.

Blumenthal KG, Freeman EE, Saff RR, Robinson LB, Wolfson AR, Foreman RK, et al. Delayed large local reactions to mRNA-1273 vaccine against SARS-CoV-2. N Engl J Med. 2021;384(13):1273–7.

Borg L, Mercieca L, Mintoff D, Micallef D, Pisani D, Betts A, et al. Pfizer-BioNTech SARS-CoV-2 mRNA vaccine-associated erythema multiforme. J Eur Acad Dermatol Venereol. 2022;36(1):e22–e4.

Cappel JA, Wetter DA. Clinical characteristics, etiologic associations, laboratory findings, treatment, and proposal of diagnostic criteria of pernio (chilblains) in a series of 104 patients at Mayo Clinic, 2000 to 2011. Mayo Clin Proc. 2014;89(2):207–15.

Català A, Muñoz-Santos C, Galván-Casas C, Roncero Riesco M, Revilla Nebreda D, Solá-Truyols A, et al. Cutaneous reactions after SARS-COV-2 vaccination: a cross-sectional Spanish nationwide study of 405 cases. Br J Dermatol. 2022;186:142.

CDC. Interim considerations: preparing for the potential management of anaphylaxis after COVID-19 vaccination. 2022. https://www.cdc.gov/vaccines/covid-19/clinical-considerations/managing-anaphylaxis.html#:~:text=Patients%20who%20experience%20a%20severe,either%20Pfizer%2DBioNTech%20or%20Moderna.

Center for Disease Control and Prevention. The moderna COVID-19 vaccine's local reactions, systemic reactions, adverse events, and serious adverse events. 2022 [updated 21 June 2022]. https://www.cdc.gov/vaccines/covid-19/info-by-product/moderna/reactogenicity.html#18-local-reactions.

Chu DK, Abrams EM, Golden DBK, Blumenthal KG, Wolfson AR, Stone CA Jr, et al. Risk of second allergic reaction to SARS-CoV-2 vaccines: a systematic review and meta-analysis. JAMA Intern Med. 2022;182(4):376–85.

Chuh A, Zawar V, Sciallis G, Kempf W. A position statement on the management of patients with pityriasis rosea. J Eur Acad Dermatol Venereol. 2016;30(10):1670–81.

Ciccarese G, Drago F, Boldrin S, Pattaro M, Parodi A. Sudden onset of vitiligo after COVID-19 vaccine. Dermatol Ther. 2022;35(1):e15196.

Corbeddu M, Diociaiuti A, Vinci MR, Santoro A, Camisa V, Zaffina S, et al. Transient cutaneous manifestations after administration of Pfizer-BioNTech COVID-19 vaccine: an Italian single-centre case series. J Eur Acad Dermatol Venereol. 2021;35(8):e483–e5.

Czech T, Sugihara S, Nishimura Y. Characteristics of hair loss after COVID-19: a systematic scoping review. J Cosmet Dermatol. 2022;21(9):3655–62.

Dahl H, Marcoccia J, Linde A. Antigen detection: the method of choice in comparison with virus isolation and serology for laboratory diagnosis of herpes zoster in human immunodeficiency virus-infected patients. J Clin Microbiol. 1997;35(2):347–9.

Decates TS, Velthuis PJ, Schelke LW, Lardy N, Palou E, Schwartz S, et al. Increased risk of late-onset, immune-mediated, adverse reactions related to dermal fillers in patients bearing HLA-B*08 and DRB1*03 haplotypes. Dermatol Ther. 2021;34(1):e14644.

Drago F, Ciccarese G, Javor S, Parodi A. Vaccine-induced pityriasis rosea and pityriasis rosea-like eruptions: a review of the literature. J Eur Acad Dermatol Venereol. 2016;30(3):544–5.

Fathy RA, McMahon DE, Lee C, Chamberlin GC, Rosenbach M, Lipoff JB, et al. Varicella-zoster and herpes simplex virus reactivation post-COVID-19 vaccination: a review of 40 cases in an international dermatology registry. J Eur Acad Dermatol Venereol. 2022;36(1):e6–9.

Freeman EE, Sun Q, McMahon DE, Singh R, Fathy R, Tyagi A, et al. Skin reactions to COVID-19 vaccines: an American Academy of Dermatology/International League of Dermatological Societies registry update on reaction location and COVID vaccine type. J Am Acad Dermatol. 2022;86(4):e165–e7.

Furer V, Zisman D, Kibari A, Rimar D, Paran Y, Elkayam O. Herpes zoster following BNT162b2 mRNA COVID-19 vaccination in patients with autoimmune inflammatory rheumatic diseases: a case series. Rheumatology (Oxford). 2021;60(Si):SI90–SI5.

Fusano M, Zerbinati N, Bencini PL. Alopecia areata after COVID-19 vaccination: two cases and review of the literature. Dermatol Rep. 2022;14(4):9495.

Ganjei Z, Yazdan Panah M, Rahmati R, Zari Meidani F, Mosavi A. COVID-19 vaccination and alopecia areata: a case report and literature review. Clin Case Rep. 2022;10(9):e6039.

Gidudu J, Kohl KS, Halperin S, Hammer SJ, Heath PT, Hennig R, et al. A local reaction at or near injection site: case definition and guidelines for collection, analysis, and presentation of immunization safety data. Vaccine. 2008;26(52):6800–13.

Hiltun I, Sarriugarte J, Martínez-de-Espronceda I, Garcés A, Llanos C, Vives R, et al. Lichen planus arising after COVID-19 vaccination. J Eur Acad Dermatol Venereol. 2021;35(7):e414–e5.

Huang X, Liang X, Zhang J, Su H, Chen Y. Pemphigus during the COVID-19 epidemic: infection risk, vaccine responses and management strategies. J Clin Med. 2022;11(14):3968.

Huff JC. Erythema multiforme. Dermatol Clin. 1985;3(1):141–52.

Hussain N, Agarwala P, Iqbal K, Omar HMS, Jangid G, Patel V, et al. A systematic review of acute telogen effluvium, a harrowing post-COVID-19 manifestation. J Med Virol. 2022;94(4):1391–401.

James WD, Elston DM, Treat JR, Rosenbach MA. Andrews' diseases of the skin : clinical dermatology. 10th ed. Philadelphia: Saunders Elsevier; 2006.

Jedlowski PM, Jedlowski MF. Morbilliform rash after administration of Pfizer-BioNTech COVID-19 mRNA vaccine. Dermatol Online J. 2021;27(1):13030/qt4xs486zg.

Judd A, Samarakoon U, Wolfson A, Banerji A, Freeman EE, Blumenthal KG. Urticaria after COVID-19 vaccination and vaccine hesitancy. J Allergy Clin Immunol Pract. 2022;149:AB56.

Kalantari Y, Aryanian Z, Mirahmadi SM, Alilou S, Hatami P, Goodarzi A. A systematic review on COVID-19 vaccination and cosmetic filler reactions: a focus on case studies and original articles. J Cosmet Dermatol 2022;21(7): 2713–24.

Karatas E, Nazim A, Patel P, Vaidya T, Drew GS, Amin SA, et al. Erythema multiforme reactions after Pfizer/BioNTech (BNT162b2) and Moderna (mRNA-1273) COVID-19 vaccination: a case series. JAAD Case Rep. 2022;32:55.

Kasperkiewicz M, Woodley DT. Association between vaccination and immunobullous disorders: a brief, updated systematic review with focus on COVID-19. J Eur Acad Dermatol Venereol. 2022a;36(7):e498–500.

Kasperkiewicz M, Woodley DT. Association between vaccination and autoimmune bullous diseases: a systematic review. J Am Acad Dermatol. 2022b;86(5):1160–4.

Katsikas Triantafyllidis K, Giannos P, Mian IT, Kyrtsonis G, Kechagias KS. Varicella zoster virus reactivation following COVID-19 vaccination: a systematic review of case reports. Vaccines (Basel). 2021;9(9):1013.

Kempf W, Kettelhack N, Kind F, Courvoisier S, Galambos J, Pfaltz K. 'COVID arm' – histological features of a delayed-type hypersensitivity reaction to Moderna mRNA-1273 SARS-CoV2 vaccine. J Eur Acad Dermatol Venereol. 2021;35(11):e730–e2.

Kha C, Itkin A. New-onset chilblains in close temporal association to mRNA-1273 vaccination. JAAD Case Rep. 2021;12:12–4.

King B, Ohyama M, Kwon O, Zlotogorski A, Ko J, Mesinkovska NA, et al. Two phase 3 trials of baricitinib for alopecia areata. N Engl J Med. 2022;386(18):1687–99.

Klein SL, Jedlicka A, Pekosz A. The Xs and Y of immune responses to viral vaccines. Lancet Infect Dis. 2010;10(5):338–49.

Kroumpouzos G, Paroikaki ME, Yumeen S, Bhargava S, Mylonakis E. Cutaneous complications of mRNA and AZD1222 COVID-19 vaccines: a worldwide review. Microorganisms. 2022;10(3):624.

Lavery MJ, Nawimana S, Parslew R, Stewart L. A flare of pre-existing erythema multiforme following BNT162b2 (Pfizer-BioNTech) COVID-19 vaccine. Clin Exp Dermatol. 2021;46(7):1325–7.

Lee C, Cotter D, Basa J, Greenberg HL. 20 post-COVID-19 vaccine-related shingles cases seen at the Las Vegas dermatology clinic and sent to us via social media. J Cosmet Dermatol. 2021;20(7):1960–4.

Lopez S, Vakharia P, Vandergriff T, Freeman EE, Vasquez R. Pernio after COVID-19 vaccination. Br J Dermatol. 2021;185:445.

Martinez-Reviejo R, Tejada S, Adebanjo GAR, Chello C, Machado MC, Parisella FR, et al. Varicella-zoster virus reactivation following severe acute respiratory syndrome coronavirus 2 vaccination or infection: new insights. Eur J Intern Med. 2022;104:73–9.

Martora F, Ruggiero A, Battista T, Fabbrocini G, Megna M. Bullous pemphigoid and COVID-19 vaccination: management and treatment reply to 'Bullous pemphigoid in a young male after COVID-19 mRNA vaccine: a report and brief literature review' by Pauluzzi et al. J Eur Acad Dermatol Venereol. 2022;37:e35.

May Lee M, Bertolani M, Pierobon E, Lotti T, Feliciani C, Satolli F. Alopecia areata following COVID-19 vaccination: vaccine-induced autoimmunity? Int J Dermatol. 2022;61(5):634–5.

McMahon DE, Amerson E, Rosenbach M, Lipoff JB, Moustafa D, Tyagi A, et al. Cutaneous reactions reported after Moderna and Pfizer COVID-19 vaccination: a registry-based study of 414 cases. J Am Acad Dermatol. 2021;85(1):46–55.

McMahon DE, Kovarik CL, Damsky W, Rosenbach M, Lipoff JB, Tyagi A, et al. Clinical and pathologic correlation of cutaneous COVID-19 vaccine reactions including V-REPP: a registry-based study. J Am Acad Dermatol. 2022;86(1):113–21.

Munavalli GG, Guthridge R, Knutsen-Larson S, Brodsky A, Matthew E, Landau M. COVID-19/SARS-CoV-2 virus spike protein-related delayed inflammatory reaction to hyaluronic acid dermal fillers: a challenging clinical conundrum in diagnosis and treatment. Arch Dermatol Res. 2022;314(1):1–15.

Ohsawa R, Sano H, Ikeda M, Sano S. Clinical and histopathological views of morbilliform rash after COVID-19 mRNA vaccination mimic those in SARS-CoV-2 virus infection-associated cutaneous manifestations. J Dermatol Sci. 2021;103(2):124–7.

Panda M, Patro N, Jena M, Dash M, Mishra S. Pityriasis rosea like drug rash - a need to identify the disease in childhood. J Clin Diagn Res. 2014;8(8):Yd01-2.

Pardi N, Hogan MJ, Porter FW, Weissman D. mRNA vaccines — a new era in vaccinology. Nat Rev Drug Discov. 2018;17(4):261–79.

Pescosolido E, Muller YD, Sabaté-Brescó M, Ferrer M, Yerly D, Caubet JC, et al. Clinical and immunological data from chronic urticaria onset after mRNA SARS-CoV-2 vaccines. Clin Exp Allergy. 2022;52(11):1343–6.

Picone V, Napolitano M, Martora F, Guerriero L, Fabbrocini G, Patruno C. Urticaria relapse after mRNA COVID-19 vaccines in patients affected by chronic spontaneous urticaria and treated with antihistamines plus omalizumab: a single-center experience. Dermatol Ther. 2022;35(11):e15838.

Polack FP, Thomas SJ, Kitchin N, Absalon J, Gurtman A, Lockhart S, et al. Safety and efficacy of the BNT162b2 mRNA Covid-19 vaccine. N Engl J Med. 2020;383(27):2603–15.

Prasad S, McMahon DE, Tyagi A, Ali R, Singh R, Rosenbach M, et al. Cutaneous reactions following booster dose administration of COVID-19 mRNA vaccine: a first look from the American Academy of Dermatology/International League of Dermatologic Societies registry. JAAD Int. 2022;8:49–51.

Rice SM, Ferree SD, Mesinkovska NA, Kourosh AS. The art of prevention: COVID-19 vaccine preparedness for the dermatologist. Int J Womens Dermatol. 2021;7(2):209–12.

Rodríguez-Jiménez P, Chicharro P, Cabrera LM, Seguí M, Morales-Caballero Á, Llamas-Velasco M, et al. Varicella-zoster virus reactivation after SARS-CoV-2 BNT162b2 mRNA vaccination: report of 5 cases. JAAD Case Rep. 2021;12:58–9.

Rosenblatt AE, Stein SL. Cutaneous reactions to vaccinations. Clin Dermatol. 2015;33(3):327–32.

Safir A, Samuelov L, Sprecher E, Daniely D, Artzi O. Association between BNT162b2 vaccination and the development of delayed inflammatory reactions to hyaluronic acid-based dermal fillers-a nationwide survey. J Cosmet Dermatol. 2022;21(10):4107–13.

Sahin U, Muik A, Derhovanessian E, Vogler I, Kranz LM, Vormehr M, et al. COVID-19 vaccine BNT162b1 elicits human antibody and TH1 T cell responses. Nature. 2020;586(7830):594–9.

Sharif N, Alzahrani KJ, Ahmed SN, Dey SK. Efficacy, immunogenicity and safety of COVID-19 vaccines: a systematic review and meta-analysis. Front Immunol. 2021;12:714170.

Singh R, Cohen JL, Astudillo M, Harris JE, Freeman EE. Vitiligo of the arm after COVID-19 vaccination. JAAD Case Rep. 2022;28:142–4.

Singh R, Ali R, Prasad S, Chen ST, Blumenthal K, Freeman EE. Proposing a standardized assessment of COVID-19 vaccine-associated cutaneous reactions. J Am Acad Dermatol. 2023;88(1):237–41.

Strahan A, Ali R, Freeman E. Chronic spontaneous urticaria after COVID-19 primary vaccine series and boosters. JAAD Case Rep. 2022;25:63.

Sun Q, Freeman EE. Chilblains and COVID-19-an update on the complexities of interpreting antibody test results, the role of interferon α, and COVID-19 vaccines. JAMA Dermatol. 2022;158(2):217–8.

Takci Z, Vahaboglu G, Eksioglu H. Epidemiological patterns of perniosis, and its association with systemic disorder. Clin Exp Dermatol. 2012;37(8):844–9.

Tassone F, Cappilli S, Antonelli F, Zingarelli R, Chiricozzi A, Peris K. Alopecia areata occurring after COVID-19 vaccination: a single-center, cross-sectional study. Vaccines (Basel). 2022;10(9):1467.

Tomayko MM, Damsky W, Fathy R, McMahon DE, Turner N, Valentin MN, et al. Subepidermal blistering eruptions, including bullous pemphigoid, following COVID-19 vaccination. J Allergy Clin Immunol. 2021;148(3):750–1.

Trüeb RM. Systematic approach to hair loss in women. J Dtsch Dermatol Ges. 2010;8(4):284–97, 298.

U.S. Food and Drug Administration. Emergency Use Authorization (EUA) for an Unapproved Product Review Memorandum [Memorandum]. 2020. https://www.fda.gov/emergency-preparedness-and-response/coronavirus-disease-2019-covid-19/covid-19-vaccines.

Wolff K, Johnson RA, Saavedra AP, Roh EK. Fitzpatrick's color atlas and synopsis of clinical dermatology. 7th ed. New York: McGraw-Hill Medical; 2006.

World Health Organization. WHO Coronavirus (COVID-19) Dashboard 2023. https://covid19.who.int/.

Zuberbier T, Asero R, Bindslev-Jensen C, Walter Canonica G, Church MK, Giménez-Arnau AM, et al. EAACI/GA(2)LEN/EDF/WAO guideline: management of urticaria. Allergy. 2009;64(10):1427–43.

Cutaneous Reactions to Non-mRNA COVID-19 Vaccines

4

Pawinee Rerknimitr, Chanudda Washrawirul, and Jidapa Triwatcharikorn

Introduction

Prompt vaccination against SARS-CoV-2 plays a major role in controlling the COVID-19 pandemic. The urgent need for mass COVID-19 vaccination has sped up the research and development of COVID-19 vaccines. To date, there are various platforms of COVID-19 vaccines being used and under development; inactivated whole-virus vaccines such as Sinovac Life Sciences (CoronaVac) and Sinopharm (WIV04 and HB02): protein subunit vaccine: Novavax (NVX-CoV2373): viral vector vaccines: Oxford-AstraZeneca (ChAdOx1 nCoV-19) and Johnson and Johnson (Ad26. CoV2.S): messenger ribonucleic acid (mRNA)-based vaccines: Pfizer-BioNTech (BNT162b2) and Moderna (mRNA-1273): Deoxyribonucleic Acid (DNA) vaccines: Zydus Cadila (ZyCoV-D) (Rabaan et al. 2022). At the time of this writing, 176 vaccines are in clinical development while 199 are in preclinical phase (https://www.who. int/publications/m/item/draft-landscape-of-COVID-19-candidate-vaccines; (Rabaan et al. 2022; Lamb 2021; Robinson et al. 2021; Rerknimitr et al. 2022)).

P. Rerknimitr (✉) · C. Washrawirul
J. Triwatcharikorn
Division of Dermatology, Department of Internal Medicine, Faculty of Medicine, Skin and Allergy Research Unit, Chulalongkorn University, Bangkok, Thailand
e-mail: pawinee.r@chula.ac.th

Incidence, Prevalence, and Type of Cutaneous Adverse Reactions Following Non-mRNA COVID-19 Vaccination

COVID-19 vaccination started in December 2020, after the approval of emergency use authorization mRNA vaccines (Lamb 2021). Until now, approximately 12,248,795,623 doses have been administered worldwide (Rabaan et al. 2022). A number of cases with cutaneous adverse reactions (CARs) from the vaccine have gradually emerged, and that number continues to grow. However, considering their widely use, CARs are not common. The incidence of cutaneous reactions following mRNA vaccines was 1.9% after the first dose and 2.3% after the second dose (Robinson et al. 2021), whereas those from inactivated virus vaccine, CoronaVac, was 0.94% and 0.70% from the first and second doses, and those of viral vector, ChAdOx1 nCoV-19 were 1% and 0.52%, respectively (Rerknimitr et al. 2022). A recent systematic review and meta-analysis indicated that the pooled incidence of overall CARs was 5%. The studies involving the mRNA vaccines alone showed the incidence of 3%, whereas when other platforms were combined, the incidence was 5% (Bellinato et al. 2022).

In addition, we have conducted a systematic review and meta-analysis of CARs following COVID-19 vaccination. Of the 946,366 vaccine doses administered, we found that the pooled

© The Author(s), under exclusive license to Springer Nature Switzerland AG 2023
H. H. Oon, C. L. Goh (eds.), *COVID-19 in Dermatology*, Updates in Clinical Dermatology,
https://doi.org/10.1007/978-3-031-45586-5_4

prevalence of overall cutaneous adverse reactions was 3.8%. Interestingly, comparing the various platforms, the mRNA vaccines exhibited the highest prevalence, followed by the viral vector-based vaccines and the inactivated SARS-CoV-2 vaccine (at 6.9%, 3.5%, and 0.9%, respectively) (Washrawirul et al. 2022). The fact that CARs occur most frequently from the mRNA vaccine administration was also confirmed by others systematic reviews and/or meta-analysis (Kroumpouzos et al. 2022; Bostan et al. 2022; Avallone et al. 2022; Seirafianpour et al. 2022). However, it is important to note that mRNA vaccine is the first platform being used. This allows a greater number of administered doses and more reported cases. Intriguingly, a meta-analysis in which CARs from mRNA were compared with those of viral vector platform, indicated that overall relative risk ratio for development of local side effects was greater with the mRNA vaccine while for non-local side effects, rash, urticaria, and angioedema, the risk was higher with the viral vector vaccine group (Shafie'ei et al. 2022).

The common CARs following the non-mRNA vaccines were acute local injection site reactions, rash/dermatitis, or unspecified skin eruption, urticaria or angioedema, maculopapular rash, herpes zoster, delayed large-local reactions, petechiae/purpura/ecchymosis, pityriasis rosea/pityriasis rosea-like eruption, vasculitis/vasculitis-like lesion, vesiculobullous lesion, and chilblains/chilblains-like lesion. Less common conditions included exacerbation of preexisting dermatosis, erythema multiforme, and severe cutaneous adverse drug reactions (SCARs) (Bellinato et al. 2022; Washrawirul et al. 2022; Avallone et al. 2022). The types of CARs remain similar across the vaccine platforms. However, certain findings such as delayed large local reactions are found far more frequent with the mRNA vaccines (Washrawirul et al. 2022; Kroumpouzos et al. 2022). Interestingly, the rate of CARs was not different between the first and second doses of vaccination (Bellinato et al. 2022; Washrawirul et al. 2022) and usually more reported in female (Kroumpouzos et al. 2022).

Cutaneous Adverse Reactions from Non-mRNA COVID-19 Vaccine

CARs following non-mRNA vaccines are like those of mRNA platforms, but a lower number of cases are reported, as discussed earlier. CARs can be categorized by the underlying immuno-pathogenesis as follows; type 1 hypersensitivity, type IV hypersensitivity, autoimmune-mediated, and other reactions (Shafie'ei et al. 2022).

Type 1 Hypersensitivity Reactions

Type 1, also known as immediate-type hypersensitivity reaction, includes urticaria, angioedema, and anaphylaxis.

Urticaria and angioedema are common CARs. Almost half of the reported cases were from the mRNA vaccine, leaving inactivate viral and viral vector vaccines the second and the third culprit agents (Washrawirul et al. 2022). From our study where CoronaVac and ChAdOx1 nCoV-19 were administered in healthcare personnel, urticaria was the most skin reactions observed, reported in 92 of 29,907 CoronaVac and 12 of 5322 ChAdOx1 nCoV-19 injections. The overall incidence of urticaria was $n = 104/35,229$ (0.3%) (Rerknimitr et al. 2022). The median onset (IQR) of urticaria was 6 (1.5, 24) h, and the duration was 2 (0.2, 8) h. Of 104 reports of urticaria, 3 (0.99%) were observed with angioedema and 2 (0.66%) were with anaphylaxis. Among urticaria following CoronaVac injections, a number of reactions with onset less than 4 h was 40 (40/92). Among these 40, there were only two reactions that the wheals presented in more than one site of the body. Recurrent eruption was found in one of these two cases with a decrease in severity, when the second dose of CoronaVac was administered. No case of anaphylaxis occurred in those with urticaria from the first dose vaccination. Therefore, we speculate that urticaria alone post CoronaVac injection is quite benign (Rerknimitr et al. 2022). From a recent perspective observational study on CARs following Sinopharm vac-

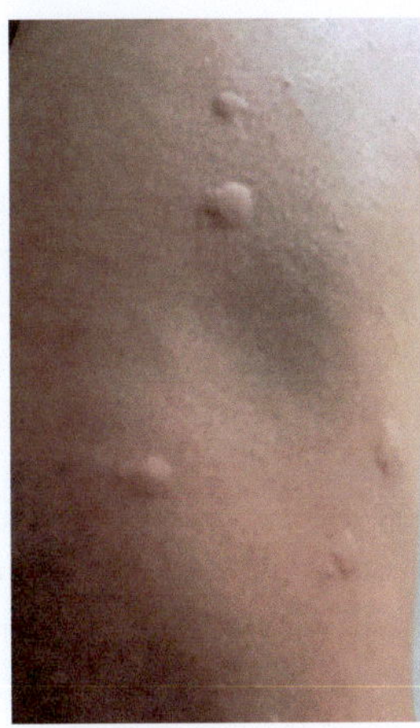

Fig. 4.1 Acute urticaria following CoronaVac vaccination

cination, it was shown that urticaria and angioedema occurred in 4.6 and 2.3% of the vaccine recipients, respectively (Shawky et al. 2023). Figure 4.1 shows urticaria following CoronaVac.

Regarding the treatments, 26% of the patients with urticaria and angioedema were treated with oral antihistamine followed by intravenous antihistamine and systemic steroid (at 20% and 17%, respectively). Spontaneous improvement was observed in 40% of the patients. The mean duration of the condition was for 24.28 ± 34.38 h (Washrawirul et al. 2022).

Anaphylaxis is a life-threatening reaction that occurs rarely from COVID-19 vaccination (Washrawirul et al. 2022; Banerji et al. 2021). The clinical symptoms include generalized urticaria, angioedema, diarrhea, respiratory distress, and possibility of anaphylactic shock in some patients. This type of hypersensitivity develops within 4 h after the vaccines are administered. Further dosage of the vaccine is contraindicated in patients with a history of anaphylaxis to the vaccine (Banerji et al. 2021; Alpalhão et al. 2021). The incidence of anaphylaxis following the vaccine was 7.91 cases per million (n = 41,000,000 vaccinations; 95% confidence interval [95% CI] 4.02–15.59; 26, with no report of fatalities. Compared to mRNA, the adenoviral vector (OR 0.47; 95% CI 0.33–0.68) and inactivated virus vaccines (OR 0.31; 95% CI 0.18–

0.53) showed lower anaphylaxis rates (Greenhawt et al. 2021). In participants receiving CoronaVac, the reported incidence rate of anaphylaxis was 0.007–0.09% (Rerknimitr et al. 2022; Öztürk et al. 2022). The onset of the reaction was 12 ± 6 min (range, 3–15 min) after vaccination. Associated systemic symptoms are shortness of breath (75%) and alteration of consciousness (75%) (Öztürk et al. 2022). A case series from Thailand reported 12 cases of anaphylaxis following CoronaVac vaccination (Laisuan et al. 2021). The mean interval from the vaccination to the onset of symptoms was 30 min (range, 6–180 min). One-third of the patients had onset within 15 min, and two-thirds within 30 min. Fifty percent of the patients had associated urticaria and/or angioedema. Ten out of 12 patients underwent skin testing. Interestingly, only two exhibited positive skin tests. Moreover, serum tryptase was not elevated in these patients. These findings suggested that anaphylaxis following CoronaVac might be mediated through various mechanisms; possibly through IgE/FcεR1-dependent mast cell activation or not (Laisuan et al. 2021). The excipients of the vaccines, not the viral antigen, is thought to be responsible for the immediate-type hypersensitivity reactions. For CoronaVac, aluminum is the most likely allergen, while polysorbate 80, also known as Tween 80, was responsible for the viral vector, ChAdOx1 nCoV-19, and Johnson & Johnson COVID-19 vaccines (Laisuan et al. 2021; Kounis et al. 2021). For those who experience anaphylaxis from CoronaVac, it is recommended to consider the alternative vaccine platforms, if the patients wish to have further COVID-19 vaccination (Laisuan et al. 2021).

Type IV Hypersensitivity

Examples of type IV or delayed-type hypersensitivity reactions are delayed large local (COVID arm), delayed inflammatory reactions (DIR) to hyaluronic acid dermal filler, maculopapular eruption, and erythema multiforme (Nakashima et al. 2023).

The most common CAR from vaccines is local reaction including erythema, edema, and tenderness at the injection site (Alpalhão et al. 2021). From phase 1/2 clinical trial of CoronaVac in healthy adults aged 18–59 years (Zhang et al. 2021) and 60 years and older (Wu et al. 2021), injection site reactions were found in 11–18.8%, and mucocutaneous eruption was found in 4% of the volunteers (Zhang et al. 2021; Wu et al. 2021). Similarly, the most common CAR of ChAdOx1 nCoV-19 is local reaction. Itch, redness, and swelling were observed in 2–12%, 0–2%, and 0–2% respectively from phase 1/2 and 2/3 clinical trials (Folegatti et al. 2020; Ramasamy et al. 2021).

Nonetheless, delayed large local reaction (COVID arm) is different from the acute local injection site reaction in that the former takes place approximately 1 week after vaccination. This usually manifests as tender, indurated erythematous subcutaneous nodule at the injection site with possible extension to upper arm. Figure 4.2 denotes delayed large local reaction from ChAdOx1 nCoV-19. The onset was 7 days after the first vaccination and 2 days after the second dose (McMahon et al. 2021). The most common associated platform was the mRNA vaccine, followed by the viral vectors. The symptoms are usually mild. The main treatment was topical corticosteroids and oral antihistamines (Washrawirul et al. 2022; Kroumpouzos et al. 2022). Interestingly, DIR to hyaluronic acid dermal filler was reported mainly in the mRNA vaccine recipients (Washrawirul et al. 2022). Only three reported cases were associated with non-mRNA vaccines: two with ChAdOx1 nCoV-19 and one case with Sinopharm (Ortigosa et al. 2022). The reported clinical presentation was edematous inflammatory erythematous papules and nodules over the injected areas (Munavalli et al. 2022; Safir et al. 2022).

Maculopapular eruptions and erythema multiforme can be observed after the mRNA, viral vector, and inactivated virus vaccines administration (the number of reported cases in descending order) (Washrawirul et al. 2022). The distribution of maculopapular rashes can be generalized, acral, and extremities predominant (Nakashima et al. 2023).

Autoimmune-Mediated Reaction

The spike protein of COVID-19 vaccines may induce immune reactions in human via molecular mimicry. For that reason, new onset and exacerbation of autoimmune diseases have been reported after the vaccination (Nakashima et al. 2023). Examples of autoimmune diseases that were reported to be aggravated by the vaccination are cutaneous lupus erythematosus, vasculitis, bullous pemphigoid, pemphigus vulgaris, vitiligo, lichen planus, and adult-onset Still's a disease (Washrawirul et al. 2022).

Though the exact causes of vasculitis in almost half of patients cannot be identified, it is known that drugs, vaccines, and infectious agents are major triggering factors (Antiga et al. 2015). Almost all available COVID-19 vaccines are associated with vasculitis. The highest number of reported cases were induced by mRNA vaccines, followed by viral vector, and inactivated vaccines (Washrawirul et al. 2022; Azzazi et al. 2022; Corrà et al. 2022; Bencharattanaphakhi and

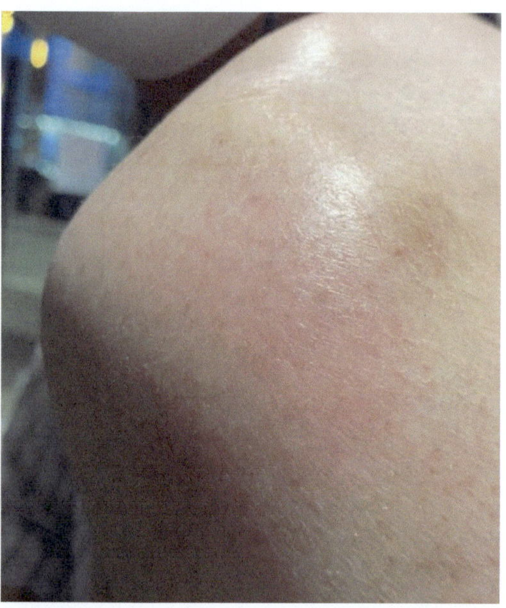

Fig. 4.2 Delayed large local reaction from ChAdOx1 nCoV-19

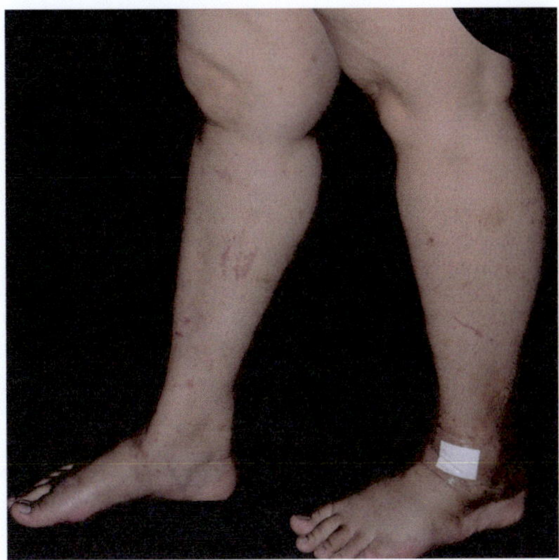

Fig. 4.3 Leukocytoclastic vasculitis following CoronaVac vaccination

Rerknimitr 2021). In a review article that focused on cutaneous vasculitis, predominantly leukocytoclastic vasculitis (LCV), 39 cases were identified. The temporal relationship between vaccination and development of lesions ranged from 36 h to 20 days. Most manifested as multiple palpable purpuric papules on the legs. Figure 4.3 shows LCV associated with CoronaVac. Direct immunofluorescence (DIF) was available in 18 (46.2%) cases; 13/18 cases showed positive results. In those with positivity, heterogeneous findings were found, 12.8% with IgA and 7.7% with C3 deposition around blood vessels (Corrà et al. 2022). Our systematic review also identified newly developed and flaring of existing vasculitis cases. If presented, concomitant systemic findings were arthralgia, fever, myalgia, fatigue, diarrhea, abdominal pain, and hematuria. Most were treated with systemic corticosteroids, and the mean duration of the illness was 15.21 (13.70) days (Washrawirul et al. 2022).

In addition to LCV, a global pharmacovigilance study described 330 cases of de novo IgA vasculitis. Eighty-five percent (280/330) of patients were associated with mRNA vaccines. Moreover, there was no significant difference between mRNA and viral vector vaccines (Ramdani et al. 2023). Interestingly, skin biopsy specimens from the IgA vasculitis lesions were examined for the presence of neutrophil extracellular traps (NETs) in the dermis in a study to investigate the differences among COVID-19, COVID-19-vaccine-induced, and non-COVID-19-related IgA vasculitis. NETs deposition is thought to underlie the pathogenesis of COVID-19. From this study, there were no differences in NETs deposition among the three groups. The author concluded that it was not the directly coronavirus-induced NETs that were responsible for the development of the lesions. On the other hand, various environmental triggers including infectious agents, drugs, and vaccines might similarly trigger the development of IgA vasculitis leading to NETs deposition (Kawakami et al. 2023).

Autoimmune bullous diseases (AIBDs) have also been reported following COVID-19 vaccination either as de novo or flaring of the diseases. The reported AIBDs were mostly non-identified AIBDs, followed by bullous pemphigoid, pemphigus vulgaris, linear IgA bullous dermatosis, and pemphigus foliaceus. The mRNA vaccines were responsible in 81.1%, viral vectors in 15.5%, and inactivated vaccine in 1.8%. The onset ranged from 1 day to 6 weeks following the vaccination. The symptoms can be controlled with traditional immunosuppressive therapy (Kasperkiewicz and Woodley 2022).

Others

Pityriasis rosea (PR) was reported after all vaccine platforms. The mean onset was 9.64 (6.11) days after the vaccination and last for 49 (24.09) days. The patients may manifest with a typical herald patch followed by minute erythematous patches with collarette scale or atypical lesions. The lesion appeared on the trunk (79.17%), extremities (70.83%), and generalized (8.33%) with pruritus. This condition can be self-limited, but several patients were treated with topical corticosteroids, systemic corticosteroids, and antihistamines (Washrawirul et al. 2022). Multiple viral reactivations including human herpesvirus-6 (HHV-6), HHV-7, and Epstein-Barr virus have been demonstrated in COVID-19 infection

(Drago et al. 2021). The reactivation might also play an important role in the development of PR post vaccination.

Herpes zoster reactivation is triggered by COVID-19 vaccination and is reported in all administered vaccine platforms. The mean onset was 7.76 (6.38) days after the vaccination and lasted for 12.46 ± 6.81 days. The reactivation may present after the first, second, and both doses of injections (58.73, 38.10, and 3.17, orderly). The lesions were located along the dermatome, mostly thoracic (50.88%), cranial (31.58%), lumbar (15.79%), and sacral (5.26%). Two cases were diagnosed with herpes zoster ophthalmicus (Bernardini et al. 2021). Most of the cases were treated with antiviral agents: acyclovir or valacyclovir (89.06%). Gabapentin was given in case of neuropathic pain (18.75%) simultaneously with analgesics drug (14.06%) (Washrawirul et al. 2022).

Vaccine-induced immune thrombotic thrombocytopenia (VITT) is an emerging syndrome from adenoviral-based platform vaccines, especially with ChAdOx1 nCoV-19. It is characterized by thrombocytopenia and thrombosis of the unusual sites, namely cerebral and/or splanchnic veins (Arepally and Ortel 2021). In addition to systemic symptoms, skin findings such as multiple small ecchymosis, purpura, and petechiae may be found (Bogdanov et al. 2021). In our study in which ChAdOx1 nCoV-19 was administered in healthcare personnel, we found no case of VITT. However, a case of secondary immune thrombotic thrombocytopenia (ITP) post ChAdOx1 nCoV-19 with multiple ecchymosis was observed (Rerknimitr et al. 2022). This is in keeping with the ongoing reports in the literature of newly developed ITP post COVID-19 vaccination (Welsh et al. 2021). Dermatologists should be aware of the importance of these skin findings, and prompt investigations should be undertaken in suspected cases.

Severe cutaneous adverse reactions to drug (SCARs) encompass Stevens–Johnson syndrome/toxic epidermal necrolysis (SJS/TEN), drug reaction with eosinophilia and systemic symptoms (DRESS), acute generalized exanthematous pustulosis (AGEP), and generalized bullous fixed drug eruptions (GBFDE). These conditions are life-threatening resulting in mortality and morbidity. Few cases of SCARs due to COVID-19 vaccination have been reported. These included AGEP ($n = 4$), SJS-TEN ($n = 4$), DRESS ($n = 1$), GBFDE ($n = 1$), bullous drug eruption with features of SJS ($n = 1$), and inconclusive diagnosis (differential diagnosis to AGEP, DRESS, or AGEP/DRESS overlap) ($n = 1$). All vaccine platforms were capable of inducing these severe reactions (ChAdOx1-S 42%, BNT162b2 17%, mRNA-1273 17%, Ad26.COV2.S 8%, BBiBP 8%, and unidentified vaccines 8%). Six cases occurred in the first dose only, three cases in the second dose, and one case in both doses of vaccination. The mean onset was 9.34 (15.38) days following the vaccination, and the duration was 20.83 (9.56) days (Drago et al. 2021; Aimo et al. 2022). Other minor drug eruptions, such as fixed drug eruption, systemic drug-related intertriginous, and flexural exanthema (SDRIFE), were also stated in publications (Washrawirul et al. 2022).

Table 4.1 summarized the various cutaneous reactions to non mRNA-COVID-19 vaccines. The number of the cases from the table came from our recent meta-analysis and systematic review that included case reports, case series, case–control studies, retrospective/prospective cohort studies, and randomized controlled trials published between January 1, 2019 and December 31, 2021 (Washrawirul et al. 2022).

Table 4.1 Cutaneous manifestations to non-mRNA COVID-19 vaccines (n = number of cases)

Cutaneous manifestations (n)	Total of non-mRNA COVID-19 vaccines	Viral vector vaccine	Inactivated viral vaccine	Protein subunit vaccine
Acute injection site reaction	12,492	12,110	382	0
Rash/unspecified skin eruption	2207	1803	404	0
Urticaria and/or angioedema	1085	920	165	0
Pruritus without skin lesion	10	6	4	0
Delayed large local reactions	24	24	0	0
Maculopapular rash	53	36	17	0
Herpes zoster	40	28	12	0
Oral blister/ulcer/vesicle	38	38	0	0
PR/PR-like lesion[a]	38	12	26	0
Vesiculobullous lesion	10	7	3	0
Petechiae/purpura/ecchymosis	41	22	19	0
Chilblains/chilblains-like lesion	10	7	3	0
Vasculitis/vasculitic-like lesion	18	9	9	0
CLE[a]	2	2	0	0
Eczema/eczematous lesion	23	5	18	0
Papulovesicular lesion	16	9	7	0
Erythema multiforme	8	4	4	0
Psoriasis	12	10	2	0
Oral white/red plaque	5	5	0	0
Anaphylaxis	20	5	15	0
Herpes simplex virus infection	7	7	0	0
Angular cheilitis	1	1	0	0
Lichen planus	2	1	0	1
Bullous pemphigoid	2	1	1	0
SCARs[a]	7	5	1	1
Alopecia	4	4	0	0
ITP[a]	2	2	0	0
Papulosquamous/pityriasiform lesion	8	0	8	0
Pemphigus Vulgaris	2	2	0	0
Acne/acneiform lesion	6	1	5	0
Sweet's syndrome	3	3	0	0
PRP/PRP-like lesion[a]	2	2	0	0
SDRIFE[a]	2	1	1	0
Vitiligo	1	0	1	0
Reaction to breast implant	1	1	0	0
Alopecia areata	3	3	0	0
Erythema nodosum	2	2	0	0
Skin necrosis	1	1	0	0
Still's disease	1	1	0	0
Multisystem inflammatory syndrome	1	1	0	0
Radiation recall dermatitis	2	1	1	0
Papulopustular lesion	1	1	0	0
Palmar erythema	2	0	2	0
Erythema annulare centrifugum	1	1	0	0
Viral warts	1	1	0	0
Darier's disease	1	1	0	0
Lipschütz ulcer	1	1	0	0

(continued)

Table 4.1 (continued)

Cutaneous manifestations (*n*)	Total of non-mRNA COVID-19 vaccines	Viral vector vaccine	Inactivated viral vaccine	Protein subunit vaccine
Acute localized exanthematous pustulosis	1	1	0	0
Superficial venous thrombosis	1	1	0	0
Serum sickness-like reaction	1	0	1	0
Eosinophilic dermatosis	1	1	0	0
Linear IgA bullous dermatosis	1	1	0	0
Exuberant lichenoid eruption	1	1	0	0
Insect bite	1	1	0	0
Folliculitis	1	0	1	0

[a] *PR* pityriasis rosea, *CLE* cutaneous lupus erythematosus, *DIR* delayed inflammatory reactions, *SCARs* severe cutaneous adverse reactions, *ITP* idiopathic thrombocytopenic purpura, *PRP* pityriasis rubra pilaris, *SDRIFE* systemic drug-related intertriginous and flexural exanthema

Conclusions

The most common CARs from non-mNRA vaccines are injection site reaction, followed by urticaria and/or angioedema, maculopapular rash, and COVID arm. Flare-up of autoimmune and preexisting dermatosis was also observed, presumably due to immune dysregulation induced by the vaccination. Delayed large local reactions and DIRs to hyaluronic dermal fillers were much more common in the mRNA platform. Skin reactions should not prevent individuals from the scheduled vaccinations.

Funding Sources None.

Conflicts of Interest None.

References

Aimo C, Mariotti EB, Corrà A, Cipollini E, Le Rose O, Serravalle C, et al. Stevens-Johnson syndrome induced by Vaxvetria (AZD1222) COVID-19 vaccine. J Eur Acad Dermatol Venereol. 2022;36(6):e417–e9. https://doi.org/10.1111/jdv.17988.

Alpalhão M, Maia-Silva J, Filipe P. Severe acute respiratory syndrome coronavirus 2 vaccines and cutaneous adverse reactions: a review. Dermatitis. 2021;32(3):133–9. https://doi.org/10.1097/der.0000000000000755.

Antiga E, Verdelli A, Bonciani D, Bonciolini V, Quintarelli L, Volpi W, et al. Drug-induced cutaneous vasculitides. G Ital Dermatol Venereol. 2015;150(2):203–10.

Arepally GM, Ortel TL. Vaccine-induced immune thrombotic thrombocytopenia (VITT): what we know and Don't know. Blood. 2021;138:293. https://doi.org/10.1182/blood.2021012152.

Avallone G, Quaglino P, Cavallo F, Roccuzzo G, Ribero S, Zalaudek I, et al. SARS-CoV-2 vaccine-related cutaneous manifestations: a systematic review. Int J Dermatol. 2022;61(10):1187–204. https://doi.org/10.1111/ijd.16063.

Azzazi Y, Abdelkader HA, Khedr H, El-Komy MHM. Extensive cutaneous leukocytoclastic vasculitis after Sinopharm vaccine: case report and review of the literature. J Cutan Pathol. 2022;49(8):736–42. https://doi.org/10.1111/cup.14235.

Banerji A, Wickner PG, Saff R, Stone CA Jr, Robinson LB, Long AA, et al. mRNA vaccines to prevent COVID-19 disease and reported allergic reactions: current evidence and suggested approach. J Allergy Clin Immunol Pract. 2021;9(4):1423–37. https://doi.org/10.1016/j.jaip.2020.12.047.

Bellinato F, Fratton Z, Girolomoni G, Gisondi P. Cutaneous adverse reactions to SARS-CoV-2 vaccines: a systematic review and meta-analysis. Vaccines (Basel). 2022;10(9):1475. https://doi.org/10.3390/vaccines10091475.

Bencharattanaphakhi R, Rerknimitr P. Sinovac COVID-19 vaccine-induced cutaneous leukocytoclastic vasculitis. JAAD Case Rep. 2021;18:1–3. https://doi.org/10.1016/j.jdcr.2021.10.002.

Bernardini N, Skroza N, Mambrin A, Proietti I, Marchesiello A, Marraffa F, et al. Herpes zoster ophthalmicus in two women after Pfizer-BioNTech (BNT162b2) vaccine. J Med Virol. 2021;94:817. https://doi.org/10.1002/jmv.27366.

Bogdanov G, Bogdanov I, Kazandjieva J, Tsankov N. Cutaneous adverse effects of the available COVID-19 vaccines. Clin Dermatol. 2021;39:523. https://doi.org/10.1016/j.clindermatol.2021.04.001.

Bostan E, Yel B, Karaduman A. Cutaneous adverse events following 771 doses of the inactivated and mRNA COVID-19 vaccines: a survey study among health care providers. J Cosmet Dermatol. 2022;21(9):3682–8. https://doi.org/10.1111/jocd.15203.

Corrà A, Verdelli A, Mariotti EB, Ruffo di Calabria V, Quintarelli L, Aimo C, et al. Cutaneous vasculitis: lessons from COVID-19 and COVID-19 vaccination. Front Med. 2022;9:1013846. https://doi.org/10.3389/fmed.2022.1013846.

Drago F, Ciccarese G, Rebora A, Parodi A. Human herpesvirus-6, -7, and Epstein-Barr virus reactivation in pityriasis rosea during COVID-19. J Med Virol. 2021;93(4):1850–1. https://doi.org/10.1002/jmv.26549.

Folegatti PM, Ewer KJ, Aley PK, Angus B, Becker S, Belij-Rammerstorfer S, et al. Safety and immunogenicity of the ChAdOx1 nCoV-19 vaccine against SARS-CoV-2: a preliminary report of a phase 1/2, single-blind, randomised controlled trial. Lancet. 2020;396(10249):467–78. https://doi.org/10.1016/s0140-6736(20)31604-4.

Greenhawt M, Abrams EM, Shaker M, Chu DK, Khan D, Akin C, et al. The risk of allergic reaction to SARS-CoV-2 vaccines and recommended evaluation and management: a systematic review, meta-analysis, GRADE assessment, and international consensus approach. J Allergy Clin Immunol Pract. 2021;9(10):3546–67. https://doi.org/10.1016/j.jaip.2021.06.006.

Kasperkiewicz M, Woodley DT. Association between vaccination and immunobullous disorders: a brief, updated systematic review with focus on COVID-19. J Eur Acad Dermatol Venereol. 2022;36(7):e498–500. https://doi.org/10.1111/jdv.18030.

Kawakami T, Yokoyama K, Ikeda T, Nishibata Y, Masuda S, Tomaru U, et al. Similar deposition of neutrophil extracellular traps in the dermis among COVID-19-associated IgA vasculitis, post-COVID-19 vaccination IgA vasculitis, and COVID-19-unrelated IgA vasculitis. J Dermatol. 2023;50:e151. https://doi.org/10.1111/1346-8138.16673.

Kounis NG, Koniari I, de Gregorio C, Velissaris D, Petalas K, Brinia A, et al. Allergic reactions to current available COVID-19 vaccinations: pathophysiology, causality, and therapeutic considerations. Vaccines (Basel). 2021;9(3):221. https://doi.org/10.3390/vaccines9030221.

Kroumpouzos G, Paroikaki ME, Yumeen S, Bhargava S, Mylonakis E. Cutaneous complications of mRNA and AZD1222 COVID-19 vaccines: a worldwide review. Microorganisms. 2022;10(3):624. https://doi.org/10.3390/microorganisms10030624.

Laisuan W, Wongsa C, Chiewchalermsri C, Thongngarm T, Rerkpattanapipat T, Iamrahong P, et al. CoronaVac COVID-19 vaccine-induced anaphylaxis: clinical characteristics and revaccination outcomes. J Asthma Allergy. 2021;14:1209–15. https://doi.org/10.2147/jaa.s333098.

Lamb YN. BNT162b2 mRNA COVID-19 vaccine: first approval. Drugs. 2021;81(4):495–501. https://doi.org/10.1007/s40265-021-01480-7.

McMahon DE, Amerson E, Rosenbach M, Lipoff JB, Moustafa D, Tyagi A, et al. Cutaneous reactions reported after Moderna and Pfizer COVID-19 vaccination: a registry-based study of 414 cases. J Am Acad Dermatol. 2021;85(1):46–55. https://doi.org/10.1016/j.jaad.2021.03.092.

Munavalli GG, Guthridge R, Knutsen-Larson S, Brodsky A, Matthew E, Landau M. COVID-19/SARS-CoV-2 virus spike protein-related delayed inflammatory reaction to hyaluronic acid dermal fillers: a challenging clinical conundrum in diagnosis and treatment. Arch Dermatol Res. 2022;314(1):1–15. https://doi.org/10.1007/s00403-021-02190-6.

Nakashima C, Kato M, Otsuka A. Cutaneous manifestations of COVID-19 and COVID-19 vaccination. J Dermatol. 2023;50:280. https://doi.org/10.1111/1346-8138.16651.

Ortigosa LCM, Lenzoni FC, Suárez MV, Duarte AA, Prestes-Carneiro LE. Hypersensitivity reaction to hyaluronic acid dermal filler after COVID-19 vaccination: a series of cases in São Paulo, Brazil. Int J Infect Dis. 2022;116:268–70. https://doi.org/10.1016/j.ijid.2022.01.024.

Öztürk B, Akdemir İ, Azap A, Çelik G, Bavbek S, Mungan D. Anaphylaxis is rare due to CoronaVac in a population of healthcare workers. Asia Pac Allergy. 2022;12(4):e35. https://doi.org/10.5415/apallergy.2022.12.e35.

Rabaan AA, Mutair AA, Hajissa K, Alfaraj AH, Al-Jishi JM, Alhajri M, et al. A comprehensive review on the current vaccines and their efficacies to combat SARS-CoV-2 variants. Vaccines (Basel). 2022;10(10):1655. https://doi.org/10.3390/vaccines10101655.

Ramasamy MN, Minassian AM, Ewer KJ, Flaxman AL, Folegatti PM, Owens DR, et al. Safety and immunogenicity of ChAdOx1 nCoV-19 vaccine administered in a prime-boost regimen in young and old adults (COV002): a single-blind, randomised, controlled, phase 2/3 trial. Lancet. 2021;396(10267):1979–93. https://doi.org/10.1016/s0140-6736(20)32466-1.

Ramdani Y, Largeau B, Jonville-Bera A-P, Maillot F, Audemard-Verger A, Ramdani Y, et al. COVID-19 vaccination as a trigger of IgA vasculitis: a global pharmacovigilance study. J Rheumatol. 2023;50:564. https://doi.org/10.3899/jrheum.220629.

Rerknimitr P, Puaratanaarunkon T, Wongtada C, Wittayabusarakam N, Krithin S, Paitoonpong L, et al. Cutaneous adverse reactions from 35,229 doses of Sinovac and AstraZeneca COVID-19 vaccination: a prospective cohort study in healthcare workers. J Eur Acad Dermatol Venereol. 2022;36(3):e158–61. https://doi.org/10.1111/jdv.17761.

Robinson LB, Fu X, Hashimoto D, Wickner P, Shenoy ES, Landman AB, et al. Incidence of cutaneous reactions after messenger RNA COVID-19 vaccines. JAMA Dermatol. 2021;157(8):1000–2. https://doi.org/10.1001/jamadermatol.2021.2114.

Safir A, Samuelov L, Sprecher E, Daniely D, Artzi O. Association between BNT162b2 vaccination and the development of delayed inflammatory reactions to hyaluronic acid-based dermal fillers—a nationwide survey. J Cosmet Dermatol. 2022;21(10):4107–13. https://doi.org/10.1111/jocd.15260.

Seirafianpour F, Pourriyahi H, Gholizadeh Mesgarha M, Pour Mohammad A, Shaka Z, Goodarzi A. A systematic review on mucocutaneous presentations after COVID-19 vaccination and expert recommendations about vaccination of important immune-mediated dermatologic disorders. Dermatol Ther. 2022;35(6):e15461. https://doi.org/10.1111/dth.15461.

Shafie'ei M, Jamali M, Akbari Z, Sarvipour N, Ahmadzade M, Ahramiyanpour N. Cutaneous adverse reactions following COVID-19 vaccinations: a systematic review and meta-analysis. J Cosmet Dermatol. 2022;21(9):3636–50. https://doi.org/10.1111/jocd.15261.

Shawky A, Elrewiny EM, Gharib K, Sallam M, Mansour M, Rageh MA. A prospective multicenter study on cutaneous reactions reported after Sinopharm COVID-19 vaccination. Int J Dermatol. 2023;62(2):221–4. https://doi.org/10.1111/ijd.16391.

Washrawirul C, Triwatcharikorn J, Phannajit J, Ullman M, Susantitaphong P, Rerknimitr P. Global prevalence and clinical manifestations of cutaneous adverse reactions following COVID-19 vaccination: a systematic review and meta-analysis. J Eur Acad Dermatol Venereol. 2022;36(11):1947–68. https://doi.org/10.1111/jdv.18294.

Welsh KJ, Baumblatt J, Chege W, Goud R, Nair N. Thrombocytopenia including immune thrombocytopenia after receipt of mRNA COVID-19 vaccines reported to the Vaccine Adverse Event Reporting System (VAERS). Vaccine. 2021;39(25):3329–32. https://doi.org/10.1016/j.vaccine.2021.04.054.

Wu Z, Hu Y, Xu M, Chen Z, Yang W, Jiang Z, et al. Safety, tolerability, and immunogenicity of an inactivated SARS-CoV-2 vaccine (CoronaVac) in healthy adults aged 60 years and older: a randomised, double-blind, placebo-controlled, phase 1/2 clinical trial. Lancet Infect Dis. 2021;21(6):803–12. https://doi.org/10.1016/s1473-3099(20)30987-7.

Zhang Y, Zeng G, Pan H, Li C, Hu Y, Chu K, et al. Safety, tolerability, and immunogenicity of an inactivated SARS-CoV-2 vaccine in healthy adults aged 18-59 years: a randomised, double-blind, placebo-controlled, phase 1/2 clinical trial. Lancet Infect Dis. 2021;21(2):181–92. https://doi.org/10.1016/s1473-3099(20)30843-4.

Evaluation of the Patient with a Coronavirus Disease (COVID-19) Vaccine Cutaneous Reaction

Tricia Y. R. Chong, Yee Kiat Heng, and Yen Loo Lim

Introduction

Coronavirus disease (COVID-19) vaccines prevent severe disease, hospitalisation and death (CDC 2023). However, as vaccination drives commenced, there have been multiple reports of cutaneous reactions following COVID-19 vaccination and resultant vaccine hesitancy (McMahon et al. 2021; Avallone et al. 2022; Judd et al. 2022). This chapter provides evidence-based guidance on the evaluation of patients with cutaneous reactions following COVID-19 vaccination. An accurate evaluation will enable physicians to risk stratify patients based on their reaction pattern and guide patients to complete recommended COVID-19 vaccinations, where possible.

History, Examination and Preliminary Investigation(s) to Determine the Cutaneous Reaction Pattern

The first step in the evaluation is to obtain information about the cutaneous reaction including the type of COVID-19 vaccine administered, time to reaction and morphology of the cutaneous reaction. Review of past medical history should include any prior adverse reactions to drugs/vaccines/foods/personal care products/excipients, pre-existing dermatological diseases and other co-morbidities. A full list of medications including herb and supplement intake should be noted, especially if newly initiated prior to the onset of the cutaneous reaction. The clinician should also enquire about pro re nata use of non-steroidal anti-inflammatory drugs for symptomatic relief immediately pre/post-vaccination.

If the patient consents, photographs of the cutaneous reaction should be obtained. Severity of the reaction should be assessed based on a validated disease severity score. Singh et al. propose adopting the National Cancer Institute's Common Terminology Criteria for Adverse Events version 5.0 criteria to grade severity of all COVID-19 vaccine-associated cutaneous reactions, to facilitate clinical care and research (Singh et al. 2023).

A skin biopsy may be performed to aid in identification of a reaction pattern, such as in cases of Vaccine-Related Eruption of Papules and Plaques, or support the diagnosis in all cases of vasculitis, severe cutaneous adverse reactions, pemphigoid and pemphigus. Full blood count, renal panel, liver function tests and urinalysis to screen for systemic involvement may be performed, if the reaction pattern is suggestive of vasculitis or severe cutaneous adverse reactions.

T. Y. R. Chong (✉) · Y. K. Heng · Y. L. Lim
National Skin Centre, Singapore, Singapore
e-mail: triciachong@nsc.com.sg;
ykheng@nsc.com.sg; yllim@nsc.com.sg

© The Author(s), under exclusive license to Springer Nature Switzerland AG 2023
H. H. Oon, C. L. Goh (eds.), *COVID-19 in Dermatology*, Updates in Clinical Dermatology,
https://doi.org/10.1007/978-3-031-45586-5_5

Assessing Causality

There are currently no validated criteria to determine if a cutaneous reaction is caused by COVID-19 vaccination.

Some authors suggest that cutaneous reactions can be attributed to a COVID-19 vaccine only if it occurs within 21 days of vaccine administration (Singh et al. 2023; Català et al. 2021). This is in line with adverse events analysed by the Centers for Disease Control and Prevention Immunization Safety Office (Singh et al. 2023).

The World Health Organization recommends considering additional factors when determining whether an adverse event has a consistent, indeterminate or inconsistent causal association to immunisation. An algorithm is provided in its user manual for causality assessment of an adverse event following immunisation. Criteria that support a consistent causal association to immunisation are as follows: (1) the patient's medical history, examination or investigations do not provide evidence for another cause; (2) there are peer-reviewed publications of similar events and biological plausibility that the vaccine may cause such an event; (3) there is no published literature to refute the causal association between the vaccine and the event (World Health Organization 2019).

Further Evaluation and Management Based on Cutaneous Reaction Pattern

Anaphylaxis

Anaphylaxis is a potentially life-threatening reaction where there is a sudden onset of symptoms and signs involving two or more organ systems. Various definitions for anaphylaxis are currently used in the literature, as summarised by the position paper by the World Allergy Organization (Cardona et al. 2020). Reported incidence rates of COVID-19 vaccine–associated anaphylaxis vary from 1.07 to 11.1/million doses (Toledo-Salinas et al. 2022; CDC 2021). Some of this discrepancy can be attributed to use of differ-

ent case definitions and over-diagnosis due to clinical mimics of anaphylaxis such as vasovagal syncope, inducible laryngeal obstruction and vocal cord dysfunction, as elaborated by Gold et al. (2023).

In a systematic review and meta-analysis on the risk of a second allergic reaction to a COVID-19 vaccine, 78 persons were noted to have severe (defined as anaphylaxis or requiring epinephrine use) immediate (occurring <4 h after vaccination) allergic reactions to their first COVID-19 messenger ribonucleic acid (mRNA) vaccination. Amongst this group of 78 persons, 4 people had a second severe immediate reaction and 15 had non-severe reactions. No deaths were recorded. In the analyses, graded vaccine dosing, skin testing and premedication as risk-stratification strategies did not alter the findings (Chu et al. 2022). Similarly, another systemic review and meta-analysis analysed 317 individuals who had immediate reactions with their first dose and underwent 578 skin tests (to mRNA COVID-19 vaccine, polyethylene glycol (PEG) or polysorbate 80 alone or in combination), concluded that skin testing had low sensitivity in predicting all-severity immediate reactions upon re-vaccination. Sensitivity was 0.2 for mRNA COVID-19 vaccine, 0.02 for polyethylene glycol, 0.03 for polysorbate 80 and 0.03 for combination of any of the three agents (Greenhawt et al. 2023). Amongst 57 patients with immediate reactions to their first dose of mRNA COVID-19 vaccine and negative skin tests to polyethylene glycol, two of these patients required adrenaline when they received their second dose of the same COVID-19 vaccine (Wolfson et al. 2021). These studies suggest that in patients with immediate reactions to their first dose of COVID-19 vaccination, skin testing cannot accurately predict second dose outcomes.

Both the American Academy of Allergy, Asthma & Immunology (AAAAI) and European Academy of Allergy and Clinical Immunology (EAACI) caution that while skin testing protocols to vaccine excipients such as polysorbate and PEG have been published, the sensitivity and specificity of these tests have not been validated. Additionally, as COVID-19 vaccine stocks may be limited, skin testing to COVID-19 vaccines should only be performed with residue in a vial, if at all (American Academy of Allergy 2022; Barbaud et al. 2022).

The role of allergy testing to COVID-19 vaccines and excipients is limited, and skin tests are not routinely recommended in practice guidelines (American Academy of Allergy 2022; Vander Leek et al. 2021). EAACI propose the following groups of patients undergo prick testing to excipients including PEG 3500 or 4000, PEG 2000, polysorbate 80 and the implicated COVID-19 vaccine:

1—anaphylaxis to injectable drug or vaccine containing PEG or derivatives;
2—anaphylaxis to oral/topical PEG-containing products;
3—recurrent anaphylaxis of unknown cause;
4—suspected or confirmed allergy to any mRNA vaccine; and.
5—confirmed allergy to PEG or derivatives.

Depending on the results of these prick tests, the EAACI practice guideline provides algorithms to guide clinicians on administration of further doses of COVID-19 vaccine for each patient. Management options listed include use of COVID-19 vaccines free from the implicated excipient (if available) and graded administration of a COVID-19 vaccine. As algorithms were constructed based on expert consensus, EAACI adds that these algorithms require further evaluation in prospective studies (Barbaud et al. 2022).

AAAAI recommends that besides undergoing evaluation with skin testing, options to omit further vaccine doses or receive further vaccine doses under physician supervision should be discussed with the patient (American Academy of Allergy 2022).

The World Allergy Organization and Centers for Disease Control and Prevention recommend that those who developed anaphylaxis with a COVID-19 vaccine should not receive further doses of that same type of vaccine or other COVID-19 vaccines with the same excipients. Of note, polyethylene glycol is found in both mRNA-1273 and BNT162b2. Polysorbate is an excipient in NVX-CoV2373 (Turner et al. 2021; CDC 2022). CoronaVac has neither polyethylene

glycol nor polysorbate, but it contains aluminium hydroxide (Health Sciences Authority 2021). When receiving further doses, all individuals with suspected anaphylaxis to a previous COVID-19 dose should be vaccinated in healthcare setting that is able to manage anaphylaxis (Chu et al. 2022; CDC 2022) and monitored for at least 30 min following vaccination (CDC 2022).

Non-Severe Immediate Reactions

Individuals with an immediate reaction (occurring <4 h after vaccination) that was not severe (does not meet the diagnostic criteria for anaphylaxis) may receive another dose of the same COVID-19 vaccine. However, such individuals should be vaccinated in a healthcare setting that is able to manage anaphylaxis and monitored for at least 30 min following vaccination (CDC 2022). As discussed in the anaphylaxis section, skin testing may be offered to selected groups of patients, but the limitations of these tests should also be considered.

Urticaria/Angio-oedema

Occurrence of urticaria has been reported following COVID-19 vaccination. In a survey of 271 patients, majority (67%) of patients developed urticaria within 1–2 weeks following COVID-19 vaccination. One in five cases progressed to chronic (>6 weeks) urticaria (Judd et al. 2022).

Individuals who develop urticaria/angio-edema, without features of anaphylaxis, may continue to receive further doses of the same COVID-19 vaccine (Barbaud et al. 2022; CDC 2022; Robinson et al. 2021; Wolfson et al. 2022). European Network for Drug Allergy and the European Academy of Allergy and Clinical Immunology recommend continuing the usual antihistamine treatment on the day of vaccination or starting antihistamines 3 days before vaccination if the individual is not on regular antihistamines (Barbaud et al. 2022).

Vasculitis

Leukocytoclastic vasculitis was the most common type of vasculitis reported following COVID-19 vaccination. A few cases of IgA vasculitis, lymphocytic vasculitis, anti-neutrophil cytoplasmic antibodies (ANCA)-associated vasculitis and urticarial vasculitis have also been reported. The time to onset was 1–20 days (average of 6.2 days) following COVID-19 vaccination (Abdelmaksoud et al. 2022).

Majority of the cases recovered without sequelae over an average period of 2.5 weeks, leading some authors to conclude that vasculitis should not be a contraindication to vaccination (Abdelmaksoud et al. 2022). However, Missoum et al. report a case of leukocytoclastic vasculitis with acute tubulointerstitial nephritis requiring dialysis. Despite resolution of his cutaneous lesions, this patient had residual renal impairment (Missoum et al. 2022). In cases of vasculitis with systemic involvement, it may be prudent to avoid further doses of the same type of COVID-19 vaccine.

Severe Cutaneous Adverse Reactions (SCARs)

SCARs include Stevens–Johnson Syndrome (SJS)/Toxic Epidermal Necrolysis (TEN), drug reaction with eosinophilia and systemic symptoms syndrome (DRESS) and acute generalised exanthematous pustulosis (AGEP). SCARs are regarded as Type IV hypersensitivity reactions to drugs, but the exact pathogenesis of COVID-19 vaccine–associated SCARs remains unknown (Wu et al. 2023; Phillips et al. 2019).

SJS/TEN has been reported following COVID-19 vaccination. The latency between vaccination and the onset of symptoms varied between 1 and 20 days (Zou and Daveluy 2022a). A flare of SJS was noted in a patient when she was re-challenged with the same BBIBP COVID-19 vaccine (Wu et al. 2023).

DRESS has been reported after COVID-19 vaccination. For these cases, the latency period varied between 3 and 7 weeks from the first dose of COVID-19 vaccination (Schroeder et al. 2022; O'Connor et al. 2022).

AGEP has been reported 3 weeks after first dose (Kang et al. 2021). The localised variant of AGEP, acute localised exanthematous pustulosis was noted 2 days after the first dose of AZD1222 vaccine. The patient was advised to further doses of AZD1222 and consider alternative brands of COVID-19 instead (Wu and Lin 2021).

DRESS-AGEP overlap has been reported following COVID-19 vaccination. These cases occurred 3 days to 11 weeks from the first dose of COVID-19 vaccination (Lospinoso et al. 2021; Ikeda et al. 2022; Tay et al. 2022).

Delayed Large Local Reaction

Delayed large local reactions (Fig. 5.1) occur near the injection site after full resolution of initial

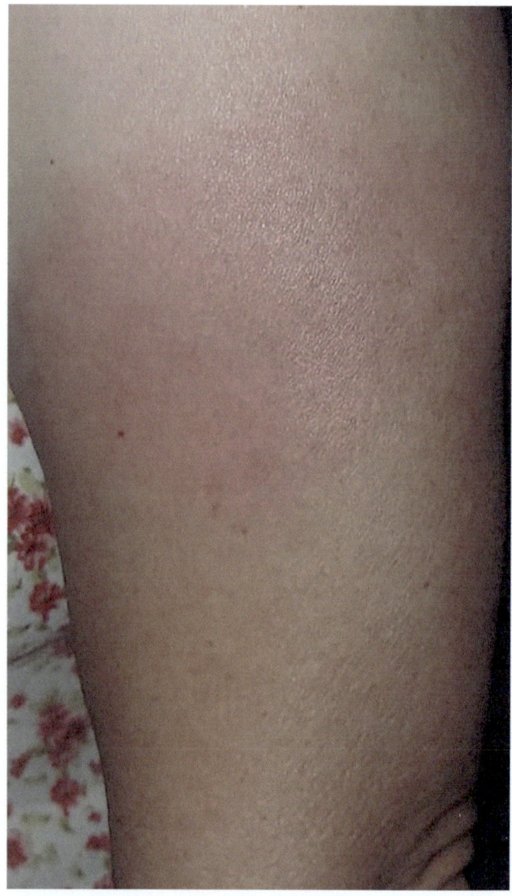

Fig. 5.1 Typical delayed large local reaction near the vaccination site

local symptoms associated with COVID-19 vaccination. Majority of cases were noted following vaccination with the mRNA-1273 COVID-19 vaccine (Papadimitriou et al. 2022; Blumenthal et al. 2022). Delayed large local reactions usually occur 4 or more days after vaccination, with a median onset on day 8 after vaccination. These reactions are typically erythematous, indurated and tender. Spontaneous resolution is usually noted 4–5 days later (Blumenthal et al. 2022).

Delayed large local reactions are not a contraindication to further doses of the same COVID-19 vaccination. However, patients should be counselled about the risk of recurrence. In a case series of 12 patients with delayed large local reactions to mRNA-1273 COVID-19 vaccine, the recurrence rate was 50% for the second dose and 33% for the third dose (booster). One of the patients in the series switched to the BNT162b2 COVID-19 vaccine for his third dose but also developed a delayed large local reaction with BNT162b2 (Blumenthal et al. 2021, 2022).

Vaccine-Related Eruption of Papules and Plaques (V-REPP)

McMahon et al. propose the term V-REPP to describe the spectrum of cutaneous lesions ranging from crusted papules, to pityriasis-rosea like eruptions, to pink papules with fine scaling reported following COVID-19 vaccination. Features of spongiotic dermatitis were noted on skin biopsies of all these cases (Missoum et al. 2022). Pityriasis rosea (PR)/ PR-like eruption (PR-LE) reactions were usually distributed over the trunk and extremities (Fig. 5.2). Facial, head and neck involvement was not common (McMahon et al. 2022; Buckley et al. 2022). The time to onset of PR/ PR-like reactions ranged from 1 to 21 days. These reactions are self-limiting, and the average time to resolution was 5.6 weeks (Buckley et al. 2022).

PR/PR-LE is not regarded as a hypersensitivity reaction. It is postulated that the post-vaccine

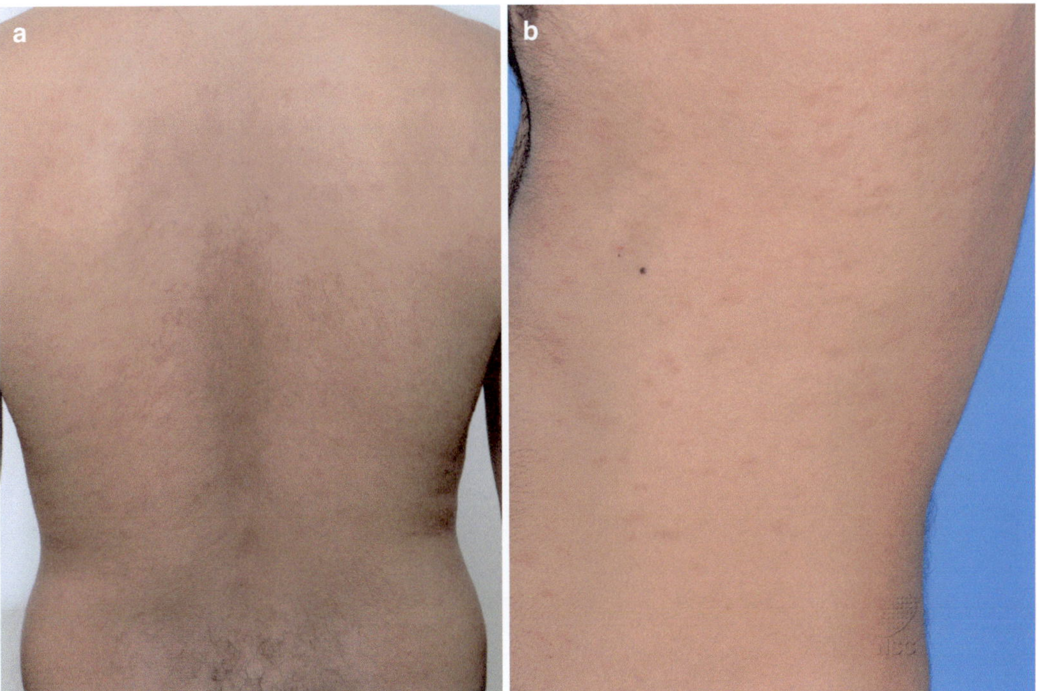

Fig. 5.2 Scaly patches over the trunk, showing a "fir-tree" distribution, of a patient with a pityriasis rosea-like eruption

inflammatory response may impair normal T-cell-mediated immune control of latent human herpes virus (HHV)-6 or HHV-7 and HHV reactivation causes PR/PR-LE reactions. Therefore, individuals with PR/PR-LE eruptions may proceed with further doses of the same COVID-19 vaccine without any allergy testing (Buckley et al. 2022).

Pemphigoid and Pemphigus

Pemphigoid and pemphigus (Fig. 5.3) are autoimmune blistering conditions. A case of de novo pemphigus was reported 5 days following the first dose of BNT162b2 with rapid disease progression noted 3 days after the second dose of BNT162b2 (Solimani et al. 2021). De novo subepidermal blistering eruptions, including bullous pemphigoid, have also been reported. The latency between vaccination and onset of blisters ranged between 12 and 21 days (Tomayko et al. 2021).

The International Pemphigus and Pemphigoid Foundation surveyed 495 patients in their database for post-booster disease aggravation. Fifty-four patients required additional treatment for disease flares and four patients required hospitalisation. Majority (50%) of disease flares were noted 1–4 weeks after vaccination. In total, 55.9% of those with disease flares for all three doses reported a milder flare compared to their initial dose(s) (Falcinelli et al. 2022).

De novo or aggravation of pre-existing pemphigus/pemphigoid is not an absolute contraindication to receiving further doses of the same COVID-19 vaccine. However, Damiani et al. remarked that in patients who experience disease aggravation following COVID-19 vaccination and require additional immunosuppression to allow for completion of the recommended vaccination series, the impact of such immunosuppression on SARS-CoV-2 S1/RBD IgG antibodies in the long term warrants further study (Damiani et al. 2021).

Varicella-Zoster Virus (VZV) Reactivation

VZV reactivation has been reported following COVID-19 vaccination. The median time from vaccination to the first reported VZV symptom was 7 days (Fathy et al. 2022).

Individuals that experience VZV reactivation may proceed with further doses of the same COVID-19 vaccine. It is recommended that individuals with active zoster defer a scheduled vaccine dose to minimise complications such as disseminated zoster (Lim et al. 2022). Majority (77%) of individuals had VZV reactivation after

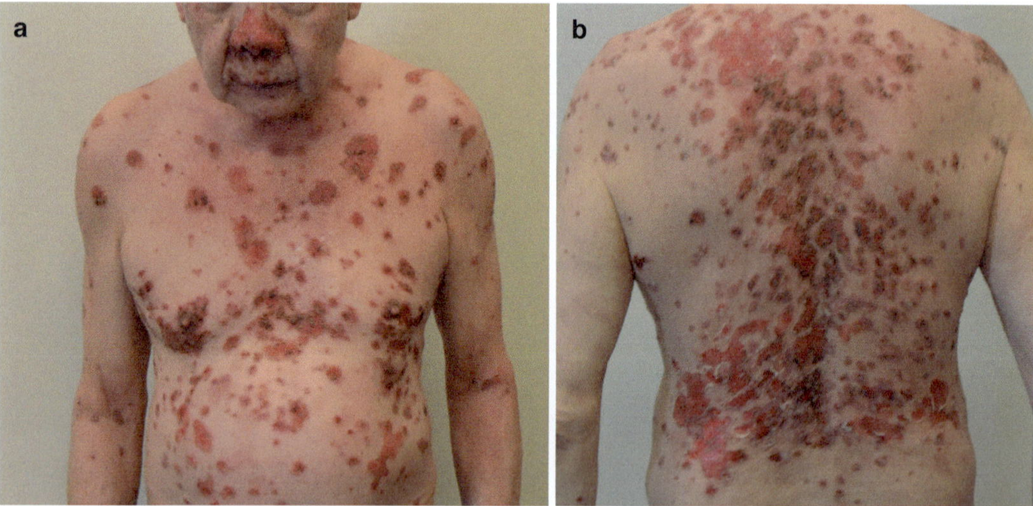

Fig. 5.3 Extensive erosions in a patient that experienced a flare of pemphigus following COVID-19 vaccination

the first vaccine dose only. None of the patients had VZV reactivations with more than one vaccine dose (Fathy et al. 2022).

Other Cutaneous Reactions

Flares of eczema have been reported following COVID-19 vaccination, with some individuals requiring initiation of systemic glucocorticoids for disease control. Eczema flares were reported between 1 and 14 days following vaccination (Phuan et al. 2022; Leasure et al. 2021; Potestio et al. 2022). Recurrent flares with further doses of the same COVID-19 vaccine were also noted, but disease control was achieved either with initiation of topical or oral glucocorticoids (Leasure et al. 2021).

De novo and flare of pre-existing psoriasis have also been reported. Amongst the cases of new-onset psoriasis, there were cases of plaque, guttate, generalised pustular psoriasis (GPP) and nail psoriasis. New-onset psoriasis was noted between 2 and 21 days following vaccination. One case of GPP was commenced on acitretin and was able to receive her second COVID-19 vaccine dose without a flare. Another case of GPP was prescribed methotrexate which resulted in improvement. However, she experienced a flare with her second COVID-19 dose. Flares of pre-existing psoriasis were reported 1–90 days following vaccination. Seven percent of patients who experienced disease flares required additional prescription of topical therapies, phototherapy, systemic immunomodulator or biologics. Some patients experienced psoriasis flares with only their first dose of COVID-19 vaccine while others noted flares with both their first and second doses of COVID-19 vaccine (Wu et al. 2022).

Apart from dupilumab, patients prescribed systemic immunomodulators post-vaccination should be counselled that their immune response to vaccination may be attenuated (Haddad et al. 2022; Di Bona et al. 2022).

A multitude of other less common cutaneous reactions including swelling around soft tissue filler sites (FDA 2021), morphea (Paolino et al. 2022), alopecia areata (Fusano et al. 2022), lichen planus (Zou and Daveluy 2022b) and systemic drug-related intertriginous and flexural exanthema-like eruption (Di Bona et al. 2022) have been reported to occur following COVID-19 vaccination.

Conclusion

The initial evaluation of a patient with a possible COVID-19 vaccine cutaneous reaction involves confirming causality to the COVID-19 vaccination. Further evaluation and management of the cutaneous reaction would be determined by the morphology, reaction pattern and the diagnosis of the cutaneous eruption. For cutaneous reactions that are potentially life-threatening such as anaphylaxis, severe cutaneous adverse reactions and systemic vasculitis, it would be prudent to avoid further doses of same type of COVID-19 vaccine. Patients with other reactions such as urticaria/angioedema without features of anaphylaxis, delayed large location reactions, pemphigoid/pemphigus, V-REPP, VZV reactivation, flares of eczema and psoriasis may continue to receive further doses of the same COVID-19 vaccine. In this latter group of patients, vaccine hesitancy may be present. The clinician should have a balanced discussion about the benefits of completing the recommended vaccination series versus the possibility that there may be a recurrence of their cutaneous reaction.

References

Abdelmaksoud A, Wollina U, Temiz SA, Hasan A. SARS-CoV-2 vaccination-induced cutaneous vasculitis: report of two new cases and literature review. Dermatol Ther. 2022;35(6):e15458. https://doi.org/10.1111/dth.15458.

American Academy of Allergy AI: AAAAI COVID-19 response task force guidance on administration of COVID-19 vaccines related to concerns of allergic reactions. 2022. https://education.aaaai.org/resources-for-a-i-clinicians/reactionguidance_COVID-19. Accessed 24 April 2023.

Avallone G, Quaglino P, Cavallo F, Roccuzzo G, Ribero S, Zalaudek I, et al. SARS-CoV-2 vaccine-related cutaneous manifestations: a systematic review. Int J Dermatol. 2022;61(10):1187–204. https://doi.org/10.1111/ijd.16063.

Barbaud A, Garvey LH, Arcolaci A, Brockow K, Mori F, Mayorga C, et al. Allergies and COVID-19 vaccines: an ENDA/EAACI position paper. Allergy. 2022;77(8):2292–312. https://doi.org/10.1111/all.15241.

Blumenthal KG, Freeman EE, Saff RR, Robinson LB, Wolfson AR, Foreman RK, et al. Delayed large local reactions to mRNA-1273 vaccine against SARS-CoV-2. N Engl J Med. 2021;384(13):1273–7. https://doi.org/10.1056/NEJMc2102131.

Blumenthal KG, Ahola C, Anvari S, Samarakoon U, Freeman EE. Delayed large local reactions to Moderna COVID-19 vaccine: a follow-up report after booster vaccination. JAAD Int. 2022;8:3–6. https://doi.org/10.1016/j.jdin.2022.03.017.

Buckley JE, Landis LN, Rapini RP. Pityriasis rosea-like rash after messenger RNA COVID-19 vaccination: a case report and review of the literature. JAAD Int. 2022;7:164–8. https://doi.org/10.1016/j.jdin.2022.01.009.

Cardona V, Ansotegui IJ, Ebisawa M, El-Gamal Y, Fernandez Rivas M, Fineman S, et al. World allergy organization anaphylaxis guidance 2020. World Allergy Organ J. 2020;13(10):100472. https://doi.org/10.1016/j.waojou.2020.100472.

Català A, Muñoz-Santos C, Galván-Casas C, Roncero Riesco M, Revilla Nebreda D, Solá-Truyols A, et al. Cutaneous reactions after SARS-COV-2 vaccination: a cross-sectional Spanish nationwide study of 405 cases. Br J Dermatol. 2021;186:142. https://doi.org/10.1111/bjd.20639.

CDC. Allergic reactions including anaphylaxis after receipt of the first dose of Pfizer-BioNTech COVID-19 vaccine - United States, December 14-23, 2020. MMWR Morb Mortal Wkly Rep. 2021;70(2):46–51. https://doi.org/10.15585/mmwr.mm7002e1.

CDC: Allergic reactions after COVID-19 vaccination. 2022. https://www.cdc.gov/coronavirus/2019-ncov/vaccines/safety/allergic-reaction.html. Accessed 24 Jan 2023.

CDC: COVID-19 vaccine effectiveness monthly update. 2023. https://covid.cdc.gov/covid-data-tracker/#vaccine-effectiveness. Accessed 1 Feb 2022.

Chu DK, Abrams EM, Golden DBK, Blumenthal KG, Wolfson AR, Stone CA Jr, et al. Risk of second allergic reaction to SARS-CoV-2 vaccines: a systematic review and meta-analysis. JAMA Intern Med. 2022;182(4):376–85. https://doi.org/10.1001/jamainternmed.2021.8515.

Damiani G, Pacifico A, Pelloni F, Iorizzo M. The first dose of COVID-19 vaccine may trigger pemphigus and bullous pemphigoid flares: is the second dose therefore contraindicated? J Eur Acad Dermatol Venereol. 2021;35(10):e645–e7. https://doi.org/10.1111/jdv.17472.

Di Bona D, Miniello A, Nettis E. Systemic drug-related intertriginous and flexural exanthema-like eruption after Oxford-AstraZeneca COVID-19 vaccine. Clin Mol Allergy. 2022;20(1):13. https://doi.org/10.1186/s12948-022-00179-8.

Falcinelli F, Lamberti A, Cota C, Rubegni P, Cinotti E. Reply to 'development of severe pemphigus vulgaris following SARS-CoV-2 vaccination with BNT162b2' by Solimani F et al. J Eur Acad Dermatol Venereol. 2022;36(12):e976–e8. https://doi.org/10.1111/jdv.18398.

Fathy RA, McMahon DE, Lee C, Chamberlin GC, Rosenbach M, Lipoff JB, et al. Varicella-zoster and herpes simplex virus reactivation post-COVID-19 vaccination: a review of 40 cases in an International Dermatology Registry. J Eur Acad Dermatol Venereol. 2022;36(1):e6–9. https://doi.org/10.1111/jdv.17646.

FDA: vaccines and related biological products Advisory Committee Meeting. https://www.fda.gov/media/144434/download. Accessed 23 Jan 2021.

Fusano M, Zerbinati N, Bencini PL. Alopecia areata after COVID-19 vaccination: two cases and review of the literature. Dermatol Rep. 2022;14(4):9495. https://doi.org/10.4081/dr.2022.9495.

Gold MS, Amarasinghe A, Greenhawt M, Kelso JM, Kochhar S, Yu-Hor Thong B, et al. Anaphylaxis: revision of the Brighton collaboration case definition. Vaccine. 2023;41(15):2605–14. https://doi.org/10.1016/j.vaccine.2022.11.027.

Greenhawt M, Shaker M, Golden DBK, Abrams EM, Blumenthal KG, Wolfson AR, et al. Diagnostic accuracy of vaccine and vaccine excipient testing in the setting of allergic reactions to COVID-19 vaccines: a systematic review and meta-analysis. Allergy. 2023;78(1):71–83. https://doi.org/10.1111/all.15571.

Haddad I, Kozman K, Kibbi A-G. Navigating patients with atopic dermatitis or chronic spontaneous urticaria during the COVID-19 pandemic. Front Allergy. 2022;3:809646. https://doi.org/10.3389/falgy.2022.809646.

Health Sciences Authority: COVID-19 vaccine (Vero Cell), inactivated. https://www.hsa.gov.sg/docs/default-source/hprg-tpb/psar/coronavac-covid-19-vaccine-package-insert-(syringe).pdf. Accessed 22 Dec 2021.

Ikeda T, Yokoyama K, Kawakami T. Overlapping acute generalized exanthematous pustulosis drug reaction with eosinophilia and systemic symptoms induced by a second dose of the Moderna COVID-19 vaccine. J Dermatol. 2022;49(12):e446–e7. https://doi.org/10.1111/1346-8138.16541.

Judd A, Samarakoon U, Wolfson A, Banerji A, Freeman EE, Blumenthal KG. Urticaria after COVID-19 vaccination and vaccine hesitancy. J Allergy Clin Immunol Pract. 2022;11:958. https://doi.org/10.1016/j.jaip.2022.12.010.

Kang SY, Park SY, Kim JH, Lee SM, Lee SP. COVID-19 vaccine-induced acute generalized exanthematous pustulosis. Korean J Intern Med. 2021;36(6):1537–8. https://doi.org/10.3904/kjim.2021.198.

Leasure AC, Cowper SE, McNiff J, Cohen JM. Generalized eczematous reactions to the Pfizer-BioNTech COVID-19 vaccine. J Eur Acad

Dermatol Venereol. 2021;35(11):e716–e7. https://doi.org/10.1111/jdv.17494.

Lim ZV, Kanagalingam J, Heng YK. Response to "varicella-zoster virus reactivation after SARS-CoV-2 BNT162b2 mRNA vaccination: report of 5 cases". JAAD Case Rep. 2022;23:141–2. https://doi.org/10.1016/j.jdcr.2021.09.044.

Lospinoso K, Nichols CS, Malachowski SJ, Mochel MC, Nutan F. A case of severe cutaneous adverse reaction following administration of the Janssen Ad26.COV2.S COVID-19 vaccine. JAAD Case Rep. 2021;13:134–7. https://doi.org/10.1016/j.jdcr.2021.05.010.

McMahon DE, Amerson E, Rosenbach M, Lipoff JB, Moustafa D, Tyagi A, et al. Cutaneous reactions reported after Moderna and Pfizer COVID-19 vaccination: a registry-based study of 414 cases. J Am Acad Dermatol. 2021;85(1):46–55. https://doi.org/10.1016/j.jaad.2021.03.092.

McMahon DE, Kovarik CL, Damsky W, Rosenbach M, Lipoff JB, Tyagi A, et al. Clinical and pathologic correlation of cutaneous COVID-19 vaccine reactions including V-REPP: a registry-based study. J Am Acad Dermatol. 2022;86(1):113–21. https://doi.org/10.1016/j.jaad.2021.09.002.

Missoum S, Lahmar M, Khellaf G. [Leukocytoclastic vasculitis and acute renal failure following inactivated SARS-CoV-2 vaccine]. Nephrol Ther. 2022;18(4):287–90. https://doi.org/10.1016/j.nephro.2021.10.006.

O'Connor T, O'Callaghan-Maher M, Ryan P, Gibson G. Drug reaction with eosinophilia and systemic symptoms syndrome following vaccination with the AstraZeneca COVID-19 vaccine. JAAD Case Rep. 2022;20:14–6. https://doi.org/10.1016/j.jdcr.2021.11.028.

Paolino G, Campochiaro C, Di Nicola MR, Mercuri SR, Rizzo N, Dagna L, et al. Generalized morphea after COVID-19 vaccines: a case series. J Eur Acad Dermatol Venereol. 2022;36(9):e680–e2. https://doi.org/10.1111/jdv.18249.

Papadimitriou I, Bakirtzi K, Sotiriou E, Vakirlis E, Hatzibougias D, Ioannides D. Delayed localized hypersensitivity reactions to COVID-19 mRNA vaccines: a 6-month retrospective study. Clin Exp Dermatol. 2022;47(1):157–8. https://doi.org/10.1111/ced.14856.

Phillips EJ, Bigliardi P, Bircher AJ, Broyles A, Chang YS, Chung WH, et al. Controversies in drug allergy: testing for delayed reactions. J Allergy Clin Immunol. 2019;143(1):66–73. https://doi.org/10.1016/j.jaci.2018.10.030.

Phuan CZY, Choi EC, Oon HH. Temporary exacerbation of pre-existing psoriasis and eczema in the context of COVID-19 messenger RNA booster vaccination: a case report and review of the literature. JAAD Int. 2022;6:94–6. https://doi.org/10.1016/j.jdin.2021.11.004.

Potestio L, Napolitano M, Bennardo L, Fabbrocini G, Patruno C. Atopic dermatitis exacerbation after Covid-19 vaccination in Dupilumab-treated patients. J Eur Acad Dermatol Venereol. 2022;36(6):e409–e11. https://doi.org/10.1111/jdv.17964.

Robinson LB, Fu X, Hashimoto D, Wickner P, Shenoy ES, Landman AB, et al. Incidence of cutaneous reactions after messenger RNA COVID-19 vaccines. JAMA Dermatol. 2021;157(8):1000–2. https://doi.org/10.1001/jamadermatol.2021.2114.

Schroeder JW, Gamba C, Toniato A, Rongioletti F. A definite case of Drug Reaction with Eosinophilia and Systemic Symptoms (DRESS) induced by administration of the Pfizer/BioNTech BNT162b2 vaccine for SARS-CoV2. Clin Dermatol. 2022;40(5):591–4. https://doi.org/10.1016/j.clindermatol.2022.02.018.

Singh R, Ali R, Prasad S, Chen ST, Blumenthal K, Freeman EE. Proposing a standardized assessment of COVID-19 vaccine-associated cutaneous reactions. J Am Acad Dermatol. 2023;88(1):237–41. https://doi.org/10.1016/j.jaad.2022.05.011.

Solimani F, Mansour Y, Didona D, Dilling A, Ghoreschi K, Meier K. Development of severe pemphigus vulgaris following SARS-CoV-2 vaccination with BNT162b2. J Eur Acad Dermatol Venereol. 2021;35(10):e649–e51. https://doi.org/10.1111/jdv.17480.

Tay WC, Lee JSS, Chong WS. Tozinameran (Pfizer-BioNTech COVID-19 vaccine)-induced AGEP-DRESS syndrome. Ann Acad Med Singap. 2022;51(12):796–7. https://doi.org/10.47102/annals-acadmedsg.2022338.

Toledo-Salinas C, Scheffler-Mendoza SC, Castano-Jaramillo LM, Ortega-Martell JA, Del Rio-Navarro BE, Santibáñez-Copado AM, et al. Anaphylaxis to SARS-CoV-2 vaccines in the setting of a Nationwide Passive Epidemiological Surveillance Program. J Clin Immunol. 2022;42(8):1593–9. https://doi.org/10.1007/s10875-022-01350-1.

Tomayko MM, Damsky W, Fathy R, McMahon DE, Turner N, Valentin MN, et al. Subepidermal blistering eruptions, including bullous pemphigoid, following COVID-19 vaccination. J Allergy Clin Immunol. 2021;148(3):750–1. https://doi.org/10.1016/j.jaci.2021.06.026.

Turner PJ, Ansotegui IJ, Campbell DE, Cardona V, Ebisawa M, El-Gamal Y, et al. COVID-19 vaccine-associated anaphylaxis: a statement of the World Allergy Organization Anaphylaxis Committee. World Allergy Organ J. 2021;14(2):100517. https://doi.org/10.1016/j.waojou.2021.100517.

Vander Leek TK, Chan ES, Connors L, Derfalvi B, Ellis AK, Upton JEM, et al. COVID-19 vaccine testing & administration guidance for allergists/immunologists from the Canadian Society of Allergy and Clinical Immunology (CSACI). Allergy Asthma Clin Immunol. 2021;17(1):29. https://doi.org/10.1186/s13223-021-00529-2.

Wolfson AR, Robinson LB, Li L, McMahon AE, Cogan AS, Fu X, et al. First-dose mRNA COVID-19 vaccine allergic reactions: limited role for excipient skin testing. J Allergy Clin Immunol Pract. 2021;9(9):3308–20.e3. https://doi.org/10.1016/j.jaip.2021.06.010.

Wolfson AR, Freeman EE, Blumenthal KG. Urticaria 12 days after COVID-19 mRNA booster vaccination. JAMA. 2022;327(17):1702–3. https://doi.org/10.1001/jama.2022.5247.

World Health Organization. Causality assessment of an adverse event following immunization (AEFI): user manual for the revised WHO classification. 2nd, 2019 update edn. Geneva: World Health Organization; 2019.

Wu RW, Lin TK. Oxford-AstraZeneca COVID-19 vaccine-induced acute localized exanthematous pustulosis. J Dermatol. 2021;48(11):e562–e3. https://doi.org/10.1111/1346-8138.16138.

Wu PC, Huang IH, Wang CW, Tsai CC, Chung WH, Chen CB. New onset and exacerbations of psoriasis following COVID-19 vaccines: a systematic review. Am J Clin Dermatol. 2022;23(6):775–99. https://doi.org/10.1007/s40257-022-00721-z.

Wu PC, Huang IH, Wang CW, Chung WH, Chen CB. Severe cutaneous adverse reactions after COVID-19 vaccination: a systematic review. Allergy. 2023;78:1383. https://doi.org/10.1111/all.15642.

Zou H, Daveluy S. Toxic epidermal necrolysis and Stevens-Johnson syndrome after COVID-19 infection and vaccination. Australas J Dermatol. 2022a;64:e1. https://doi.org/10.1111/ajd.13958.

Zou H, Daveluy S. Lichen planus after COVID-19 infection and vaccination. Arch Dermatol Res. 2022b;315:139. https://doi.org/10.1007/s00403-022-02497-y.

Personal Protective Equipment (PPE)-Related Occupational Dermatoses During COVID 19

Hwee Chyen Lee and Chee Leok Goh

Introduction

The World Health Organization (WHO) first declared COVID-19 as a pandemic on March 12, 2020. Since then, the CDC (Centers for Disease Control and Prevention) and WHO have recommended personal protective equipment (PPE) for frontline healthcare workers (HCWs) to prevent transmission of the virus. These include N95 (or equivalent) respirators/masks, protective goggles, and isolation gowns. There is a high incidence of occupational skin disease due to PPE among HCWs all over the world, especially when PPE is used over prolonged periods of time (Elston 2020; Lin et al. 2020; Lee and Goh 2021). During the Severe Acute Respiratory Syndrome (SARS) epidemic, high rates of adverse skin reactions in HCWs were reported (Foo et al. 2006). To date, there has been a sharp rise in the incidence of PPE-related occupational dermatoses globally due to the ongoing COVID-19 pandemic (Lin et al. 2020; Lee and Goh 2021). These skin reactions are a significant occupational hazard that can affect quality of life, staff morale, and PPE compliance. In the event of such PPE failure or noncompliance, the HCWs become vulnerable to COVID-19 transmission at work. The COVID-19 era has brought the critical importance of prevention and early recognition of these PPE-related occupational skin diseases to our attention. In this chapter, we discuss various PPE-related occupational dermatoses and suggest measures to prevent, mitigate, and manage these conditions.

Facial PPE Occupational Dermatoses

These are facial dermatoses and skin reactions developed secondary to facial PPE that includes surgical masks, N95 respirators, goggles, face shields.

Acne and Rosacea

Acne is a common facial dermatosis seen among frontline HCWs wearing PPE regularly and for prolonged durations. This is also proverbially known as "mask-related acne" or "maskne" (Fig. 6.1). The use of facial protection devices such as masks and goggles creates a hot and humid "micro-climate" on the face, resulting in accumulation of sweat and seborrhea. This also promotes bacterial growth and thus, acne. Working in hot, humid, tropical climates and having a pre-existing history of acne vulgaris are

H. C. Lee (✉)
Dermatology Department, KK Women's and Children's Hospital, Singapore, Singapore

C. L. Goh
National Skin Centre, Singapore, Singapore

© The Author(s), under exclusive license to Springer Nature Switzerland AG 2023
H. H. Oon, C. L. Goh (eds.), *COVID-19 in Dermatology*, Updates in Clinical Dermatology,
https://doi.org/10.1007/978-3-031-45586-5_6

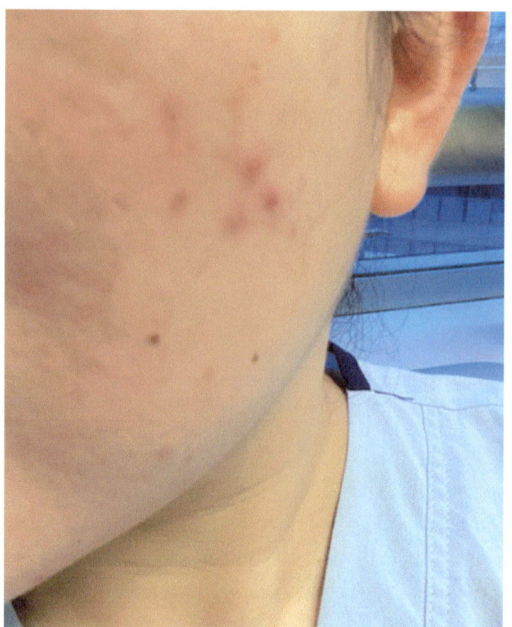

Fig. 6.1 "Maskne" in a HCW, reported after wearing N95 respirators for long hours during shift work

risk factors for PPE-related acne. Those with no prior history of acne can also develop acne mechanica, in which the mask and goggles cause constant friction and repetitive pressure, rupturing the micro-comedones and resulting in inflammatory acne.

Rosacea due to facial PPE has also been reported. HCWs have reported new-onset episodes or aggravations of previously controlled rosacea after prolonged use of facial PPE. The papulopustular and erythematotelangiectatic variants of rosacea were the most common forms reported. Like "Maskne", "Mask Rosacea" is a rising new phenomenon triggered by prolonged mask wearing during this pandemic. *Demodex folliculorum*, a known trigger of rosacea, is believed to accumulate easily due to the microclimate created by the mask on the face, resulting in more inflammation and erythema and subsequent flares of rosacea.

Recommendations

We recommend regular breaks from PPE in a safe, well-ventilated area. Gentle facial cleansers containing comedolytic agents like salicylic acid (SA) and benzoyl peroxide (BPO) can be used

before and after donning PPE. The inflammatory papules of maskne can be treated with topical antibiotics, BPO 2.5% cream or gel, or combination creams. Comedolytic agents like topical retinoids can be used at night for prevention. Lower concentration of retinoids or retinols may be preferred to minimize the risk of skin irritation. Noncomedogenic, oil-free facial moisturizers are recommended for barrier protection.

For those with predominantly mask-induced rosacea, rosacea-targeted topicals can be prescribed. These include 1% ivermectin cream, metronidazole gel, or azelaic acid gel/cream.

In general, we recommend that all topicals should be applied at least 30–60 minutes before donning PPE. If there is concomitant skin irritation or intolerance to topical treatment, additional anti-inflammatory agents in the form of topical calcineurin inhibitors such as pimecrolimus cream can be applied. Severe cases should be referred to dermatologists or occupational dermatology clinics as they may require further treatment in the form of systemic agents. These may include oral antibiotics or systemic retinoids, depending on the condition and status of the patient.

Skin Indentations, Pressure Injuries (PIs)

N95 respirators and goggles require a tight seal to achieve adequate protection. The nasal bridge and malar cheeks are constant contact points with these PPEs and are thus the most common sites vulnerable to developing skin indentations and subsequent PIs, also known as "Device-related Pressure Ulcers" (DRPUs). Skin indentations and erythema over these sites are early warning signs of PIs and should not be dismissed. If not attended to promptly, the constant pressure to these areas will eventually progress to blistering, erosions, and even ulcers. A hot and humid environment, especially in the tropics, may inadvertently cause excess moisture and eventual skin maceration. PIs can also result in secondary infections, subsequent breach of PPE compliance, and subsequent viral transmission.

Recommendations

It has been found that prolonged mask use of more than 6 hours daily is a risk factor for facial dermatoses, particularly for PIs. We recommend scheduled "mask breaks" for 15 minutes every 2–3 hours to ensure regular pressure relief. The first step is to prepare the skin prior to donning PPE by using a gentle, pH-balanced facial cleanser. This is followed by applying a topical skin-protectant over potential sites of pressure and friction. Silicone or dimethicone barrier creams, 3M™ Cavilon™ No Sting barrier film are examples of safe topical skin protectants that can be used prior to donning PPE that reduce friction and decrease the coefficient of friction (COF) between the skin and PPE. These should be rubbed gently into the skin, and the skin should be fully dry before donning the mask or other facial PPE.

It is important to choose the right skin-protective topicals; greasy ointments like petrolatum jelly and mineral oils are not advisable as these will cause mask slippage and compromise the integrity and seal of the mask. Thick and bulky dressings are also discouraged for the same reason.

Usage of prophylactic thin hydrocolloid dressings with N95 respirators remains controversial due to concerns that they may compromise mask fitting. We recommend that this is to be assessed on a case-by-case basis; the National Pressure Injury Advisory Panel (NPIAP) states that if they are to be used, regular seal checks and mask fittings should be done to ensure that there is no breach of PPE (National Pressure Injury Advisory Panel n.d.; Gefen and Ousey 2020). As the welfare of the HCW remains a priority, if they do decide to proceed with prophylactic thin dressings, the latter should be changed regularly, and mask fitting should be done frequently to ensure that their safety is not compromised in any way.

Severe and/or infected PIs may need specialized wound dressing, and specialist medical advice should be sought. Depending on the severity, temporary excuse from PPE and work may be required. The skin barrier should be allowed to recover completely before resuming facial PPE at work.

Contact and Delayed Pressure Urticaria

N95 respirators and goggles, along with their accompanying straps, may cause contact or delayed pressure urticaria as they create a tight seal on facial skin.

Recommendations

Regular, scheduled breaks from PPE every 2–3 hours are recommended to minimize pressure to these areas. Non-sedating oral antihistamines can also be taken prophylactically, at least 1–2 hours prior to shift duty. Decreased exposure time to PPE or job reassignment may be considered if therapeutic measures are unsuccessful.

Contact Dermatitis (CD)

Irritant contact dermatitis (ICD) is one of the most common PPE-related dermatoses encountered by HCWs (Babino et al. 2022; Sarfraz et al. 2022). This can be due to the mask or goggle linings and/or their accompanying straps, resulting in frictional or irritant contact dermatitis on the external ear or other areas of contact. Heat and humidity in tropical climates or the working environment can also result in hyperhydration effects making one more prone to skin barrier dysfunction and subsequent ICD.

Recommendations

The first step in preventing ICD is to focus on preventing constant friction and pressure, while maintaining the integrity of PPE for the wearer. Regular cleansing with a gentle pH-balanced facial cleanser is important. Moisturizers and/or barrier creams on cleansed skin should be applied regularly. If there is active dermatitis, topical steroids should be administered. Secondary infections should be treated with antimicrobial therapy where appropriate. Donning of PPE should only resume after the skin has completely healed and the skin barrier has recovered.

The risk of developing ICD can be reduced by alternating between masks with loops and those with manually tied straps over the back of the head. Thin dressings or skin protectants can be applied to contact areas around the ear or other areas on the face to minimize contact and friction. This pandemic has prompted many to explore the use of 3D-printed respirators and unique mask designs as possible alternatives to conventional N95 masks (Levine et al. 2022; Ohara et al. 2022). Some have also proposed novel ear-independent mask designs, including headbands with plastic 3D-printed straps, thereby avoiding constant friction on the ears. While the latter proves to be acceptable for surgical masks, it is still controversial with respect to N95 respirators (and their equivalents) as it might compromise the fit and integrity of the latter. Another option is to consider covering these areas with a surgical cap before wearing ear-dependent facial protection devices, thereby minimizing pressure from any of the straps of these devices.

Allergic Contact Dermatitis (ACD)

Rarely, ACD due to mask components (metal clips, rubber straps, adhesives, etc.) can occur. ACD to thiuram in the elastic straps of masks, goggles, and rubber-compounding materials such as carba mix and acrylates in mask adhesives have been reported (Kosann et al. 2003; Al Badri 2017; Hamann et al. 2003). Dibromodicyanobutane, found in surgical face mask adhesives, has been reported to cause ACD in a HCW (Al Badri 2017). With regard to textile ACD, HCWs have developed ACD to free formaldehyde and formaldehyde-releasing agents found in N95 respirators (Donovan and Skotnicki-Grant 2007).

Recommendations
If ACD is suspected, comprehensive patch testing and repeat open application tests (ROAT) of potential allergens should be carried out. Where necessary, the facial protection devices can be deconstructed, and individual components of the PPE (e.g. metal clips, layers of mask, straps, buckles, etc.) can be isolated for testing. This is done by placing the component on the skin directly with a drop of saline followed by application of tape and

standard patch test protocols. If an occupational-related ACD is confirmed through these tests, appropriate substitution is mandatory. If this is not possible, then a change in designation or job reassignment may be necessary.

Cheilitis and Other Skin Reactions

Lip licker's dermatitis or cheilitis has been reported in frontline HCWs. This is due to frequent licking of lips due to dehydration and reduced fluid intake while at the frontline and can be exacerbated by hot and humid environments and long working hours.

Irritant rhinitis to FFP masks during the pandemic has also been recently reported (Klimek et al. 2020).

Recommendations
We recommend regular application of allergen-free, lip protectants and scheduled "mask breaks" and regular hydration in safe, non-contaminated areas.

Facial pigmentation has also been reported among HCWs. This is commonly due to post inflammatory hyperpigmentation following frictional or contact dermatitis or rarely, from pigmented ICD. Seborrheic dermatitis (SD) is also another facial PPE-related dermatosis that has been reported among HCWs.

Mild topical steroids should be applied to all inflamed areas, and regular emollients should be used to protect the skin barrier from further damage. The skin should be cleansed, and all topicals should be applied at least 30–60 minutes before donning PPE.

Skin Reactions Related to Hand Hygiene and Gloves

Hand Hygiene and Irritant Hand Dermatitis

Occupational dermatoses due to excessive and frequent hand hygiene is the most common skin reaction during the COVID-19 pandemic among frontline HCWs. A Chinese cohort of HCWs

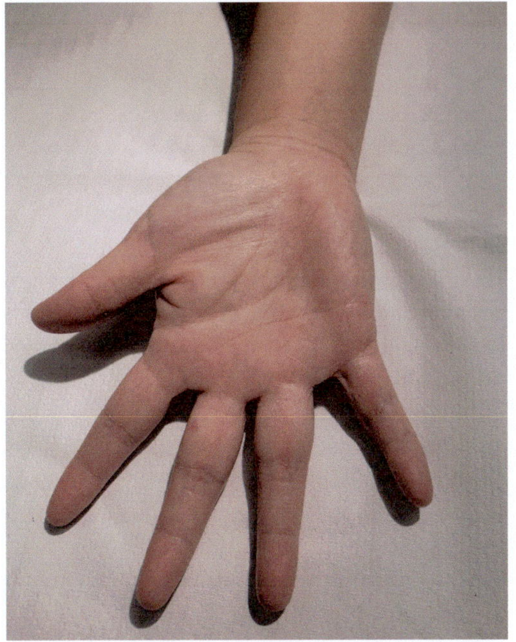

Fig. 6.2 Hand eczema developed after overzealous hand hygiene in a healthcare worker in the emergency department during the pandemic

reported 84.6% had adverse skin reactions due to hand hygiene practices (Lin et al. 2020). While hand hygiene remains critical for the prevention of any viral transmission, overzealous hand hygiene amongst HCWs with no regular hand protection or barrier repair has commonly led to hand dermatitis (Guertler et al. 2020). Constant friction, rubbing, water, surfactants, and defatting chemicals from frequent hand hygiene cause barrier dysfunction and resultant hand dermatitis (Fig. 6.2). Furthermore, this skin damage also provides a potential route of entry for COVID-19 and other viruses. It is important to highlight the importance of "rational hand hygiene" and regular skin barrier protection to all frontline HCWs.

CDC recommends that HCWs use hand sanitizers containing at least 60% ethanol or 70% isopropyl alcohol instead of soap and water unless there is visible soilage (Kratzel et al. 2020; CDC n.d.). Alcohol-based hand rubs (ABHR) can not only inactivate the virus, they are also more convenient and have been shown to improve compliance to hand hygiene among HCWs. They are also believed to cause less skin damage than conventional hand washes, and they tend to contain emol-lients and moisturizers that help to protect or repair the skin barrier. However, indiscriminate, frequent use of ABHR without subsequent skin barrier repair can also cause skin dryness and ICD.

Recommendations

It is recommended that all HCWs practice rational hand hygiene and remember to use moisturizers and/or barrier creams after hand hygiene. Application of moisturizers does not compromise the efficacy of ABHRs. Hand accessories such as rings and watches should not be worn at work as potential allergens or irritants may accumulate underneath them during hand hygiene practices, resulting in ACD or ICD, respectively.

ICD of the hands should be treated with topical steroids, and secondary infections should be treated with antimicrobials where appropriate. The skin barrier must be fully recovered before resuming duties to prevent recurrence.

Allergic Contact Dermatitis (ACD)

The preservatives, fragrances, and surfactants used in the antiseptic hand soaps and washes are potential contact allergens that may cause ACD of the hands.

True allergic reactions to ABHRs are uncommon but have been reported. Cases of ACD to components in different brands of ABHRs such as iodopropynyl butylcarbamate, isopropanol have been reported (Toholka and Nixon 2014). Positive patch tests to isopropanol in a case series of 44 patients was shown to have an 84% relevance rate, but it has been postulated that these patch test reactions are more likely toxic skin reactions to 100% isopropanol rather than true allergic reactions (García-Gavín et al. 2011). Most other allergic reactions to ABHRs, if ever, are more likely caused by the preservatives in the ABHRs. In a review of healthcare hand sanitizers, tocopherol (Vitamin E), fragrance, propylene glycol, benzoates, and cetyl stearyl alcohol were the top five allergens listed (Voller et al. 2020).

Recommendations

To confirm ACD, a patch test must be done. In the evaluation of isopropanol allergy, this should be done with a dilution of 10% isopropanol, as 100% isopropanol under occlusion is highly likely to result in a toxic skin reaction, which will be misinterpreted as a true allergy.

Alcohol-free hand sanitizers are available, and these often contain benzalkonium chloride (BAC). While approved for the formulation of hand rubs for HCWs, there are limited data on the efficacy of BAC against certain microbes compared to that of AHBRs. BAC is also a common irritant and in some cases, a contact allergen. As it is commonly found in disinfectants in the healthcare setting, BAC should also be considered in the evaluation of occupational contact dermatitis in HCWs.

Glove-Related Skin Reactions

Rubber gloves provide an additional layer of protection for HCWs on the frontline.

However, excessive glove use can also damage the skin barrier and result in hand dermatitis. This includes both ICD and ACD.

Irritant Contact Dermatitis

ICD is the most common skin reaction to wearing gloves among HCWs. This is caused by occlusive effects of gloves, glove powder, soaps, and moisture from incomplete hand drying before donning gloves and perspiration.

Long-term, prolonged use of gloves may also lead to occlusion and hyperhydration effects on the stratum corneum, thereby resulting in maceration and skin barrier damage. This makes the skin more vulnerable to irritation due to the components of medical gloves. In total, 88.5% of frontline HCWs wearing rubber latex gloves during the pandemic for an average of 10 hours a day for 3.5 months complained of skin reactions, including xerosis, itching, and rashes (Hu et al. 2020); 12.4% of HCWs in another cohort reported wearing three layers of gloves to reduce the risk of viral contamination, and this significantly increases the risk of ICD (Yan et al. 2020).

Recommendations

It should be reinforced that a single layer of latex gloves is adequate for prevention of viral trans-

mission. An additional layer of gloves should only be considered in special circumstances where there is potential breach in hand PPE in the presence of preexisting skin damage, heavy soilage, or torn gloves.

Glove-Related Occupational Allergic Skin Reactions

Medical-grade latex gloves are composed of rubber accelerators and natural rubber latex proteins (NRL), both of which can cause glove-related occupational allergic skin reactions.

Medical glove-induced ACD is the most common cause of occupational hand dermatitis in HCWs (Hamnerius et al. 2018). Such Type IV delayed hypersensitivity reactions are caused by rubber accelerators such as thiurams, carbamates, benzothiazoles, diphenylguanidine, and mixed dialkyl thioureas.

Patch tests remain the gold standard for evaluation of occupational-related hand ACD. In suspected or confirmed cases, we recommend the use of accelerator-free medical gloves.

Immediate Type I hypersensitivity reactions to NRL or "True Latex Allergy" can present as anything from mild contact urticaria to potentially fatal anaphylaxis and should not be missed.

The prevalence of latex sensitization among HCWs in a cohort study in Singapore was found to be 9.6% (Tang et al. 2005). Of these latex-sensitized HCWs, only 26.7% had glove-related symptoms, while the rest remained asymptomatic. NRLs present in medical glove powder can also be potential aeroallergens and cause systemic allergic reactions in latex-sensitive HCWs.

Recommendations

The gold standard for diagnosing Type 1 latex allergy is in the form of skin prick tests. The latter should be performed in the hospital setting where latex-free resuscitation equipment and trained medical staff are available.

Such investigations may not be readily available during the pandemic. The following measures may help to decrease to the rate of sensitization in HCWs and reduce the rate of NRL allergic reactions in sensitized individuals:

1. The use of powder-free, reduced protein and low-allergen latex gloves by all workers.

2. The use of latex-free (nitrile or vinyl) gloves by sensitized individuals.

In the event that resources are limited, simple measures like wearing plastic or cotton gloves beneath latex gloves can be adopted temporarily until evaluation at the occupational health clinic is available.

General Management for Hand Dermatitis

Treatment includes topical steroids for inflamed areas and skin barrier repair in the form of intensive emollients. All topicals should be applied at least 1 h before donning PPE to avoid occlusion or paradoxical hyper-hydration effects that can cause maceration and skin barrier dysfunction. Petrolatum-based protectants or oil should be avoided before donning PPE as they may cause glove deterioration. These thick petrolatum-based emollients should instead be applied nightly on the hands under occlusion with white cotton gloves overnight till the next morning. In evaluation of suspected ACD, it is important to remember that the causative allergens are not limited to medical gloves alone. Potential allergens in the soaps, cleansers, and moisturizers used by HCWs should also be considered.

Textile-Related Skin Reactions

Surgical caps and disposable medical gowns provide an additional barrier to protect HCWs from viral transmission in the hospital or frontline setting.

Surgical caps can cause itch, folliculitis and aggravate seborrheic dermatitis on the scalp.

Protective clothing and gowns have been reported to be the top non-glove PPE responsible for ICD in HCWs. Repeated wearing of disposable gowns (and their accompanying straps) can cause ICD, frictional dermatitis, urticaria, and truncal acne. Many HCWs reported itch and dermatitis at their wrists following repeated wearing of disposable gowns during the SARS pandemic in Singapore.

Heat injuries are potential occupational hazards for HCWs working in the tropics. Overheating has been reported with all forms of PPE among HCWs (Davey et al. 2021; Zhu et al. 2022). New-onset dermatitis or flares of preexisting inflammatory skin conditions such as atopic dermatitis, psoriasis, and seborrheic dermatitis can develop in HCWs due to PPE (Fig. 6.3). Perspiration, occlusion, and friction due to the disposable gowns and caps are potential exacerbating factors for these skin reactions (Fig. 6.4). Other skin conditions such as miliaria, choliner-

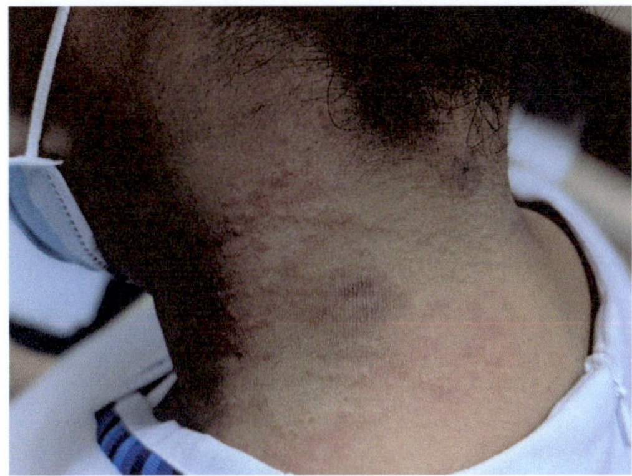

Fig. 6.3 Persistent flare of atopic dermatitis reported over the neck, worsened by sweat, perspiration, and humidity due to prolonged donning of surgical gowns and straps while on 8 h shift work

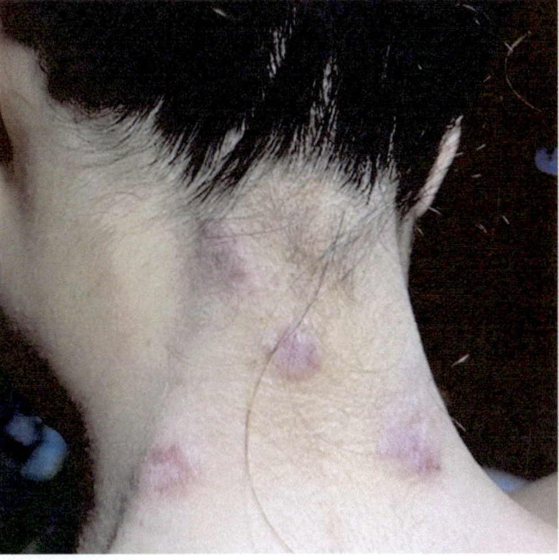

Fig. 6.4 Recurrent irritant contact dermatitis over the nape of the neck, caused the friction from surgical caps and gown straps during long shift work

gic urticaria, and superficial fungal infections tend to occur in tropical climates.

Hospital uniforms and non-woven fabric in disposable medical gowns and masks may contain free formaldehyde and formaldehyde textile resins (FTRs). These may potentially cause textile ACD. Suspected cases should be thoroughly evaluated with patch testing.

Recommendations

To mitigate these risks, HCWs should be given frequent hydration breaks along with the scheduled "mask breaks" during their shift in well ventilated, non-contaminated areas with cooling devices. For those working long hours in hot and humid environments, thin, cool, moisture-wicking garments beneath the PPE gowns are recommended.

Non-sedating antihistamines can be taken for cholinergic urticaria or itch. Topical steroids can be used for miliaria, and flares of eczema, psoriasis, and seborrheic dermatitis. Topical antifungals should be used for superficial fungal infections.

Gentle soap-free cleansers and regular application of moisturizers before and after shifts and as much as possible at home should be encouraged.

Scalp hair can be kept trim and short to facilitate easy decontamination and cleansing, which also reduces the chance of sweat accumulation and occlusion under surgical caps. This reduces the overall risk of developing skin reactions.

Facial hair may increase the risk of mask-related skin reactions including acne, folliculitis, and ICD. Thick and long facial hair may also compromise the seal and integrity of N95 masks. We recommend regular shaving and cleansing to mitigate these risks.

Conclusion

In this chapter, we have discussed common types of occupational dermatoses related to various PPE and hygiene practices used by frontline

HCWs during the era of the COVID-19 pandemic. At the time of writing, the COVID-19 virus and its emerging variants still remain at large globally. While there has been much improvement in the handling of health emergencies over the last decade since the global SARS outbreak, the world still needs to better prepare ourselves for future waves and other global outbreaks. There is a constant, growing need to update PPE guidelines and improve the design and materials of PPE to reduce the risk of these PPE-related occupational dermatoses. More preventive measures and appropriate training and/or guidelines to counter these adverse skin reactions are recommended for all HCWs. Relevant authorities should recognize PPE-related occupational dermatoses as a critical occupational hazard and work towards applying measures to mitigate the risks of these dermatoses and to improve the overall morale and welfare of HCWs.

References

Al Badri F. Surgical mask contact dermatitis and epidemiology of contact dermatitis in healthcare workers. Curr Allergy Clin Immunol. 2017;30:183–8.

Babino G, Argenziano G, Balato A. Impact in contact dermatitis during and after SARS-CoV2 pandemic. Curr Treat Options Allergy. 2022;9(1):19–26.

Davey SL, Lee BJ, Robbins T, Randeva H, Thake CD. Heat stress and PPE during COVID-19: impact on healthcare workers' performance, safety and well-being in NHS settings. J Hosp Infect. 2021;108:185–8.

Donovan J, Skotnicki-Grant S. Allergic contact dermatitis from formaldehyde textile resins in surgical uniforms and nonwoven textile masks. Dermatitis. 2007;18(1):40–4.

Elston DM. Occupational skin disease among health care workers during the coronavirus (COVID-19) epidemic. J Am Acad Dermatol. 2020;82(5):1085–6.

Foo CC, Goon AT, Leow YH, Goh CL. Adverse skin reactions to personal protective equipment against severe acute respiratory syndrome—a descriptive study in Singapore. Contact Derm. 2006;55(5):291–4.

García-Gavín J, Lissens R, Timmermans A, Goossens A. Allergic contact dermatitis caused by isopropyl alcohol: a missed allergen? Contact Dermatitis. 2011;65(2):101–6.

Gefen A, Ousey K. Update to device-related pressure ulcers: SECURE prevention. COVID-19, face masks and skin damage. J Wound Care. 2020;29(5):245–59.

Guertler A, Moellhoff N, Schenck TL, et al. Onset of occupational hand eczema among healthcare workers during the SARS-CoV-2 pandemic: comparing a single surgical site with a COVID-19 intensive care unit. Contact Dermatitis. 2020;83(2):108–14.

Hamann CP, Rodgers PA, Sullivan K. Allergic contact dermatitis in dental professionals: effective diagnosis and treatment. J Am Dent Assoc. 2003;134(2):185–94.

Hamnerius N, Svedman C, Bergendorff O, et al. Hand eczema and occupational contact allergies in health-care workers with a focus on rubber additives. Contact Dermatitis. 2018;79(3):149–56.

Hand hygiene recommendations, guidance for health care providers and COVID-19. CDC guidelines. https://www.cdc.gov/hicpac/recommendations/core-practices.html.

Hu K, Fan J, Li X, et al. The adverse skin reactions of health care workers using personal protective equipment for COVID-19. Medicine (Baltimore). 2020;99(24):e20603.

Klimek L, Huppertz T, Alali A, et al. A new form of irritant rhinitis to filtering facepiece particle (FFP) masks (FFP2/N95/KN95 respirators) during COVID-19 pandemic. World Allergy Organ J. 2020;13(10):100474.

Kosann MK, Brancaccio R, Cohen D. Occupational allergic contact dermatitis in an obstetrics and gynecology resident. Dermatitis. 2003;14(4):217–8.

Kratzel A, Todt D, V'kovski P, et al. Inactivation of severe acute respiratory syndrome coronavirus 2 by WHO-recommended hand rub formulations and alcohols. Emerg Infect Dis. 2020;26:1592.

Lee HC, Goh CL. Occupational dermatoses from personal protective equipment during the COVID-19 pandemic in the tropics - a review. J Eur Acad Dermatol Venereol. 2021;35(3):589–96.

Levine M, Levine L, Xun H, et al. Face off: 3D-printed masks as a cost-effective and reusable alternative to N95 respirators: a feasibility study. Am J Med. 2022;135(9):1109–15.

Lin P, Zhu S, Huang Y, et al. Adverse skin reactions among healthcare workers during the coronavirus disease 2019 outbreak: a survey in Wuhan and its surrounding regions. Br J Dermatol. 2020;183(1):190–2.

National Pressure Injury Advisory Panel (NPIAP) Position statements on preventing injury with with N95 masks. https://cdn.ymaws.com/npiap.com/resource/resmgr/position_statements/Mask_Position_Paper_FINAL_fo.pdf.

Ohara Y, Kanie J, Hori K. Fabrication of a highly protective 3D-printed mask and evaluation of its viral filtration efficiency using a human head mannequin. HardwareX. 2022;11:e00314.

Sarfraz Z, Sarfraz A, Sarfraz M, et al. Contact dermatitis due to personal protective equipment use and hygiene practices during the COVID-19 pandemic: a systematic review of case reports. Ann Med Surg (Lond). 2022;74:103254.

Tang MB, Leow YH, Ng V, Koh D, Goh CL. Latex sensitisation in healthcare workers in Singapore. Ann Acad Med Singap. 2005;34(5):376–82.

Toholka R, Nixon R. Suspected allergic contact dermatitis to iodopropynyl butylcarbamate in an alcohol hand rub commonly used in Australian health-care settings. Australas J Dermatol. 2014;55(1):70–1.

Voller LM, Schlarbaum JP, Hylwa SA. Allergenic ingredients in health care hand sanitizers in the United States. Dermatitis. 2020;10:1097.

Yan Y, Chen H, Chen L, et al. Consensus of Chinese experts on protection of skin and mucous membrane barrier for health-care workers fighting against coronavirus disease 2019. Dermatol Ther. 2020;33:e13310.

Zhu Y, Qiao S, Wu W, Li Y, Jian H, Lin S, Tang T, Zheng Z, Mao Y, Chen X, Fang Z. Thermal discomfort caused by personal protective equipment in health-care workers during the delta COVID-19 pandemic in Guangzhou, China: a case study. Case Stud Therm Eng. 2022;34:101971.

COVID-19 Outbreak Response in Dermatology

Nancy Garcia-Tan and Nicole Marella G. Tan

Introduction

The impact of COVID-19 on the healthcare system transcended many fields. Dermatologists, pulled to the frontlines, were well positioned to identify and manage emerging cutaneous manifestations of COVID-19, reactions from personal protective equipment (PPE), vaccinations, and treatment. Healthcare facilities experienced a drastic shift in patient volume and restraints in procedures, impacting patient care in both urban and rural areas, albeit more severely in the latter. Dermatologists went beyond borders, utilizing telemedicine and social media, to leverage these disparities. Online platforms were effectively harnessed to continue on with medical training.

As COVID-19 restrictions were lifted, patients gradually returned for in-office consultations and dermatologic procedures. Cognizant of the risk of transmission that may occur within the medical facility, it is imperative that COVID-proof environments were provided for the safety of our patients, our health workers, and the community as a whole.

Global Dermatology Perspective of COVID-19

With the SARS-CoV-2 outbreak and its eventual declaration as a global pandemic, COVID-19 infection posed an unprecedented challenge to the entire healthcare system. Dermatologists have evolved alongside the developing pandemic, learning to deal with new challenges and situations.

Dramatic Transition from Face to Face to Teledermatology Consultations

In the global spirit of minimization of COVID-19 transmission, dermatologic practices took a backseat during the first wave of the pandemic. Dermatology clinics were closed to reduce transmission of the disease by preventing overcrowding in shared medical spaces (e.g., outpatient areas, wards, laboratories, and surgical units) (Bhargava et al. 2021). Elective procedures were rescheduled and reduced so that medical resource utilization could be optimized. This led to a dramatic decrease of in-person dermatologic consul-

N. Garcia-Tan
Department of Internal Medicine - Section of Dermatology, Cardinal Santos Medical Center, Manila, Philippines

MedDERM Asia Laser & Surgicentre, Manila, Philippines

N. M. G. Tan (✉)
MedDERM Asia Laser & Surgicentre, Manila, Philippines

Department of Dermatology, University of the Philippines - Philippine General Hospital, Manila, Philippines
e-mail: ngtan1@alum.up.edu.ph

© The Author(s), under exclusive license to Springer Nature Switzerland AG 2023
H. H. Oon, C. L. Goh (eds.), *COVID-19 in Dermatology*, Updates in Clinical Dermatology,
https://doi.org/10.1007/978-3-031-45586-5_7

tations and procedures. In a survey of 678 dermatologists from 52 different countries, 49.26% of respondents reported a reduction of over 75% in their daily work activities (Conforti et al. 2021). Minor procedures such as biopsies, cryotherapy, and electrosurgery significantly decreased, and removal of benign lesions and cosmetic procedures were postponed until after lockdowns were lifted (Bhargava et al. 2021).

Dermatology clinics adapted as the pandemic continued, incorporating preventive and protective measures. However, factors such as strict public health regulations, transportation and logistics issues, even mass media reports on infection rates and reports of exhausted healthcare workers, affected patients' anxiety and ability to return to outpatient clinics (Alfieri and Yogianti 2021). In the United Kingdom, the National Health Service was concerned that patient censuses did not return to baseline numbers post-lockdown (Ibrahim et al. 2021). A university dermatology outpatient clinic in Germany reported a 39.2% decrease in consultations in March 2020 compared to March 2019, with higher no-show rates in the elderly, those with malignancies, chronic inflammatory, and infectious skin diseases. In the post-COVID era, identification and targeted follow-up of these patients may be a challenge (Wang et al. 2020).

A significant proportion of doctors and patients shifted to teledermatology. A global survey of 733 dermatologists noted an almost threefold increase in the number of dermatologists practicing teledermatology, as compared to before the pandemic. In total, 68.6% also expected to continue practicing teledermatology in the future as part of their regular practice (Bhargava and Sarkar 2020). However, disparities in economy, technological and physical infrastructure, legal restrictions, and reimbursements may limit the implementation of teledermatology (Pala et al. 2020).

Dermatologists on the Frontlines: Cutaneous Manifestations Associated with the COVID-19 Pandemic

As the number of COVID-19 cases rose, so did the need for more frontline physicians. Dermatology residents and consultants were deployed to wards, emergency departments, and intensive care units, managing COVID-19 cases alongside colleagues from other specialties. Seeing COVID-19 patients face-to-face enabled dermatologists to study emerging cutaneous manifestations. The largest meta-analysis to date pooled 61,089 COVID-19 patients from 33 studies. In total, 5.6% presented with cutaneous manifestations, including: maculopapular rashes, livedoid lesions, petechial lesions, urticaria, pernio-like lesions, and vesicular lesions. Petechial and livedoid lesions were seen in a higher proportion of patients with severe disease (Li et al. 2022). Dermatologists on the frontlines could greatly assist in prompt recognition and assessment of generalized skin eruptions, including drug-adverse events, chronic underlying skin diseases, viral infections, and systemic conditions, differentiating them from known cutaneous COVID-19 manifestations (Lee 2020).

Importantly, dermatologists treated not only the patients affected with COVID-19 but also the healthcare workers caring for these patients. Over 90% of healthcare workers experienced friction/pressure injuries and allergic contact dermatitis from personal protective equipment (PPE), irritant contact dermatitis from frequent hand hygiene, and facial dermatoses (e.g., "maskne") from prolonged mask wearing (Feldman et al. n.d.). Therapeutic strategies against COVID-19 also caused cutaneous reactions, necessitating dermatologic support to differentiate and manage these side effects. Side effects of nirmatrelvir/ritonavir are commonly mild, but caution is still warranted as these have still been documented to cause Stevens–Johnson syndrome (Albrecht et al. 2023). Cutaneous symptoms from allergic reactions to convalescent plasma range from mild pruritus to urticaria and flushing (Selvi 2020). Vaccines against COVID-19 may cause local injection site reactions, delayed local reactions, and urticaria, most commonly by mRNA-based vaccines (Wei 2022).

Strict quarantine measures, prolonged isolation, stresses of employment and loss of income, and bereavement of loved ones made unquantifiable burdens to society and individuals. Psychosocial stressors have been linked to acute flares and exacerbations of known stress-responsive dermatoses like psoriasis, alopecia areata, telogen effluvium, atopic dermatitis, and acne (Pendlebury et al. 2022; Rossi et al. 2021; Turkmen et al. 2020; Rivetti and Barruscotti 2020; Mahil et al. 2021; Brishkoska-Boshkovski et al. 2020), adding to the collateral damage of the pandemic.

Dermatology and Education

Prioritizing safety, numerous global events were canceled last minute. Virtual e-learning platforms were implemented for the first time, allowing world-class dermatologic education to reach thousands of global participants simultaneously. A positive outcome of the shift to virtual conventions was costs saved from travel, registration, and accommodation (Bhargava and Sarkar 2020). Online education was similarly implemented across medical schools, residency programs, and hospital departments, utilizing modalities such as live streaming of lectures, webinars, on-demand videos, adaptive tutorials, audio clips, and virtual models. Participants had greater control in selecting learning activities that matched their needs, at a time and location of their preference. A blend of traditional medical education with the e-learning approach may have a significant impact on the learning environment of students (Vasavda et al. 2021).

Dermatologists Beyond Borders

Dermatologists on Rural Grounds

Rural patients have experienced a long-standing lack of access to health care. Geographical, financial, and cultural factors strongly influence healthcare access and utilization (Golembiewski et al. 2022). Globally, dermatologists are concentrated in urban populations (Gaffney and Rao 2015), while rural, uninsured/underinsured, racial minorities, and ethnic minorities have limited access (Vaidya et al. 2018). These disparities only continue to increase with time (Feng et al. 2018). In the United States, only 1.8% of board-certified dermatologists practice in the 100 least dense area codes, while some areas do not have any dermatologist at all (Glazer et al. 2017).

The exponential expansion of telemedicine during the COVID-19 pandemic created avenues to reach more underserved populations. Use of telemedicine in outpatient care was estimated to have risen by 154% in 2020 (Koonin et al. 2020). The issuance of the 1135 Waiver by the Centers for Medicare and Medicaid Services in the United States eliminated numerous barriers, specifically those pertaining to licensing restrictions, lack of reimbursement, and health insurance compliance (Centers for Medicare and Medicaid Services 2023). However, low- and lower-middle income countries face more primal problems—absence of national policies and lack of government support, perceived high costs of telemedicine implementation, underdeveloped infrastructure (including low quality of connectivity and frequent power outages), lack of technical expertise and support, and digital illiteracy (Gaffney and Rao 2015; Ahuja et al. 2022; World Health Organization 2010; Faye et al. 2018).

For lower-income populations, "direct-to-patient" teledermatology was frequently impossible. A commonplace practice is for general practitioners or family physicians to make informal referrals to dermatology colleagues and friends on various online platforms, to provide support to communities where specialists are out of reach (Morris et al. 2022; Koh et al. 2022).

Recent studies have documented the benefits of a formal teledermatology partnership across various aspects. In Central Northern India, primary care physicians stationed in areas classified as "very low" on the United Nations Human Development Index were connected with dermatologists via the WhatsApp messaging platform. Teledermatology consultations were conducted via the store-and-forward method, with the dermatologists taking turns to respond to various cases. Over 80% of the consultations were successfully managed at local peripheral hospitals (Thomas et al. 2022). A similar asynchronous teledermatology service between primary care physicians and dermatology specialists conducted in Catalonia estimated that about 51,164 euros were saved by utilizing teledermatology (Vidal-Alaball et al. 2018).

Educational benefit was observed in many of these partnerships. In French Guiana, Delocalized Centers for Prevention and Care were spread over remote rainforest areas to ameliorate access to health care. General physicians and nurses stationed at these peripheral centers would coordinate with the few specialists at the main hospital to treat dermatologic conditions, including neglected conditions like leishmaniasis and leprosy. Ninety-three percent of the non-specialist healthcare workers reported that regular teledermatology improved their knowledge and served as continuing medical education (Messagier et al. 2019).

A group of dermatologists in the Philippines tapped and trained over a hundred *"Doctors to the Barrios,"* general physicians already integrated into local health units across the Philippines. On a weekly basis, a reported 10–30% of their consults were for a primary dermatologic condition. Investigators conducted a week-long basic dermatology course, a hybrid of synchronous online activities and asynchronous self-study. Participants stated that their dermatologic knowledge and confidence in diagnosis and management of skin disease increased significantly, with 80.2% stating that they would attend similar courses in the future (Salazar-Paras et al. 2021).

In Mali, West Africa, selected frontline personnel (general physicians, nurses, or minimally trained healthcare workers) were taught the algorithmic approach of common skin diseases and basic skills, including use of a teledermatology application for referrals. Overall diagnostic concordance between the dermatologists and health personnel was high at 95% after training. Interviews with both healthcare workers and patients revealed that majority were strongly satisfied with the conduct of the teledermatology service, specifically appreciating that they were locally managed, and expressed the need to sustain the initiative (Faye et al. 2018).

The landscape and experience of health care are vastly different across high- to low-income countries. Success depends heavily on strong collaborations between rural health units and urban-based dermatologic centers, complemented with cost-efficient use of resources. Optimal expansion would require support from national governments and policymakers, to provide regulations and resources to expand teledermatology access in these areas.

Dermatologists on Social Media

Social media has firmly entrenched its role in healthcare, with overlapping uses in patient education, public outreach, professional development and networking, and clinical research. Users are able to share information and ideas, whether their own created content or from other sources, and connect worldwide. Over half the world's population owns and uses at least one social media account (Cooper et al. 2022). Strict lockdowns intensified global use of social media, with many tuning in for updates on the evolving pandemic, including healthcare workers (Bhagavathula et al. 2020).

During COVID-19, dermatologists utilized social media for rapid study of emerging information. Maximization of instant messaging and crowdsourcing techniques gave rise to an express collection of COVID-19 cutaneous manifestations that could be shared, scrutinized, and reviewed by dermatologists around the world almost as soon as they were encountered (Duong et al. 2020; Freeman et al. 2020). Even with lockdown restrictions, the degree of connectivity has allowed researchers to conduct web-based research, global online surveys, and virtual clinical trials (Geist et al. 2021), continually building new knowledge on COVID-19. Many reputable dermatology journals have robust followings on social media, magnifying the reach, citations, and consequently, the impact of significant research findings (Geist et al. 2021; Laughter et al. 2020).

Dermatologists on social media promoted healthy skin through polls, blogs, videos, live

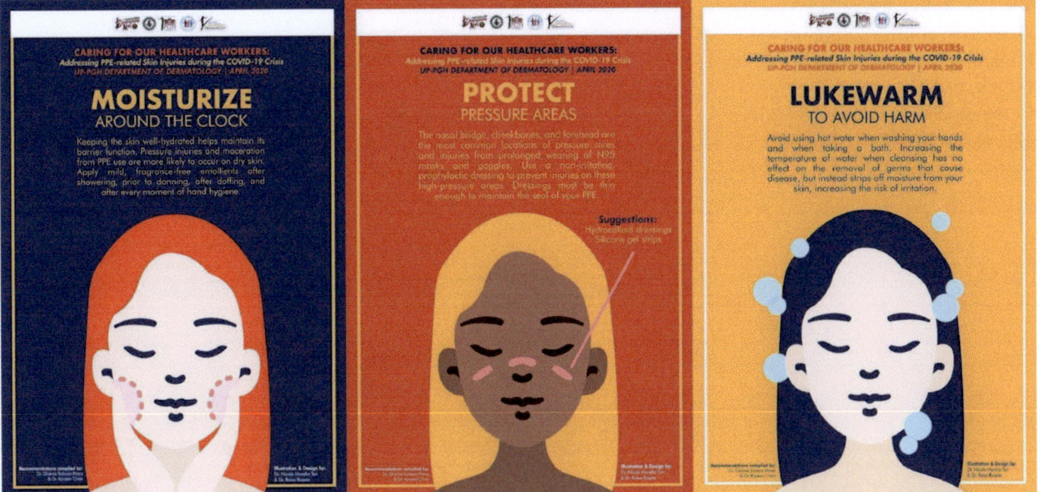

Fig. 7.1 Caring for our Healthcare Workers: Addressing PPE-related Skin Injuries during the COVID-19 Crisis. University of the Philippines – Philippine General Hospital Department of Dermatology. (Reproduced with permission)

streaming sessions, and "tweetorials" (Cooper et al. 2022; Szeto et al. 2021). Pandemic-specific educational dermatologic content centered on skin care from occupational dermatoses (Fig. 7.1).

In the Philippines, a team of dermatologists was specifically recruited to transform constantly evolving COVID-19 guidelines into infographics that could be readily comprehended by healthcare workers of all health literacy levels (Fig. 7.2). Fast-paced creation of these infographics with feedback from concerned stakeholders helped streamline hospital-wide operations, gradually evolving into an effective communication framework (Tan et al. 2021). Dermatologic communication skills, hand in hand with evidence-based guidelines, can be a powerful tool in public health and patient education.

However, networks may be easily abused in the spread of misinformation and disinformation, especially evident during the beginning of the COVID-19 pandemic. During the Munich Security Conference on February 15, 2020, the World Health Organization Director-General Dr. Tedros Adhanom Ghebreyesus was famously quoted for stating, "We're not just fighting an epidemic; we're fighting an infodemic." The general quality of health information procured online and the challenge to be critical and discerning of accuracy are often left to individual users (Swire-Thompson and Lazer 2019). Furthermore, fact-checked information tends to be propagated at a much slower rate than false information (Cha et al. 2021).

Social media is a powerful tool in the arsenal of public health and education, but optimal processes and safeguards are still wanting. Ideally, national governments and scientific organizations should take the lead in a centralized approach to data gathering and dissemination. At present, majority of "educational" postings come from users without any formal medical or dermatological training (Nguyen et al. 2021). The strong social media presence of dermatologists comes with the potential to heavily influence individual patients' health-related behavior, contributing to a more informed and healthy online population.

Fig. 7.2 Infographics from the University of the Philippines – Philippine General Hospital Information Education Communication Committee. 2020. (Reproduced with permission)

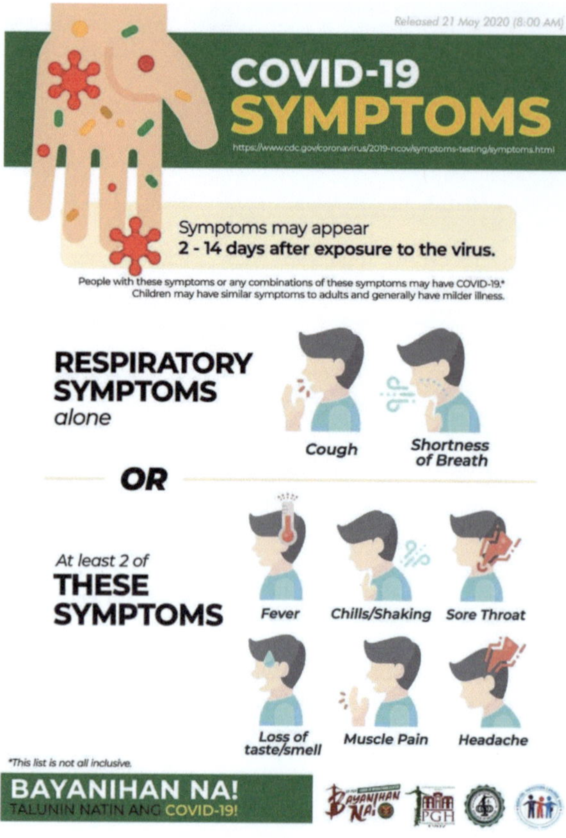

How to COVID-Proof the Small Office Dermatology Practice

What Worked, What Didn't, What Policies and Practices Should Stay

The COVID-19 pandemic has brought public health and safety concerns to the forefront. Post-pandemic, patients appreciate the new measures, structural modifications, and a scheduling system that limits the number of people they are exposed to in the facility. Updates are needed to incorporate best practices found to be effective during this pandemic.

Baseline precautions and recommendations presented here consider the safety and welfare of all stakeholders, both inside and outside the walls of the medical facility, with the caveat that as the global understanding of COVID-19 continues to progress, the perspectives, policies, and guidelines will continue to evolve.

Workplace Policies and Procedures

When planning the setup of a dermatology center, safety protocols and regulations are put in place as a matter of procedure. These guidelines should be based on internationally accepted standards and adjusted accordingly to conform to local government regulations. Crafted with the dermatology center's purpose in mind, this serves as a useful resource that should be easily accessed, read, and understood by all employees. Mandatory periodic review of these policies should be performed.

It is essential to assign a safety officer to ensure that policies are strictly observed. A staff member should be assigned to ensure that the facility is compliant with local health regulations for the safety of the whole community.

Employee Training

Staff training is mandatory whenever new personnel are hired or reassigned to a new task or division. Training sessions should be targeted to ensure optimal understanding and adherence, given that comprehension may vary based on work category, competency, and literacy level. Post-training appraisal should be made part of the employee's performance assessment.

- Training should include the following topics on workplace safety:
    - PPE for healthcare workers and patients.
    - Disinfection protocols—including types and preparation of disinfectants.
    - Risk assessment of procedures performed within the medical facility.
    - Signs and symptoms of highly infectious diseases.
    - Protocol when infection is detected in coworkers, patients, visitors.

Quick reference guides installed throughout the medical facility encourage compliance with health and safety protocols. Posters or infographics should be placed at strategic areas of the workplace.

Health Screening

Health screening is required for all personnel within the health facility, including ancillary staff, patients, companions, and third-party providers (e.g., delivery crew). Such measures are in place not only to protect the health and welfare of those within the medical facility but also to protect their families and the communities within which they interact.

1. **Employees**: Health screening processes should conform to local health regulations and adjusted as appropriate to the work environment. An online line screening tool may be utilized and employees asked to self-monitor at home. On-site, it would be ideal to have a separate entrance for employees where a staff member is stationed to perform screening prior to entry.

   Judicious testing protocol should be in place with a clear course of action following significant exposure or infection. Employees who manifest signs and symptoms should be instructed to abstain from attending work, and immediately report to their supervisor for further instructions. Self-isolation and appropriate testing may be done following local health guidelines.

2. **Third-Party Providers**: Visits for preventive maintenance, repairs, and cleaning services should be scheduled outside regular clinic hours. It would be ideal to use a separate entrance and receiving area for delivery of supplies and other clinic needs to avoid unnecessary contact with patients or staff. In the presence of symptoms or potential exposure, visitors should not be allowed entry and should be referred for proper evaluation and care.

3. **Patients**: Effective patient communication, adequate and timely information is of utmost importance, as this plays a great part in limiting transmission and exposure.

Pre-Visit

- Call patients before their scheduled visit. Confirm their appointment, perform pre-screening, and provide information on current health protocols observed in the facility, especially if they were recently updated.
- Offer teledermatology or reschedule as necessary.
- Remind patients to come strictly on time to comply with physical distancing measures.
- Advise patients to come alone. If a companion is necessary, limit to one.

During Visit

- At the height of the pandemic, allow patients to enter the premises only at the time of their scheduled appointment. Early comers and companions may wait outside or in their vehicles. Companions may be called in when needed.
- Conduct health screening tests and temperature checks at the entrance to the facility, before ushering them into the waiting area. Patients may be guided directly to the treatment room, if feasible.

- In the presence of symptoms or potential exposure, non-urgent consultations and procedures should be rescheduled and patients referred for proper evaluation and care. For urgent dermatologic concerns, it is advised to designate a specific isolation room and provide PPE for symptomatic patients.

Post-Visit

- Prepare clear post-procedure instructions to avoid lengthy discussions. Hard copies may be replaced by digital copies, provided it is ascertained that patients clearly understood the instructions and are able to ask questions.
- Provide a helpline or number that patients can call if they have any concerns post-procedure, or if they develop any signs or symptoms after the visit.
- Consider assigning a staff member to check for any signs or symptoms the patient may have developed post-visit by phone call or text message.
- Consider follow-up via teledermatology to limit the number of people visiting the facility.

Clinic Schedule Management

The number of patients for each time slot should be limited to give ample time in between patients to disinfect areas particularly in a small dermatology practice. Walk-ins should be discouraged except in cases of medical emergency.

Facility Management

Physical arrangements help regulate the number of individuals in any given area at any given time and aid in maintaining proper physical distancing throughout the facility. Provisions should be in place for room dividers or natural barriers (e.g., sliding walls, foldable partitions, planters), to make distancing easier to implement and to maintain a distance of 1.5 m between seating arrangements (Vashisht et al. 2021).

Directional flow may be enforced with use of clear signages to avoid crowding along hallways and in common areas. It would be advisable to have separate changing rooms for donning of treatment gowns with lockers for personal things

to avoid placing over counter-tops. Disinfection of barrier surfaces needs to be done at regular intervals and at the end of each clinic day.

Use of acrylic barriers varies widely in effectiveness in reducing exposure to aerosols; some barriers may even increase risk for exposure if not positioned correctly (Cadnum et al. 2022). When placing barriers, consideration should be made to the relative location of windows and vents. Attention to airflow and air quality is essential to decrease risk of transmission. There should be adequate ventilation allowing 12–15 gas exchanges per hour. Natural ventilation is preferred over closed air conditioning (Vashisht et al. 2021). Table 7.1 provides a quick summary of reminders for key areas within medical facilities.

Disinfection Procedures

Special focus is given to the type and concentration of disinfectant used, frequency of disinfection, and identification of high-touch surfaces and materials.

The ability of common coronaviruses to survive on surfaces for up to a month (Ren et al. 2020) underscores the importance of maintaining a heightened level of cleanliness throughout the day and between patient interactions. Frequent disinfection of surfaces is crucial in safeguarding

Table 7.1 Checklist and reminders for key areas

Reception	• Establish a health screening checkpoint at immediate entryway
	• Use a non-contact infrared thermometer
	• Provide spare masks for patients and staff
	• Allow only the patient into the facility; limit companions to one if necessary
Waiting area	• Ensure a well-ventilated room
	• Arrange seating area with 1.5 m distance between seats
	• Remove all unnecessary items (e.g. magazines, brochures); replace promotional items with on-screen videos
	• Avoid beverages and food service in the area

Table 7.1 (continued)

Consultation and treatment rooms	• Post door signages to signify room status for each room (e.g. occupied, procedure ongoing, disinfection in-process)
	• Provide PPE (masks, gloves, face-shield, goggles) in each room, avoid transferring from one room to another
	• Use smoke evacuators, air purifiers with high-efficiency particulate air (HEPA) filters
	• Allow only one patient into the room at a time
	• Disinfect instruments and dermatoscopes after every use
	• Remove all unnecessary items (e.g. extra pillows, blankets)
Common areas (*kitchen/pantry/ staff lounge*)	• Space out break-time schedules to avoid staff congregation
	• Limit seating area
	• Keep food individually packed
	• Wash utensils immediately after use, or replace with disposables
	• Use disposable paper towels over cloth hand towels
All areas	• Put up clear signages as reminders for all visitors and staff (e.g. proper PPE, proper cough etiquette, mask-wearing)
	• Provide alcohol-based hand sanitizers on every countertop
	• Use no-touch lidded garbage bins
	• Disinfect rooms after every use, and at the end of day
	• Sanitize doorknobs, tabletops, pens, and other administrative items after every use and at the end of the day
	• Dispose used filters as medical waste

the health of patients and staff given the contagiousness of the virus (World Health Organization 2020a).

Cleaning should include disinfecting all common, high-touch areas such as the waiting room, reception areas, kitchen and break rooms, labs, offices and workstations, computer keyboards, tablets, credit card machines, pens, bathrooms, door handles, and light switches (Dover et al. 2020).

Regular cleaning with soap and water removes dirt, debris, and organic matter such as blood, secretions, and excretions. Organic matter can impede direct contact of a disinfectant to a surface and inactivate the germicidal properties or mode of action of several disinfectants (World Health Organization 2020b). Medical-grade chemical disinfectants must be used afterward to kill any live microorganisms (Adams et al. 2008). A minimum contact time of 1 min is recommended for these disinfectants. These disinfectants may be used on environmental surfaces to achieve a >3 log (World Health Organization 2020c) reduction of human coronavirus (Kampf et al. 2020), and they are also effective against other clinically relevant pathogens in the healthcare setting (World Health Organization 2020b).

- Ethanol 70–90%.
- Chlorine-based products (e.g., hypochlorite) at 0.1% (1000 ppm) for general environmental disinfection or 0.5% (5000 ppm) for blood and body fluids large spills.
- Hydrogen peroxide >0.5%.

Use of portable air cleaners with High-Efficiency Particulate Air (HEPA) filters has proven to significantly reduce airborne SARS-CoV-2 surrogate particles. Furthermore, the use of portable HEPA purifiers can enhance other decontamination methods such as ventilation (Liu et al. 2022). Used filters should be collected and disposed of as medical waste or disinfected thoroughly to prevent secondary contamination (Zhao et al. 2020).

UVC lamps have been used to inactivate the SARS-CoV-2 virus, but effectiveness is unknown due to limited data about the optimal wavelength, dose, and duration of UVC radiation required to inactivate the virus.

Considerations for Aesthetic Procedures

During the COVID-19 outbreak, aesthetic procedures were generally discouraged, not allowed, or postponed. This had a significant impact on the mental and emotional state of patients who were not able to receive treatments amidst the stress of the pandemic; many were eager to return to the clinics for aesthetic procedures to improve their sense of well-being. In a cross-sectional online survey of 8080 Italian consumers of aesthetic medicine and surgery, the desire for aesthetic treatments was not reduced in 49% of cases despite the pandemic; almost 45% of the patients declared to be ready for rescheduling a surgical or nonsurgical aesthetic procedure, and approximately 47% would return to their physician without any need for an explanation about the security protocols (Melfa et al. 2020).

With patients eager to resume their aesthetic treatments, it is imperative that practitioners are able to provide a safe environment when performing procedures. The number of patients entering the facility per day should be managed, with consideration of the total duration the patient spends in the facility and the number of procedures done per patient, particularly those with close contact between patient and practitioner. A staff member should be assigned to prepare consent forms, room setup, and medical equipment (including smoke evacuators and air filters) prior to the patient entering the treatment room to avoid delays.

Minimize the number of people within treatment rooms. For pain management, it would be prudent to use modalities that do not involve cooling fans or other handheld devices. Disposable tips and other applicators are preferred over reusable ones. During procedures, patients are advised to keep their masks on except during treatments on the lower half of the face; a new mask should then be provided post-procedure (Dover et al. 2020).

Recommendations for the type of PPE to be worn during the pandemic were based on the nature of treatment being performed, invasiveness, and risk of aerosol exposure (Arora et al. 2020). Regardless of the practice prior to and during the pandemic, it is important to continue using appropriate PPE when performing procedures post-pandemic. Table 7.2 lists the common aesthetic procedures and the suggested PPE for the practitioner.

Table 7.2 Personal protective equipment for aesthetic procedures and treatments

Procedures	PPE
Noninvasive	Face mask
Medical facials, superficial chemical peels, IPL, LED, LLLT, HIFU, radiofrequency, cryolipolysis, non-ablative lasers (non-plume generating)	Gloves Protective eye wear
Minimally invasive	Face mask
Medium depth peels, microdermabrasion, microneedling, injectables (toxins, fillers, skin boosters, mesotherapy), thread lifts, sclerotherapy, laser hair reduction	Gloves Protective eye wear Gown
Invasive	Face mask (N95 advised)
Deep chemical peels, ablative laser treatments (plume-generating), dermabrasion, liposuction, platelet rich plasma treatment, hair transplant	Gloves Protective eye wear Gown Surgical cap Face shield

IPL intense pulsed light, *LED* light-emitting diode, *LLLT* low level light therapy, *HIFU* high-intensity focused ultrasound, *LHR* laser hair removal

Conclusion

Each country's response to the COVID-19 pandemic varied in approach, swiftness in action, and expeditiousness to adapt to emerging protocols. What we do moving forward determines if the outbreak response to another pandemic will have a more positive outcome versus COVID-19's devastating statistics—over 760 million confirmed cases worldwide, and over 6.8 million deaths as of March 2023 (World Health Organization 2023). A global coordinated response would have greatly improved the outcome. This should be the concerted goal should the threat of a pandemic loom over mankind once again.

Appendix

HOW TO COVID-PROOF THE **SMALL OFFICE DERMATOLOGY PRACTICE**

WORKPLACE POLICIES AND PROCEDURES
- **Perform a mandatory periodic review** of policies.
- **Assign a safety officer** to ensure the center is compliant with local health regulations.

EMPLOYEE TRAINING
- **Conduct regular staff training** and **assess employee comprehension** on essential topics (eg. PPE, disinfection protocols, risk assessment of procedures, signs and symptoms of disease).
- **Install quick reference guides** throughout the medical facility to encourage compliance with health and safety protocols.

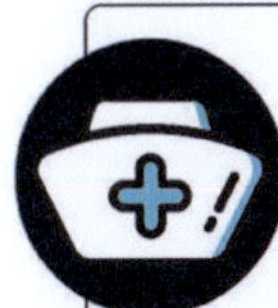

HEALTH SCREENING

1. EMPLOYEES
- **Implement an employee health screening process**.
- **Establish judicious testing protocol** and **clearly lay out the subsequent course of action** following significant exposure or infection.

2. THIRD-PARTY PROVIDERS
- **Schedule visits** for preventive maintenance, repairs, and cleaning **outside clinic hours**.
- **Use a separate entrance and receiving area** for delivery of supplies.
- If with symptoms or potential exposure, visitor/s should **not** be allowed entry and should be **referred for proper evaluation and care**.

3. PATIENTS

PRE-VISIT
- **Call patients before** their scheduled visit: 1) confirm their appointment and perform pre-screening, 2) provide information on current health protocols observed in the facility.
- **Offer teledermatology or reschedule** as necessary.
- Remind patients to **strictly come on time** and to **limit companions**.

DURING VISIT
- **Allow patients to enter the premises only during their scheduled appointment.** Early comers and companions may wait outside or in their vehicles.
- **Conduct health screening tests and temperature checks** at the entrance.
- If with symptoms or potential exposure, patients should be rescheduled, and **referred for proper evaluation and care**.

POST-VISIT
- **Prepare clear post-procedure instructions** to avoid lengthy discussions.
- **Provide a help-line or number** that patients can call if they have any concerns post-procedure, or if they develop any signs or symptoms after the visit.
- Consider assigning a staff member to **phone or message the patient for any signs or symptoms** they may have developed post-visit.
- **Consider follow-up via teledermatology.**

HOW TO COVID-PROOF THE SMALL OFFICE DERMATOLOGY PRACTICE

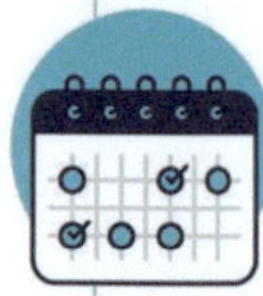

CLINIC SCHEDULE MANAGEMENT

- **Maintain an appointment system** to control the number of people going in and out of the facility.
- **Limit the number of patients** for each time slot.
- **Ensure adequate time between patient appointments.**
- **Discourage walk-ins**, except in cases of medical emergency.

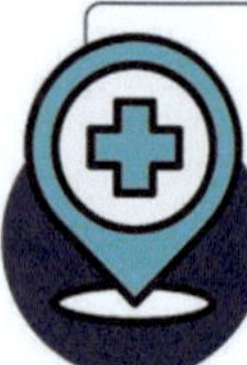

FACILITY MANAGEMENT

- **Arrange each area** to ensure adequate ventilation and maintain proper physical distancing throughout the facility.
- **Control directional flow** (ingress and egress) of patients and staff..
- **Implement check-in and check-out procedures**.
- **Post clear signages in critical areas** as reminders for all visitors and staff (eg. proper PPE, proper cough etiquette, mask-wearing)
- **Provide alcohol-based sanitizers** and **no-touch lidded garbage bins** throughout the facility.
- **Declutter spaces** and remove all unnecessary items.

See: *Table 2. Checklist for Key Areas*

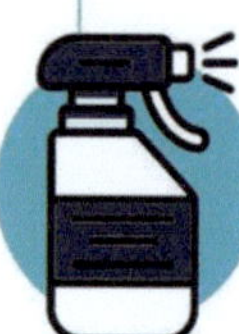

DISINFECTION PROCEDURES

- **Perform regular disinfection** after each room use and at the end of every day, especially over high-touch surfaces.
- **Use medical grade chemical disinfectant** (eg. ethanol 70-90%, 0.1% chlorine-based products, >0.5% hydrogen peroxide) to kill live microorganisms.
- **Use HEPA filters** to reduce airborne particles.

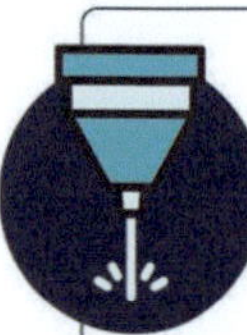

CONSIDERATIONS FOR AESTHETIC PROCEDURES

- **Prioritize safety** at all times.
- **Manage the number of patients entering the facility** per day.
- **Limit the number of procedures per patient** per visit.
- **Assign a staff member to prepare** consent forms, room set-up, and medical equipment (including smoke evacuators and air filters) prior to the patient entering the treatment room.
- **Minimize the number of people in treatment rooms**.
- **Use disposable equipment** as much as possible.

Infographic by Dr. Nancy Garcia-Tan and Dr. Nicole Marella G. Tan | 2023

References

Adams J, Bartram J, Chartier Y, editors. Essential environmental health standards for health care. World Health Organization; 2008.

Ahuja S, Briggs SM, Collier SM. Teledermatology in rural, underserved, and isolated environments: a review. Curr Dermatol Rep. 2022;20:1–8.

Albrecht JM, Cooper BR, Waller JD, Presley CL, Pulsipher KJ, Rundle CW, Dellavalle RP. Nirmatrelvir-ritonivir, COVID-19, and possible adverse cutaneous reactions. Dermatol Online J. 2023;29(1).

Alfieri A, Yogianti F. Impact of pandemic COVID-19 on dermatology and venereology outpatient clinic in a tertiary referral hospital in Yogyakarta, Indonesia. Dermatol Rep. 2021;13(3):9381.

Arora G, Arora S, Talathi A, Kandhari R, Joshi V, Langar S, Nagpal S, Shetty VH, Nair RV, Sharma D, Sharma R. Safer practice of aesthetic dermatology during the COVID-19 pandemic: recommendations by SIG aesthetics (IADVL academy). Indian Dermatol Online J. 2020;11(4):534.

Bhagavathula AS, Aldhaleei WA, Rahmani J, Mahabadi MA, Bandari DK. Knowledge and perceptions of COVID-19 among health care workers: cross-sectional study. JMIR Public Health Surveill. 2020;6(2):e19160.

Bhargava S, Sarkar R. Impact of COVID-19 pandemic on dermatology practice in India. Indian Dermatol Online J. 2020;11(5):712.

Bhargava S, Negbenebor N, Sadoughifar R, Ahmad S, Kroumpouzos G. Global impact on dermatology practice due to the COVID-19 pandemic. Clin Dermatol. 2021;39(3):479–87.

Brishkoska-Boshkovski V, Vasileva M, Dimitrovska I, Grivcheva-Panovska V. Coronavirus disease-19 pandemic and dermatology. what to expect? Open Access Macedonian J Med Sci. 2020;8(T1):290–3.

Cadnum J, Jencson A, Memic S, Osborne A, Torres-Teran M, Wilson B, Deshpande A, Donskey C. Real-world evidence on the effectiveness of Plexiglass barriers in reducing aerosol exposure. Pathog Immunity. 2022;7(2):66–77.

Centers for Medicare & Medicaid Services. Medicare telemedicine healthcare provider fact sheet: medicare coverage and payment of virtual services. https://www.cms.gov/newsroom/fact-sheets/medicare-telemedicine-health-care-provider-fact-sheet?inf_contact_key1/438ca3f198618fc3aeba4091611f5b055680f8914173f9191b1c0223e68310bb1. Accessed 10 Jan 2023.

Cha M, Cha C, Singh K, Lima G, Ahn YY, Kulshrestha J, Varol O. Prevalence of misinformation and factchecks on the COVID-19 pandemic in 35 countries: observational infodemiology study. JMIR Hum Factors. 2021;8(1):e23279.

Conforti C, Lallas A, Argenziano G, Dianzani C, Di Meo N, Giuffrida R, Kittler H, Malvehy J, Marghoob AA, Soyer HP, Zalaudek I. Impact of the COVID-19 pandemic on dermatology practice worldwide: results of a survey promoted by the International Dermoscopy Society (IDS). Dermatol Pract Concept. 2021;11(1):e2021153.

Cooper BR, Concilla A, Albrecht JM, Bhukhan A, Laughter MR, Anderson JB, Rundle CW, McEldrew EC, Presley CL. Social media as a medium for dermatologic education. Curr Dermatol Rep. 2022;11(2):103–9.

Dover JS, Moran ML, Figueroa JF, Furnas H, Vyas JM, Wiviott LD, Karchmer AW. A path to resume aesthetic care: executive summary of Project AesCert guidance supplement—practical considerations for aesthetic medicine professionals supporting clinic preparedness in response to the SARS-CoV-2 outbreak. Facial Plast Surg Aesthet Med. 2020;22(3):125–51.

Duong TA, Velter C, Rybojad M, Comte C, Bagot M, Sulimovic L, Bouaziz JD. Did Whatsapp® reveal a new cutaneous COVID-19 manifestation. J Eur Acad Dermatol Venereol. 2020;34(8):e348–50.

Faye O, Bagayoko CO, Dicko A, Cissé L, Berthé S, Traoré B, Fofana Y, Niang M, Traoré ST, Karabinta Y, Gassama M. A teledermatology pilot programme for the management of skin diseases in primary health care centres: experiences from a resource-limited country (Mali, West Africa). Trop Med Infect Dis. 2018;3(3):88.

Feldman SR, Freeman EE, Duffin KC, Corona R. COVID-19: cutaneous manifestations as issues related to dermatologic care. UpToDate, April 2023.

Feng H, Berk-Krauss J, Feng PW, Stein JA. Comparison of dermatologist density between urban and rural counties in the United States. JAMA Dermatol. 2018;154(11):1265–71.

Freeman EE, McMahon DE, Fitzgerald ME, Fox LP, Rosenbach M, Takeshita J, French LE, Thiers BH, Hruza GJ. The American Academy of Dermatology COVID-19 registry: crowdsourcing dermatology in the age of COVID-19. J Am Acad Dermatol. 2020;83(2):509–10.

Gaffney R, Rao B. Global teledermatology. Glob Dermatol. 2015;2:209–14.

Geist R, Militello M, Albrecht JM, Presley CL, Anderson JB, Laughter M, Rundle CW. Social media and clinical research in dermatology. Curr Dermatol Rep. 2021;10(4):105–11.

Glazer AM, Farberg AS, Winkelmann RR, Rigel DS. Analysis of trends in geographic distribution and density of US dermatologists. JAMA Dermatol. 2017;153(4):322–5.

Golembiewski EH, Gravholt DL, Roldan VD, Naranjo EP, Vallejo S, Bautista AG, LaVecchia CM, Patten CA, Allen SV, Jaladi S, Boehmer KR. Rural patient experiences of accessing care for chronic conditions: a systematic review and thematic synthesis of qualitative studies. Ann Fam Med. 2022;20(3):266–72.

Ibrahim LS, Venables ZC, Levell NJ. The impact of COVID-19 on dermatology outpatient services in England in 2020. Clin Exp Dermatol. 2021;46(2):377–8.

Kampf G, Todt D, Pfaender S, Steinmann E. Persistence of coronaviruses on inanimate surfaces and their inactivation with biocidal agents. J Hosp Infect. 2020;104(3):246–51.

Koh E, Maranga A, Yane T, Ndlovu K, Jereni B, Nwako-Mohamadi MK, Kovarik C, Forrestel A, Williams VL. Evaluation of WhatsApp as a platform for Teledermatology in Botswana: retrospective review and survey. JMIR Dermatol. 2022;5(3):e35254.

Koonin LM, Hoots B, Tsang CA, Leroy Z, Farris K, Jolly B, Antall P, McCabe B, Zelis CB, Tong I, Harris AM. Trends in the use of telehealth during the emergence of the COVID-19 pandemic—United States, January–March 2020. Morb Mortal Wkly Rep. 2020;69(43):1595.

Laughter MR, Zangara T, Maymone MB, Rundle CW, Dunnick CA, Hugh JM, Sadeghpour M, Dellavalle RP. Social media use in dermatology. Dermatol Sin. 2020;38(1):28.

Lee CH. Role of dermatologists in the uprising of the novel corona virus (COVID-19): perspectives and opportunities. Dermatol Sin. 2020;38(1):1.

Li J, Wen W, Mu Z, Du X, Han X. Prevalence of cutaneous manifestations in COVID-19: a meta-analysis. J Dermatol. 2022 Dec;20:622.

Liu DT, Phillips KM, Speth MM, Besser G, Mueller CA, Sedaghat AR. Portable HEPA purifiers to eliminate airborne SARS-CoV-2: a systematic review. Otolaryngol Head Neck Surg. 2022 Apr;166(4):615–22.

Mahil SK, Yates M, Yiu Z, Langan SM, Tsakok T, Dand N, Mason KJ, McAteer H, Meynell F, Coker B, et al. Describing the burden of the COVID-19 pandemic in people with psoriasis: findings from a global cross-sectional study. J Eur Acad Dermatol Venereol. 2021;35:e636–40.

Melfa F, Bovani B, Cirillo P, Tretti Clementoni M, Gennai A. Attitudes, concerns, and expectations of consumers of aesthetic medicine and surgery during the COVID-19 outbreak: an Italian online survey. Aesthet Surg J Open Forum. 2020;2(4):ojaa037.

Messagier AL, Blaizot R, Couppié P, Delaigue S. Teledermatology use in remote areas of French Guiana: experience from a long-running system. Front Public Health. 2019;7:387.

Morris C, Scott RE, Mars M. An audit and survey of informal use of instant messaging for dermatology in District Hospitals in KwaZulu-Natal, South Africa. Int J Environ Res Public Health. 2022;19(12):7462.

Nguyen M, Youssef R, Kwon A, Chen R, Park JH. Dermatology on TikTok: analysis of content and creators. Int J Womens Dermatol. 2021;7(4):488.

Pala P, Bergler-Czop BS, Gwiżdż J. Teledermatology: idea, benefits and risks of modern age–a systematic review based on melanoma. Adv Dermatol Allergol. 2020;37(2):159–67.

Pendlebury GA, Oro P, Haynes W, Merideth D, Bartling S, Bongiorno MA. The impact of COVID-19 pandemic on dermatological conditions: a novel, comprehensive review. Dermatopathology. 2022;9(3):212–43.

Ren SY, Wang WB, Hao YG, Zhang HR, Wang ZC, Chen YL, Gao RD. Stability and infectivity of coronaviruses in inanimate environments. World J Clin Cases. 2020;8(8):1391.

Rivetti N, Barruscotti S. Management of telogen effluvium during the COVID-19 emergency: psychological implications. Dermatol Ther. 2020;33:e13648.

Rossi A, Magri F, Sernicola A, Michelini S, Caro G, Muscianese M, Di Fraia M, Chello C, Fortuna MC, Grieco T. Telogen effluvium after SARS-CoV-2 infection: a series of cases and possible pathogenetic mechanisms. Skin Appendage Disord. 2021;21:1–5.

Salazar-Paras DKR, Rosete RCR, Manalo DMLM, Batac MCFR. The effectiveness of an online basic dermatology didactic course on the dermatologic knowledge of doctors to the barrios [unpublished]. Department of Dermatology, University of the Philippines - Philippine General Hospital; 2021.

Selvi V. Convalescent plasma: a challenging tool to treat COVID-19 patients—a lesson from the past and new perspectives. Biomed Res Int. 2020;2020:1.

Swire-Thompson B, Lazer D. Public health and online misinformation: challenges and recommendations. Annu Rev Public Health. 2019;41:433–51.

Szeto MD, Mamo A, Afrin A, Militello M, Barber C. Social media in dermatology and an overview of popular social media platforms. Curr Dermatol Rep. 2021;19:1–8.

Tan NMG, Molina AJR, Rosete RCR, Escandor SEE, Ke BN, Ramos VME, Berberabe AEB, Del Rosario JJD, Berba RP, Cubillan ELA, Mojica WP. Establishing a communication framework in response to the COVID-19 pandemic in a tertiary government hospital in The Philippines [unpublished]. Department of Dermatology, University of the Philippines - Philippine General Hospital; 2021.

Thomas M, Chiramel MJ, Priyanka M, Singh M, Ponraj L, Devakumar K, Balan F, Joseph AK, Joy M, Jeyaseelan L, George R. Feasibility of store-and-forward teledermatology in out-patient care: a prospective study from rural India utilising specialist referral services through an instant messaging platform-"WhatsApp". J Int Soc Telemed eHealth. 2022;10:e2–1.

Turkmen D, Altunisik N, Sener S, Colak C. Evaluation of the effects of COVID-19 pandemic on hair diseases through a web-based questionnaire. Dermatol Ther. 2020;33:e13923.

Vaidya T, Zubritsky L, Alikhan A, Housholder A. Socioeconomic and geographic barriers to dermatology care in urban and rural US populations. J Am Acad Dermatol. 2018;78(2):406–8.

Vasavda C, Ho BK, Davison A. Socially distant medical education in the face of COVID-19. Med Sci Educ. 2021;31:231–3.

Vashisht D, Neema S, Venugopalan R, Pathania V, Sandhu S, Vasudevan B. Dermatology practice in the times of the COVID-19 pandemic. Indian J Dermatol Venereol Leprol. 2021;87(5):603–10.

Vidal-Alaball J, Garcia Domingo JL, Garcia Cuyàs F, Mendioroz Peña J, Flores Mateo G, Deniel Rosanas

J, Sauch VG. A cost savings analysis of asynchronous teledermatology compared to face-to-face dermatology in Catalonia. BMC Health Serv Res. 2018;18:1–6.

Wang R, Helf C, Tizek L, Neuhauser R, Eyerich K, Zink A, Eberlein B, Biedermann T, Brockow K, Boehner A. The impact and consequences of SARS-CoV-2 pandemic on a single university dermatology outpatient clinic in Germany. Int J Environ Res Public Health. 2020;17(17):6182.

Wei TS. Cutaneous reactions to COVID-19 vaccines: a review. JAAD Int. 2022;17.

World Health Organization. Telemedicine: opportunities and developments in member states: report on the second global survey on eHealth. Global Observatory for eHealth series, vol. 2; 2010.

World Health Organization. Getting your workplace ready for COVID-19: how COVID-19 spreads, 19 March 2020. World Health Organization; 2020a.

World Health Organization. Cleaning and disinfection of environmental surfaces in the context of COVID-19: interim guidance, 15 May 2020. World Health Organization; 2020b. [cited 2023 February 01]. https://www.who.int/publications/i/item/cleaning-and-disinfection-of-environmental-surfaces-inthe-context-of-covid-19.

World Health Organization. Report of the WHO-China joint mission on coronavirus disease 2019 (COVID-19). Geneva: World Health Organization; 2020c. Google Scholar. 2020:1-40. [cited 2023 February 01]. https://www.who.int/docs/default-source/coronaviruse/who-china-joint-mission-on-covid-19-final-report.pdf. Accessed 10 May 2020.

World Health Organization. WHO Coronavirus (COVID-19) Dashboard, 2023. [cited 2023 March 16] https://covid19.who.int/?adgroupsurvey={adgroupsurvey}&gclid=Cj0KCQjw27mhBhC9ARIsAIFsETHgRvJXZH1nrAs27kJyvQQncVlbjUmZySzes_UMpiPdGkbUYmRq9CgaAhtQEALw_wcB.

Zhao B, Liu Y, Chen C. Air purifiers: a supplementary measure to remove airborne SARS-CoV-2. Build Environ. 2020;177:106918.

Leveraging on Teledermatology in the COVID-19 Pandemic

Wen Hao Tan and Haur Yueh Lee

Abbreviations

HS   Hidradenitis suppurativa
PPE   Personal protective equipment
TD   Teledermatology

Introduction

Teledermatology (TD) is the practice of using digital technology to provide dermatological care and is used for the diagnosis, assessment, and management of skin disease without the physical presence of the patient.

Models of TD

There are three main models of TD: (1) asynchronous (also known as store and forward), (2) synchronous, and (3) hybrid. The asynchronous mode uses a store-and-forward mode with digital images stored and subsequently transmitted. Synchronous mode occurs when the consultations are conducted in real time using videoconferencing tools. The hybrid mode uses both synchronous and nonsynchronous methods (Eedy and Wootton 2001). Such TD interactions can occur between patients and dermatologists or between healthcare professionals.

Platforms

Various platforms have been utilized to implement TD. These include Zoom, Skype, Facebook messaging, WhatsApp, email, and paid online portals. However, the adoption of platforms varies between countries. In a global survey of practitioners, Facebook and WhatsApp were the platforms of choice for TD (Naik 2022). These preferences for, for example, WhatsApp, were likely influenced by the familiarity with the messaging application (Naik 2022). In countries like Iran that do not have established TD platforms, WhatsApp has emerged as an effective tool to reach patients (Daneshpazhooh and Mahmoudi 2021). Although a reliable internet connection is desired, modifications to the TD work process may help circumvent the issues associated with unreliable internet access. For example, instead of continuous videoconferencing, photos were submitted using Facebook messenger for evaluation and diagnosis, and a telephone call made in real time was used to review clinical history and discuss management (Tinio et al. 2022).

W. H. Tan · H. Y. Lee (✉)
Department of Dermatology, Singapore General Hospital, Singapore, Singapore
e-mail: wenhao.tan@mohh.com.sg;
lee.haur.yueh@singhealth.com.sg

© The Author(s), under exclusive license to Springer Nature Switzerland AG 2023
H. H. Oon, C. L. Goh (eds.), *COVID-19 in Dermatology*, Updates in Clinical Dermatology,
https://doi.org/10.1007/978-3-031-45586-5_8

Usage Prior to COVID-19

TD was used primarily in the mid-1990s as a tool to improve access to specialist care for underserved populations, due to geographic and economic reasons (Perednia and Brown 1995; Whited 2015). In 2010, 38% of the countries had some form of TD service, and by 2015, 46% of the countries surveyed had an established TD service (World Health Organization 2010, 2015). Nevertheless, active TD provision is often limited to academic centers, for example, in the United States, 50% of TD consults occur in academic centers (Yim et al. 2018).

Teledermatology During COVID-19 Pandemic

Growth of TD During the Pandemic

With the COVID-19 pandemic, global health systems were burdened and health resources stretched. Healthcare providers were challenged with the need to minimize exposure to healthcare workers/patients, conserve and rationally allocate resources, while providing timely medical care for COVID and non-COVID-related conditions. Such needs were readily met by the use of TD as seen by the exponential growth during the pandemic period. Adoption rates of TD for dermatologists increased: 28% of dermatologists surveyed provided TD for the first time. In another survey of 733 dermatologists, uptake of TD increased from 26.1% before pandemic to 75.2% during the pandemic with the most favored platforms being Whatsapp (48.8%), Zoom (16%), Facetime (15.1%), Facebook messenger (11.6%), and Viber (4.2%) (Conforti et al. 2021; Bhargava et al. 2021). In the United States, a similar growth was observed; 14.1% of dermatologists ($n = 4356$) used TD before the pandemic compared to 96.9% during the pandemic (Kennedy et al. 2021).

In addition to adoption rates, TD consultation visits also showed a corresponding increase, with 60–90% of dermatologists surveyed highlighting a doubling or increase in demand over the pandemic (Conforti et al. 2021; Moscarella et al. 2020).

Barriers to TD

Although the growth of TD has been exponential, barriers to adoption remain, and these include (1) patient factors, (2) disease factors, (3) physician factors, and (4) technological factors (Table 8.1).

Poor TD adoption rates have been demonstrated in the elderly, those with lower education backgrounds, and in underserved communities. Older patients prefer in-person visits, and this may be related to technical know-how (Yi et al. 2021; Scott Kruse et al. 2018). In the United States, underserved communities, such as Spanish-speaking patients, had fewer TD visits during the pandemic, and those of Hispanic eth-

Table 8.1 Barriers to TD adoption

Patient factors	– Poor technological literacy/ education
	– Lack of awareness of such a service in underserved communities
	– Patient preference for in-person visits
Disease factors	– Dermatoses that affect sensitive areas (e.g. genitalia, breasts, buttocks.) or inaccessible regions e.g. (buccal/intra-oral, back & buttocks)
	– Inability of physicians to palpate lesions
Physician factors	– Equipment cost
	– Staff training
	– Reimbursement policies for TD (lack of support from government and insurance claim
	– Impression of TD as an inadequate tool to make a clinical diagnosis
	– Medicolegal concerns
Technological factors	– Unstable internet connection
	– Technological competencies in the use of equipment—requires a secure network for the transmission and storage of confidential information and images
	– Poor resolution of images/ videoconferencing

nicity were more reluctant to adopt TD (Yi et al. 2021; Pannu et al. 2021). This disparity was also observed between ethnic groups in the pediatric population where Black/African American and Hispanic/Latino were identified as having a lower chance of access to TD and overall access to pediatric dermatology during COVID-19 (Duan et al. 2022).

Disease factors, such as lesions or dermatoses affecting the genitalia, breasts, or buttocks, can discourage TD. Dermatologists may not adopt TD if they think that TD was inadequate to make a clinical diagnosis (Moscarella et al. 2020). Similarly, monitoring of adverse reactions to medications via a TD platform can be challenging (Bull et al. 2016). Furthermore, physicians may face concerns regarding medicolegal issues.

Technological factors, including unstable Internet, lack of adequate equipment, poor resolution of images or video, have also contributed to the poor adoption rates.

In patients who decline TD, common concerns for their reluctance include the ability of TD to address medical concerns (32%), preference for face-to-face consultations (30%), lack of technological expertise (19.2%) and personal data security (1.6%).

Utilization During Pandemic

Outpatient Setting

Most skin conditions treated in an ambulatory dermatology setting can be managed by TD. A successful transition from a completely office-based practice to a primarily TD model over 3 weeks has been reported in the United States (Perkins et al. 2020).

In Egypt, TD use during COVID-19 was perceived as effective and satisfactory for patients, and 91.5% considered TD as equal to in-person visits (Mostafa and Hegazy 2022). In addition, TD also proved helpful for patients with stable chronic diseases.

Certain conditions have been reported to be successfully managed by TD including acne, psoriasis, atopic dermatitis, rosacea, warts, and nevi. Less amenable conditions for TD include hidradenitis suppurativa and examinations of the total body skin examinations (Perkins et al. 2020).

In a study that used video call consultations for follow-up acne care, 71% (37/52) of the patients reported satisfaction with their acne treatment and 80.7% reported high well-being after treatment (Ruggiero et al. 2020). In total, 96.1% of the patients also reported that they will continue to consult the same dermatologist, while 92.3% were satisfied with the attention provided by their dermatologist, and 86.5% were satisfied with the duration of the visit (Ruggiero et al. 2020). In an Italian study, almost half (48.3%, 103/213) of the patients had chosen to continue with TD follow-up visits despite lifting restrictions on in-person visits during the pandemic. In total, 94.2% of these 103 patients who preferred TD instead had mild-to-moderate acne on topical therapy, the remaining six were treated with systemic therapy (Villani et al. 2022). Patients who preferred TD were those who lived farther away from the clinic (Villani et al. 2022).

Inflammatory Diseases

Chronic inflammatory diseases can also be safely managed in a lockdown situation using TD (Brunasso and Massone 2020). Remote monitoring using a telephone call or the store-and-forward TD approach was successful in 94% (183/195) of the patients. Of these 183 patients, 126 had moderate-to-severe psoriasis, 10 had severe acne, 11 had severe atopic dermatitis, 11 had hidradenitis suppurativa, 9 had blistering autoimmune diseases (4 pemphigus, 5 bullous pemphigoid), 16 with other autoimmune skin diseases. TD was also effective in preventing unnecessary worsening of severe chronic skin diseases and poor outcomes due to withdrawal of current therapy, with only five patients requiring a personal office visit (2.7%). Furthermore, it was also possible to switch or initiate new therapies as required (Brunasso and Massone 2020).

Patients with hidradenitis suppurativa (HS) face unique challenges during TD consultations, as patients may feel uncomfortable exposing intertriginous (especially genital) areas via videoconferencing. There is also an inability of dermatologists to palpate fluctuating lesions in a virtual setting. Therefore, even with optimized TD, patients with HS may be better suited for in-person care, as procedures (such as surgery) may be required in flares (Kang et al. 2020).

Noninflammatory Diseases

Skin Cancer

In noninflammatory skin conditions, particularly skin cancer, TD can be a useful screening tool, although an in-person review may still be required for an accurate diagnosis. COVID-19 has resulted in delays in the diagnosis and treatment of skin cancer patients due to restrictions in diagnostic capacity and/or delay in treatment (Dessinioti et al. 2021).

Despite the initial reduction in skin cancer referrals during COVID-19 in France, continued care via store-and-forward TD has been shown to be effective in skin cancer, as skin cancer diagnosis through TD did not show a decrease in 2020 compared to 2019 (Skayem et al. 2022).

However, the precision of TD in diagnosing NMSC has limitations. In Auckland, more than a quarter of the TD assessments conducted during the COVID-19 lockdown (28%) still required subsequent in-person follow-up for the diagnosis of NMSC (Cheng and Schurr 2022).

The detection of skin cancer could also continue with precision during the pandemic with asynchronous TD through a mobile phone application. This was evident in Hungary during the first wave of the COVID-19 pandemic (Jobbágy et al. 2022). In a single-center study, there was substantial agreement between malignant diagnoses determined by TD compared to face-to-face consultations or histological examination (Jobbágy et al. 2022).

Limitations of TD in the outpatient setting include the provision of total body skin examination or dermoscopic melanoma surveillance.

Asynchronous models adopted in Hungary through a mobile phone application served as a fast and accurate screening tool and provided effective skin cancer care during the first wave of the COVID-19 pandemic (Jobbágy et al. 2022). However, while the diagnostic precision for malignancies was reported to be 85.3% in this study, a nodular melanoma was misdiagnosed as hemangioma during TD consultation. But the patient was triaged as moderately urgent and attended an in person examination within a month, and the tumor was excised. This case highlighted that extra care must be taken with newly developed nodular vascularized or pinkish lesions.

The use of dermoscopic imaging can help increase diagnostic accuracy for both pigmented lesions and NMSC. Location of lesions at intimate body sites may hamper diagnosis via TD, as shown in the same study where one of the misdiagnosed SCCs was localized in the genital region (Jobbágy et al. 2022).

Utilization of TD triage services for suspected skin cancer can significantly reduce the time to reach diagnosis. In the same study, the vast majority of malignancies were identified to seek immediate help, while in the low-urgency group, 14 of 16 skin cancers were correctly diagnosed as AK, and the two remaining lesions were superficial BCC.

Diagnosis of nonmalignant pigmented lesions, such as naevi, or seborrheic keratosis, using TD was also useful during COVID-19, as most were correctly identified during TD consultations.

Infections

TD was also used to diagnose infections. Cutaneous leishmaniasis was diagnosed with TD in Nepal (Paudel 2020). Crusted scabies was also diagnosed by TD in Brazil during the pandemic (Bimbi et al. 2020).

Pediatric Population

In the pediatric population, TD through a phone consultation supported by images may not be suitable, with 52% not satisfied with the service and only 19% reported being very satisfied in one study (Lowe et al. 2022). Furthermore, while parents and patients felt virtual consultations were more convenient, parental anxiety was not adequately alleviated compared to in-person review. In the pediatric population, the majority of cases are inflammatory dermatoses (75%, 87/116), and while such conditions have been reported to be adequately managed via TD in the adult population, parental anxiety may be insufficiently addressed virtually due to concerns that the clinician may not have seen the whole picture (Lowe et al. 2022). This study also highlighted the discrepancy between the clinician's perspective and the patient's/parent's in a virtual consultation.

However, as a triaging tool, Store-and-Forward TD provided quick access to high-quality pediatric dermatologic care, with the majority of virtual consultations completed in 2 days and patients with urgent conditions seeing a dermatologist earlier (Pahalyants et al. 2021). Only a third of TD cases were referred for follow-up appointment, and only five cases resulted in clinically significant management discordance (impetigo → HSV, unclear rash → psoriasis, unclear dermatitis → verruca vulgaris, seborrheic dermatitis → perioral dermatitis, urticaria → eczema). Overall, there was 70.1% concordance in diagnosis between TD and in-person review (Pahalyants et al. 2021).

Overall, the pandemic caused a collaborative effect between primary providers and dermatologists. This was evident in Italy, where a network of dermatologists and general practitioners/pediatricians was created, and sharing clinical photos became common practice (Bergamo et al. 2020).

Inpatient Setting

TD has been shown in various studies to be an effective care delivery model in the in-patient setting during COVID-19. In the setting of a tertiary general hospital, the diagnostic concurrence between physical and TD was 90% (Tan et al. 2021).

In hospitals without access to the inpatient dermatology service, teledermatologists performed comparable to an in-person dermatologist for the diagnosis (84.9% at least partial agreement) and treatment (77.4% systemic treatment agreement) of hospitalized patients with skin conditions, further supporting the role of TD as a suitable alternative to provide in-patient care if no dermatologist is available (Keller et al. 2020). In another study, asynchronous TD using store-and-forward also showed reliable diagnoses (median 91.7% agreement between in-person

dermatologist and teledermatologist) and treatment decisions (median concordance 100%) in inpatients using non-dermatologist generated data (Gabel et al. 2021).

In dermatological emergencies such as toxic epidermal necrolysis, mobile TD served as a successful management tool to identify and stop the offending drug while directing care for rural patients who would otherwise not have access to a dermatologist during COVID-19 (Paudel and Chudal 2020).

During the pandemic, the switch to TD for inpatient care was useful at many levels; scarce personal protective equipment was preserved; reduction of exposure to COVID for both patients/physicians; processes were streamlined; and healthcare providers were able to work collaboratively (Tan et al. 2021; Rismiller et al. 2020).

Asynchronous TD for patients without access to an in-person dermatology service and in-patient TD were shown to improve diagnostic accuracy and management of erythroderma, with a 78.8% change in diagnosis and therapeutic changes in all 33 cases (Khosravi et al. 2021).

Quality of care was not significantly affected by the implementation of TD in in-patient settings, as various studies showed substantial agreement between the assessment of the diagnosis in person and by TD (Tan et al. 2021). There was also evident agreement between the primary dermatologist and the teledermatologist in differential diagnosis, laboratory evaluation decisions, imaging decisions, and biopsy decisions (Gabel et al. 2021).

Benefits of TD

There are multiple advantages to TD. Firstly, increased accessibility for patients who cannot visit in person. In addition, there is a role in triage, with an increased efficiency in the stratification of cases by dermatologists according to acuity and complexity, therefore prioritizing patients who may need earlier in-person review. Wait times have also been reduced with TD.

Table 8.2 Benefits and limitations of teledermatology

Benefits	Limitations
Increased access to care, especially in resource-poor areas	Requires access to good quality technology and internet connection
Faster, cost-effective care	Underutilization in part due to provider skepticism
Useful for patient triage before disposition	Limited by patient history and lack of physical examination
Shorter hospital stays and lower risk of readmission	May miss incidental lesions if no complete body examination is conducted
Cases can be used for education	Reimbursement is, at best, poor
No chance of exposure to disease or to the patient	Licensure restrictions may prohibit interstate consultations

- **Accessibility:** Better access for patients who cannot physically visit.
- **Convenience:** Patients can access medical consultations from the comfort of their home.
- **More efficient triaging:** Increased classification of cases by allowing dermatologists to stratify patients according to acuity and complexity, therefore prioritizing patients who may need earlier in-person review.

The benefits and limitations of TD are summarized in Table 8.2. Adapted from (Mocharnuk et al. 2022).

Limitations of TD

Although TD improved access to diagnostic care, COVID-19 restrictions on in-person consultations could delay timely biopsies. Office diagnostic tools such as KOH preparation or woods lamp cannot be used remotely to help diagnose specific problems. Therapeutic office procedures such as cryotherapy, intralesional corticosteroids, or narrow-band phototherapy can also be delayed (Berman et al. 2020).

Costly misdiagnosis can occur with the use of TD. While diagnostic lesions relevant to the main complaint may be addressed during TD, the inability to perform a full skin examination in areas such as the scalp, oral cavity, and sensitive areas, particularly the genitalia, may result in missing significant malignancies. For example, a referral for herpes infection via TD almost resulted in a missed diagnosis of malignant melanoma (unrelated to the primary complaint) had the dermatologist not reviewed in person (Deacon and Madigan 2020).

The quality of photographs or video conferences can pose a significant challenge for TD, as diagnosis heavily relies on visual clarity. Unclear photographs often occur due to poor visual resolution from poor lighting, unfocused imaging from suboptimal user technical literacy, or low camera image resolution. Videoconferencing software may also reduce image resolution to preserve bandwidth.

Furthermore, with the requirement to wear PPE while caring for COVID-19 patients, the PPE may impede clear photograph taking, and digital images taken using a phone camera stored in a protective cover may easily obstruct the lens (Tan et al. 2021).

Patients have been reported to be uncooperative during physical examination, with difficult-to-reach locations such as the buttocks cited as reasons for the lack of quality photographs (Tan et al. 2021).

The use of TD may be limited by social culture. For example, in Saudi Arabia, women may feel uncomfortable with TD consultations for cultural or religious reasons (Kaliyadan et al. 2020).

Another limitation of TD is the doubtful reliability of the physical findings of the referring provider. A significant proportion of malignant lesions were incidentally detected in addition to the specific lesion of interest. Malignant lesions were previously unrecognized by the referring physician (Viola et al. 2011).

Furthermore, despite collaborative efforts, GPs and pediatricians were not familiar with tools such as dermoscopy. Therefore, to avoid a missed diagnosis of melanoma, every pigmented or non-pigmented lesion had to be referred to a dermatologist (Jobbágy et al. 2022).

Teledermoscopy incorporated into a primary care skin cancer referral pathway during COVID-19 significantly reduced the time to dermatologist advice (Jones et al. 2021). However, the selection and subsequent imaging of the lesions were determined by the patient or generalists, who are often limited in knowledge of atypical dermoscopic features. Therefore, there is a risk of overlooking skin malignancies that would have been incidentally detected by a dermatologist during an in-person consultation (Lee et al. 2023).

Not all aspects of dermatology are suitable for TD. Critical care dermatology, such as in severe cutaneous drug reaction (Steven–Johnson Syndrome/Toxic Epidermal Necrolysis), angioedema with anaphylaxis, vasculitic conditions, or exacerbation of bullous disorders, is ideally not taken up for TD. In such cases, TD can be a tool for triage, but a physical review may still be necessary (Ashique and Kaliyadan 2020).

The challenges to the use of TD during the pandemic included poor internet connection, lack of ubiquitous access to smartphones, and poor technological knowledge. Such limitations add to existing hurdles in TD implementation, especially in countries like Sub-Saharan Africa and India (Ashique and Kaliyadan 2020; Oaku and Anaba 2022).

Cost-Effectiveness of TD

TD also provided significant cost savings by reducing personal protective equipment (PPE) and in-person encounters required in clinics and within the hospital (Rismiller et al. 2020).

The cost-effectiveness of TD is comparable to standardized patient care based on economic analysis before COVID-19 (Snoswell et al. 2016). Newer studies have shown that TD reduces costs, although most of these were analyzed before 2020 (López-Liria et al. 2022). However, the implementation of TD requires investment in healthcare and technological infrastructure, as well as training professionals and patients on the use of the tools (López-Liria et al. 2022).

Additionally, TD has a positive impact on the environment. Through TD, over 3 months, 55,737 miles of travel in cars were saved, and an average of 37.8 miles of patients were returned per trip, which equals a reduction of 15.37 tonnes of CO_2 during this period. This corresponds to 16 transatlantic flights from London to New York (O'Connell et al. 2021).

Challenges in the Setting Up of a TD Service

When setting up a TD service, there are challenges.

- **Licensing requirements**: 64.9% of a global survey reported that their medical board/council or licensing authority permitted virtual consultations or relaxed HIPAA compliance related to telehealth during the COVID-19 pandemic (Bhargava et al. 2021).
- **Technical issues and infrastructure**: The lack of a technical and legal infrastructure to support TD has also undermined the local utility of TD in countries such as Iran and Turkey (Daneshpazhooh and Mahmoudi 2021; Temiz et al. 2020). Mobile WhatsApp became a powerful tool for TD during COVID-19 in Iran due to the lack of established TD platforms (Daneshpazhooh and Mahmoudi 2021).
- **Financial reimbursement**: Poor reimbursement from teleconsultation was a significant limitation before COVID-19. The time invested in TD and the amount of financial reimbursement remained mismatched, thus providing little incentive for dermatologists to use this during COVID-19.
- **Privacy issues**: Confidentiality and privacy are a concern. Although examples like WhatsApp are end-to-end encrypted, the lack of secure HIPAA compliance may be a concern. As a result, paid online services served as a secure platform for users who are more concerned about data safety.
- **Physician buy-in**: The challenges of TD were also due in part to the stress of the practitioner. TD in COVID-19 was an important predictor of dermatologist mental distress, which could be exacerbated by the lack of a technical infrastructure to support fully functional TD services. Another reason could be the uncertainty in the reimbursement of TD consultations (Bhargava et al. 2021).

Ideal TD Service Setup

An ideal TD service setup requires the following:

- Appropriate infrastructure to conduct synchronous, asynchronous, or hybrid TD for both primary care/referring physician and teledermatologist.
- Practitioners involved in TD should be familiar with the dermatological vocabulary and be able to perform essential dermatological imaging.
- Secure system for electronic health/medical data, including digital storage of patient images, to ensure confidentiality during TD consultation.
- The image capture device must be able to record high-quality images or videos. A Madrid pilot study showed that more than half (52.1%) of the submitted images were of sufficient quality for diagnosis (Sendagorta et al. 2021).
- Stable internet connectivity to transmit data promptly. An unstable internet connection disrupts the flow of the consultation and may take longer to complete. This is even more relevant during synchronous TD reviews, where consultations are conducted in "real time."
- Clarity on legal and ethical issues, especially related to the confidentiality of patient data, must be established beyond national borders. The referring site should ensure that there is informed consent to capture images and explain to patients how the images will be used thoroughly.

Future of Teledermatology in a Post COVID-19 Era

TD has evolved and improved during the COVID-19 pandemic to treat benign skin conditions, such as skin warts in the community, with TD-guided home treatment using a cryogenic pen. The combination of face-to-face consultants for initial and final visits, with the use of TD during the treatment phase, was proposed as a model for other dermatologic conditions (Micali et al. 2022).

According to a recent survey by the American Academy of Dermatology, 70% of dermatologists who responded believe that the increased use of TD will persist even after COVID-19, while 58% (323 of 557) plan to continue using TD after COVID-19 (Kennedy et al. 2021).

How TD will evolve beyond the early phase of COVID-19 depends on the expectations of patients who have started to rely on this service during the pandemic, as TD saves time and travel.

Standardized Training for Healthcare Care Providers

Inequalities in healthcare can hinder TD's ability to provide adequate care to all (Kennedy et al. 2021).

Standardized TD training must be implemented to ensure physician confidence and patient safety. A standardized curriculum is needed to educate and assess physicians on telemedicine competencies in telemedicine (Chike-Harris et al. 2021). Dermatology residency training in the USA has begun incorporating TD in residency curriculum, especially during COVID-19 (Oldenburg and Marsch 2020). A survey among dermatology trainees across the United Kingdom showed that only 15% felt slightly confident in managing TD referrals, and almost all (96%) felt more teaching was required (Lowe et al. 2020). It would be a good idea to consider incorporating telemedicine training into medical school education.

Optimizing the TD Consult

Factors to consider in the optimization of TD are shown in Table 8.3 (Choi et al. 2021).

Conditions not recommended for TD include total body skin examination, while acne was reported to be the most appropriate condition (Kennedy et al. 2021). TD has also been considered less accurate than in-person consultation, particularly in skin cancers (Finnane et al. 2017; Chuchu et al. 2018).

Table 8.3 Challenges and solutions in optimizing the teledermatology consult (Choi et al. 2021)

Optimizing the teledermatological consult	
Challenge	Solution
Poor visual resolution of images – Poor lighting – Poor focus of the camera – User difficulty with the front-facing camera on lesions	Consider supplementing with clear photographs taken in well-lit settings – Focused close-up and far-out images – Disable phone camera software filters Utilizing device software with prompts to ensure higher resolution images Healthcare professional (for example, a nurse) vets quality of photographs prior to upload/submission to teledermatologist
Limited physical examination – Inability to palpate the lesion of interest – Lack of a dermoscopic view	Focus on taking clinical history – A pre-consult screening questionnaire focusing on pertinent details such as medical and family history, physical characteristics of the skin condition, and risk factors may be useful in skin cancer screening Photograph directly on or at an angle
	Use the zoom function on the camera to get a closer view of the lesion of interest
Privacy – Patient discomfort with the examination of sensitive body areas – Potential consequences of data leakage	Allow patients to curate their photographs instead of live video conferencing Conduct a teleconsult in a locked clinic room Provide priority for the patient to be reviewed in person for lesions involving sensitive body areas

Addressing Challenges and Obstacles

The main obstacles are technology-specific and can be overcome by training, change management techniques, and the provision of alternate consultations via TD and individual patient–provider interaction in person. A targeted policy may eliminate such barriers (Scott Kruse et al. 2018).

Increasing the uptake of TD may also require a review of the reimbursement rates to incentivise TD providers to use the system. Malpractice and liability concerns must also be addressed at the national level.

Potential solutions for dermatologists to tackle the challenges of TD include implementing a triaging system to identify and treat the most suspicious or complex lesions. Other solutions involve streamlining reimbursement protocols for clarity and simplicity.

Ethical Concerns

Licensing requirements have changed during COVID-19 to allow the practice of medicine across borders/states, which would otherwise have been difficult in person. With the increase in the use of TD during COVID-19, ethical and legal challenges must be navigated and addressed. Healthcare providers involved in TD are encouraged to participate in teleconsultation courses provided by the local medical councils, if available.

Patients should have the autonomy to be reviewed in a secure platform modality of their choice. However, as TD eliminates face-to-face interaction between dermatologists and patients, the patient–physician relationship may be affected. Patients and healthcare professionals should also know that certain conditions are more suitable for TD, while others benefit more from in-person reviews. Therefore, the appropriate modality for evaluation that acts in the patient's best interest while preserving privacy and comfort should be recommended.

Conclusion

In general, TD can effectively provide dermatological care to patients who may not have access to in-person care during the COVID-19 pandemic. It is essential to ensure that patient privacy is protected and that quality of care is not compromised by TD. The future of TD as an integral part of dermatological care is promising.

References

Ashique KT, Kaliyadan F. Teledermatology in the wake of COVID -19 scenario: an Indian perspective. Indian Dermatol Online J. 2020;11(3):301. https://doi.org/10.4103/IDOJ.IDOJ_260_20.

Bergamo S, Calacione R, Fagotti S, et al. Teledermatology with general practitioners and pediatricians during COVID-19 outbreak in Italy: preliminary data from a second-level dermatology department in north-eastern Italy. Dermatol Ther. 2020;33(6):e14040. https://doi.org/10.1111/DTH.14040.

Berman A, Shi HS, Hsiao VY, Berman HS, Shi VY, Hsiao JL. Challenges of teledermatology: lessons learned during the COVID-19 pandemic. Dermatol Online J. 2020;26(11):13030/qt7193305r. https://doi.org/10.5070/D32611048125.

Bhargava S, McKeever C, Kroumpouzos G. Impact of COVID-19 pandemic on dermatology practices: results of a web-based, global survey. Int J Womens Dermatol. 2021;7(2):217–23. https://doi.org/10.1016/J.IJWD.2020.09.010.

Bimbi C, Wollina U, Kyriakou G, Dalla Lana DF, Ramos M. Basic teledermatology solving two cases of crusted scabies. Dermatol Ther. 2020;33(6):e14214. https://doi.org/10.1111/DTH.14214.

Brunasso AMG, Massone C. Teledermatologic monitoring for chronic cutaneous autoimmune diseases with smartworking during COVID-19 emergency in a tertiary center in Italy. Dermatol Ther. 2020;33(4):e13495. https://doi.org/10.1111/dth.13695.

Bull TP, Dewar AR, Malvey DM, Szalma JL. Considerations for the telehealth systems of tomorrow: an analysis of student perceptions of telehealth technologies. JMIR Med Educ. 2016;2(2):e11. https://doi.org/10.2196/MEDEDU.5392.

Cheng HS, Schurr L. Teledermatology for suspected skin cancer in New Zealand during the COVID-19 pandemic required in-person follow-up in 28% of cases. JAAD Int. 2022;6:59–60. https://doi.org/10.1016/j.jdin.2021.11.003.

Chike-Harris KE, Durham C, Logan A, Smith G, Dubose-Morris R. Integration of telehealth education into the health care provider curriculum: a review. Telemed J E Health. 2021;27(2):137–49. https://doi.org/10.1089/TMJ.2019.0261.

Choi E, Mak WK, Law JY, Santos D, Quek SC. Optimizing teledermatology: looking beyond the COVID-19 pandemic. Int J Dermatol. 2021;60(1):119–21. https://doi.org/10.1111/IJD.15272.

Chuchu N, Dinnes J, Takwoingi Y, et al. Teledermatology for diagnosing skin cancer in adults. Cochrane Database Syst Rev. 2018;12(12):CD013193. https://doi.org/10.1002/14651858.CD013193.

Conforti C, Lallas A, Argenziano G, et al. Impact of the COVID-19 pandemic on dermatology practice worldwide: results of a survey promoted by the International Dermoscopy Society (IDS). Dermatol Pract Concept. 2021;11(1):e2021153.

Daneshpazhooh M, Mahmoudi HR. COVID-19: the experience from Iran. Clin Dermatol. 2021;39(1):23–32. https://doi.org/10.1016/J.CLINDERMATOL.2020.12.009.

Deacon DC, Madigan LM. Inpatient teledermatology in the era of COVID-19 and the importance of the complete skin examination. JAAD Case Rep. 2020;6(10):977–8. https://doi.org/10.1016/j.jdcr.2020.07.050.

Dessinioti C, Garbe C, Stratigos AJ. The impact of the COVID-19 pandemic on diagnostic delay of skin cancer: a call to restart screening activities. J Eur Acad Dermatol Venereol. 2021;35(12):e836–7. https://doi.org/10.1111/jdv.17552.

Duan GY, Ruiz De Luzuriaga AM, Schroedl LM, Rosenblatt AE. Disparities in telemedicine use during the COVID-19 pandemic among pediatric dermatology patients. Pediatr Dermatol. 2022;39(4):520–7. https://doi.org/10.1111/pde.14982.

Eedy DJ, Wootton R. Teledermatology: a review. Br J Dermatol. 2001;144(4):696–707. https://doi.org/10.1046/J.1365-2133.2001.04124.X.

Finnane A, Dallest K, Janda M, Soyer HP. Teledermatology for the diagnosis and management of skin cancer: a systematic review. JAMA Dermatol. 2017;153(3):319–27. https://doi.org/10.1001/JAMADERMATOL.2016.4361.

Gabel CK, Nguyen E, Karmouta R, et al. The use of teledermatology by dermatology hospitalists is effective in the diagnosis and management of inpatient disease. J Am Acad Dermatol. 2021;84(6):1547–53. https://doi.org/10.1016/J.JAAD.2020.04.171.

Jobbágy A, Kiss N, Meznerics FA, et al. Emergency use and efficacy of an asynchronous teledermatology system as a novel tool for early diagnosis of skin cancer during the first wave of COVID-19 pandemic. Int J Environ Res Public Health. 2022;19(5):2699. https://doi.org/10.3390/ijerph19052699. Published 2022 Feb 25.

Jones L, Jameson M, Oakley A. Remote skin cancer diagnosis: adding images to electronic referrals is more efficient than wait-listing for a nurse-led imaging clinic. Cancers (Basel). 2021;13(22):5828. https://doi.org/10.3390/cancers13225828. Published 2021 Nov 20.

Kaliyadan F, Al Ameer MA, Al Ameer A, Al Alwan Q. Telemedicine practice in Saudi Arabia during the COVID-19 pandemic. Cureus. 2020;12(12):e12004. https://doi.org/10.7759/CUREUS.12004.

Kang NC, Hsiao J, Shi V, Naik HB, Lowes MA, Alavi A. Remote management of hidradenitis suppurativa in a pandemic era of COVID-19. Int J Dermatol. 2020;59(9):e318–20. https://doi.org/10.1111/ijd.15022.

Keller JJ, Johnson JP, Latour E. Inpatient teledermatology: diagnostic and therapeutic concordance among a hospitalist, dermatologist, and teledermatologist using store-and-forward teledermatology. J Am Acad Dermatol. 2020;82(5):1262–7. https://doi.org/10.1016/j.jaad.2020.01.030.

Kennedy J, Arey S, Hopkins Z, et al. Dermatologist perceptions of Teledermatology implementation and future use after COVID-19: demographics, barriers, and insights. JAMA Dermatol. 2021;157(5):595–7. https://doi.org/10.1001/JAMADERMATOL.2021.0195.

Khosravi H, Nekooie MB, Moorhead A, English JC. Inpatient teledermatology improves diagnostic accuracy and erythroderma management in hospitalized patients. Clin Exp Dermatol. 2021;46(8):1555–7. https://doi.org/10.1111/CED.14807.

Lee C, Witkowski A, Żychowska M, Ludzik J. The role of mobile teledermoscopy in skin cancer triage and management during the COVID-19 pandemic. Indian J Dermatol Venereol Leprol. 2023;89(3):347–52. https://doi.org/10.25259/IJDVL_118_2022.

López-Liria R, Valverde-Martínez MÁ, López-Villegas A, et al. Teledermatology versus face-to-face dermatology: an analysis of cost-effectiveness from eight studies from Europe and the United States. Int J Environ Res Public Health. 2022;19(5):2534. https://doi.org/10.3390/IJERPH19052534.

Lowe A, Pararajasingam A, Goodwin R. A UK-wide survey looking at teaching and trainee confidence in teledermatology: a vital gap in a COVID-19-induced era of rapid digital transformation? Clin Exp Dermatol. 2020;45(7):876–9. https://doi.org/10.1111/ced.14358.

Lowe A, Dawood S, Al-Tayeb A, et al. Evaluating paediatric dermatology telephone clinics during COVID-19 from a dual clinician and patient perspective: a prospective study. Clin Exp Dermatol. 2022;47(3):553–60. https://doi.org/10.1111/ced.14990.

Micali G, Dall'Oglio F, Verzì AE, Platania H, Lacarrubba F. Home treatment of single cutaneous warts combining face-to-face and teledermatology consultation: a new perspective. Dermatol Ther. 2022;35(7):e15528. https://doi.org/10.1111/DTH.15528.

Mocharnuk J, Lockard T, Georgesen C, English JC. Inpatient Teledermatology: a review. Curr Dermatol Rep. 2022;11(2):52–9. https://doi.org/10.1007/s13671-022-00360-x.

Moscarella E, Pasquali P, Cinotti E, Tognetti L, Argenziano G, Rubegni P. A survey on teledermatology use and doctors' perception in times of COVID-19. J Eur Acad Dermatol Venereol. 2020;34(12):e772.

Mostafa PIN, Hegazy AA. Dermatological consultations in the COVID-19 era: is teledermatology the key to social distancing? An Egyptian experience. J Dermatolog Treat. 2022;33(2):910–5. https://doi.org/10.1080/09546634.2020.1789046.

Naik PP. Rise of teledermatology in the COVID-19 era: a pan-world perspective. Digit Health. 2022;8:8. https://doi.org/10.1177/20552076221076671.

O'Connell G, O'Connor C, Murphy M. Every cloud has a silver lining: the environmental benefit of teledermatology during the COVID-19 pandemic. Clin Exp Dermatol. 2021;46(8):1589–90. https://doi.org/10.1111/CED.14795.

Oaku I, Anaba EL. The impact of COVID-19 on the practice of dermatology in sub-Saharan Africa. Dermatol Ther. 2022;35(3):e14642. https://doi.org/10.1111/DTH.14642.

Oldenburg R, Marsch A. Optimizing teledermatology visits for dermatology resident education during the COVID-19 pandemic. J Am Acad Dermatol. 2020;82(6):e229. https://doi.org/10.1016/j.jaad.2020.03.097.

Pahalyants V, Murphy WS, Gunasekera NS, Das S, Hawryluk EB, Kroshinsky D. Evaluation of electronic consults for outpatient pediatric patients with dermatologic complaints. Pediatr Dermatol. 2021;38(5):1210–8. https://doi.org/10.1111/pde.14719.

Pannu S, Nguyen BM, Yang FSC, Rosmarin D. Predictors of patient experience with teledermatology in setting of COVID-19 pandemic in a single medical center. Int J Dermatol. 2021;60(5):626–7. https://doi.org/10.1111/IJD.15394.

Paudel V. Tele-dermatology in clinical management of suspected cutaneous leishmaniasis in COVID-19 pandemic. Nepal J Dermatol Venereol Leprol. 2020;18(1):91–2. https://doi.org/10.3126/NJDVL.V18I1.31120.

Paudel V, Chudal D. Carbamazepine-induced toxic epidermal necrolysis managed by mobile teledermatology in COVID-19 pandemic in rural Nepal. Case Rep Dermatol Med. 2020;2020:8845759. https://doi.org/10.1155/2020/8845759.

Perednia DA, Brown NA. Teledermatology: one application of telemedicine. Bull Med Libr Assoc. 1995;83(1):42. Accessed 3 Jan 2023.

Perkins S, Cohen JM, Nelson CA, Bunick CG. Teledermatology in the era of COVID-19: experience of an academic department of dermatology. J Am Acad Dermatol. 2020;83(1):e43–4. https://doi.org/10.1016/J.JAAD.2020.04.048.

Rismiller K, Cartron AM, Trinidad JCL. Inpatient teledermatology during the COVID-19 pandemic. J Dermatolog Treat. 2020;31(5):441–3. https://doi.org/10.1080/09546634.2020.1762843.

Ruggiero A, Megna M, Annunziata MC, et al. Teledermatology for acne during COVID-19: high patients' satisfaction in spite of the emergency. J Eur Acad Dermatol Venereol. 2020;34(11):e662. https://doi.org/10.1111/JDV.16746.

Scott Kruse C, Karem P, Shifflett K, Vegi L, Ravi K, Brooks M. Evaluating barriers to adopting telemedicine worldwide: a systematic review. J Telemed Telecare. 2018;24(1):4–12. https://doi.org/10.1177/1357633X16674087.

Sendagorta E, Servera G, Nuño A, Gil R, Pérez-España L, Herranz P. Direct-to-patient teledermatology during COVID-19 lockdown in a Health District in Madrid, Spain: the EVIDE-19 Pilot Study. Actas Dermosifiliogr. 2021;112(4):345–53. https://doi.org/10.1016/J.AD.2020.11.020.

Skayem C, Hua C, Zehou O, et al. Skin cancer and COVID-19: was the diagnosis safeguarded by teledermatology? A study on 1229 cases. J Eur Acad Dermatol Venereol. 2022;36(8):e615–7. https://doi.org/10.1111/jdv.18138.

Snoswell C, Finnane A, Janda M, Soyer HP, Whitty JA. Cost-effectiveness of store-and-forward teledermatology: a systematic review. JAMA Dermatol. 2016;152(6):702–8. https://doi.org/10.1001/JAMADERMATOL.2016.0525.

Tan WH, Loh CH, Chai ZT, et al. Early experience of inpatient teledermatology in Singapore during COVID-19. Ann Acad Med Singap. 2021;50(6):487–9. https://doi.org/10.47102/ANNALS-ACADMEDSG.202130.

Temiz SA, Dursun R, Daye M, Ataseven A. Evaluation of dermatology consultations in the era of COVID-19. Dermatol Ther. 2020;33(5):e13642. https://doi.org/10.1111/DTH.13642.

Tinio PA, Melendres JM, Chavez CP, et al. Clinical profile and response to treatment of patients with psoriasis seen via teledermatology during the COVID-19 pandemic in The Philippines. JAAD Int. 2022;7:35–7. https://doi.org/10.1016/J.JDIN.2022.02.001.

Villani A, Annunziata MC, Megna M, Scalvenzi M, Fabbrocini G. Long-term results of teledermatology for acne patients during COVID-19 pandemic. J Cosmet Dermatol. 2022;21(4):1356–7. https://doi.org/10.1111/jocd.14805.

Viola KV, Tolpinrud WL, Gross CP, Kirsner RS, Imaeda S, Federman DG. Outcomes of referral to dermatology for suspicious lesions: implications for teledermatology. Arch Dermatol. 2011;147(5):556–60. https://doi.org/10.1001/ARCHDERMATOL.2011.108.

Whited JD. Teledermatology. Med Clin North Am. 2015;99(6):1365–79. https://doi.org/10.1016/J.MCNA.2015.07.005.

World Health Organization. Telemedicine: opportunities and developments in member states; 2010. p. 1–96.

World Health Organization. Global diffusion of EHealth: making universal health coverage achievable: report of the Third Global Survey on EHealth; 2015.

Yi JZ, Reynolds RV, Olbricht SM, McGee JS. Moving forward with teledermatology: operational challenges of a hybrid in-person and virtual practice. Clin Dermatol. 2021;39(4):707–9. https://doi.org/10.1016/J.CLINDERMATOL.2021.05.016.

Yim KM, Florek AG, Oh DH, McKoy K, Armstrong AW. Teledermatology in the United States: an update in a dynamic era. Telemed J E Health. 2018;24(9):691–7. https://doi.org/10.1089/TMJ.2017.0253.

COVID-19 Dermatology Registries and the Impact of COVID-19 on Dermatology Research

Abrahim Abduelmula, Yuliya Lytvyn, Khalad Maliyar, Muskaan Sachdeva, Jorge R. Georgakopoulos, Asfandyar Mufti, Melinda J. Gooderham, and Jensen Yeung

Introduction

The first case of SARs-CoV2, also known as COVID-19 or "Coronavirus," was reported in December 2019. By January 2020, it spread worldwide and was declared a pandemic by the World Health Organization (WHO) on March 11th, 2020. With an estimated 659 million cases confirmed and 6.7 million deaths as of January 1st, 2023, the COVID-19 pandemic led to unprecedented changes in daily life and significantly strained our healthcare system (COVID-19 Data Explorer 2022). To tackle the COVID-19 outbreak, healthcare systems redirected most resources to urgent healthcare needs, such as emergency rooms and intensive care units. Many departments and clinics were temporarily shut down or repurposed to help the increased demands

Abrahim Abduelmula and Yuliya Lytvyn contributed equally with all other contributors.

A. Abduelmula · K. Maliyar · M. Sachdeva · J. R. Georgakopoulos
Division of Dermatology, Department of Medicine, University of Toronto, Toronto, ON, Canada
e-mail: aabduelmula2023@meds.uwo.ca;
khalad.maliyar@mail.utoronto.ca;
muskaan.sachdeva@mail.utoronto.ca;
jorge.georgakopoulos@mail.utoronto.ca

Y. Lytvyn
Temerty Faculty of Medicine, University of Toronto, Toronto, ON, Canada
e-mail: julia.lytvyn@mail.utoronto.ca

A. Mufti
Division of Dermatology, Department of Medicine, University of Toronto, Toronto, ON, Canada

Division of Dermatology, Department of Medicine, Sunnybrook Health Sciences Centre, Toronto, ON, Canada

M. J. Gooderham
Queen's University, Kingston, ON, Canada

SKiN Centre for Dermatology, Peterborough, ON, Canada

Probity Medical Research, Waterloo, ON, Canada

J. Yeung (✉)
Division of Dermatology, Department of Medicine, University of Toronto, Toronto, ON, Canada

Division of Dermatology, Department of Medicine, Sunnybrook Health Sciences Centre, Toronto, ON, Canada

Probity Medical Research, Waterloo, ON, Canada

Women's College Research Institute, Women's College Hospital, Toronto, ON, Canada
e-mail: jensen.yeung@utoronto.ca

© The Author(s), under exclusive license to Springer Nature Switzerland AG 2023
H. H. Oon, C. L. Goh (eds.), *COVID-19 in Dermatology*, Updates in Clinical Dermatology,
https://doi.org/10.1007/978-3-031-45586-5_9

in care. This had some impact on ongoing dermatology research resulting in some protocol adaptations to try and retain study participation and minimize impact on data collection.

Dermatology clinics, among many others, experienced significant halting and service disruptions (Conforti et al. 2021), which led to increased use of teledermatology and calls for COVID-19-related research. Interestingly, a rise of unusual cutaneous manifestations was reported during the COVID-19 pandemic, which brought forth a suspicion of a potential correlation between these dermatologic manifestations and the SARs-CoV2 virus (Singh et al. 2021). These unusual presentations brought about the creation of COVID-19 dermatology registries that collect information on dermatologic manifestations of COVID-19 or pre-existing dermatologic conditions affected by this virus as reported by providers and patients. These real-world databases are an important tool that fueled new areas of research in dermatology to help guide physicians in diagnosing and managing skin conditions that may be associated with the COVID-19 virus. In the era of COVID-19, new research trials and databases were developed in dermatology, and existing research trials were modified to adapt to the new circumstances to maintain data collection and integrity.

Dermatology Registries and COVID-19

Early in the pandemic, sharing cases of dermatologic manifestations of COVID-19 through informal networks was challenging (Freeman et al. 2020a). Therefore, registries were created to rapidly collect crowdsourced data in a centralized manner to help inform frontline workers (Freeman et al. 2020a). Dermatology registries are datasets containing patient information with specific dermatologic conditions, manifestations, and treatments. Moreover, these registries allow for the representation of patients with COVID-19 disparities across racial and socioeconomic groups (Freeman et al. 2020a).

There are two main methods of registry data collection: (1) provider-facing registries that include provider-entered data and (2) patient-facing registries with patient self-reported information. Multiple provider- and patient-facing registries were established during the COVID-19 pandemic through a rapidly organized international effort. These registries were launched in March 2020, amassing over 8000 patient entries by March 2021. Among these registries, seven leading international provider-facing dermatology registries as of March 2021 aimed to collect data on novel COVID-19 dermatologic manifestations and the effects of COVID-19 on patients with existing dermatologic conditions (Freeman et al. 2020b).

American Academy of Dermatology (AAD)/International League of Dermatological Societies (ILDS) COVID-19 Dermatology Registry

The AAD and the ILDS collaborated to create this registry on April 9th, 2020 to crowdsource data on patients with cutaneous manifestations of COVID-19 and those with skin conditions potentially affected by the virus. It also includes cutaneous symptoms reported weeks or months after COVID-19 exposure. In late December of 2021, the registry expanded its data eligibility to include patients with cutaneous reactions from the COVID-19 vaccine and (McMahon et al. 2021; Lopez et al. 2021) as of July 2022 includes cases of cutaneous reactions to monkeypox and the respective vaccine (Freeman et al. 2022). On March 2021, this database had collected 1875 patients from over 52 countries (Freeman et al. 2021). This registry is provider-facing and is not open for access to the public. It remained open in January 2023 for new entries, with the intent to keep the registry available for updates with new emerging infections (COVID-19 Dermatology Registry 2022) (Table 9.1).

PsoProtect

The PsoProtect registry was launched on March 27th, 2020, as a provider-facing platform for

Table 9.1 COVID-19 dermatology registries available by January 2023

Registry	Created	Patient or Provider entries	Cases [a]	Registry inclusions	COVID-19 vaccine information?	Active?[b]
AAD/ILDS	April 9th, 2022	Provider	1875[c]	Cutaneous reactions to COVID-19 and COVID-19 vaccination	Yes	Yes
				Skin conditions potentially affected by COVID-19		
				Cutaneous reactions to monkeypox and monkeypox/smallpox vaccines		
PsoProtect/PsoProtectMe	March 27th, 2020/May 4th, 2020	Both	5479[b]	People with psoriasis affected by the pandemic, regardless of COVID-19 status	No	No
				Effects of COVID-19 on psoriasis course and treatments		
SECURE-ALOPECIA	April 8th, 2020	Provider	229[c]	Effects of COVID-19 on alopecia course and treatments	No	Yes
SECURE-AD	April 1st, 2020	Both	900[c]	Effects of COVID-19 on AD course and treatments	No	Yes
SECURE-PSORIASIS	April 1st, 2020	Provider	30[c]	Effects of COVID-19 on psoriasis course and treatments	No	Yes
HS-COVID	April 5th 2020	Both	448[d]	Effects of COVID-19 on HS course and treatments	No	Yes
PeDRA REGISTRY	April 12th, 2020	Provider	467	Acral pernio-like reactions to COVID-19 in pediatric populations	No	Yes

AAD American Academy of Dermatology, *AD* atopic dermatitis, *HS* Hidradenitis suppurativa, *ILDS* International League of Dermatological Societies

[a] Latest registry entries can be obtained through a data request process

[b] As of January 2023

[c] As of March 2021

[d] As of June 2022

data on the course of COVID-19 in patients with psoriasis and its effects on treatments and adverse outcomes. This registry included patients with psoriasis and confirmed or suspected COVID-19 infection with a provider-facing data entry method. By March 2021, the PsoProtect registry collected 996 cases of patients with psoriasis and has since closed (Brumage 2016). On May 4th, 2020, the PsoProtectMe, a patient-facing registry separate from PsoProtect, was created. PsoProtectMe aims to characterize patients' experiences and behaviors (regardless of COVID-19 status) during the pandemic. A previous analysis of 2869 entries from the PsoProtectMe registry suggested that there was no increase in COVID-19 rates or severity while on immunosuppressive medications (Brumage 2016; Mahil et al. 2021a). As of January 2023, 5479 cases have been collected by the PsoProtectMe registry; however, this registry is also now closed (Brumage 2020) (Table 9.1).

Surveillance Epidemiology of Coronavirus Under Research Exclusion (SECURE)-ALOPECIA

SECURE alopecia was launched on April 8th, 2020, as a provider-facing registry to collect data on scarring and non-scarring alopecia patients with COVID-19. As of March 2021, there were 229 cases from 14 countries in the SECURE-ALOPECIA registry (Freeman et al. 2021). This registry remained open as of January 2023 for new entries with the goal of extending the data collection to the impact of vaccination on patients with alopecia (SECURE-Alopecia Registry 2020) (Table 9.1).

SECURE-Atopic Dermatitis (AD)

SECURE-AD is both a patient- and provider-facing registry created on April 1st, 2020. This registry aims to gather data regarding AD outcomes in patients with COVID-19 treated with systemic immunomodulating medications, along with gaining an understanding of essential demographic information relating to AD outcomes. This registry also aimed to measure the disease course and severity of AD with the influence of COVID-19. As of March 2021, the registered collected data on 900 patients from 22 countries (Freeman et al. 2021). As of January 2023, SECURE-AD remained active and intended to expand its dataset to allow for analysis of COVID-19 vaccination effects on AD (SECURE-AD Patient Survey 2020) (Table 9.1).

SECURE-PSORIASIS

Created April 1st 2020, the SECURE-PSORIASIS is a provider-facing registry aiming to collect COVID-19-related information on patients receiving systemic treatment for psoriasis and the effects of the virus on the disease course. As of March 2021, the registered collected data from over 30 patients (Freeman et al. 2021). This registry helps address patients' concerns regarding the use of biologic therapy for inflammatory conditions during a COVID-19 infection (Mahil et al. 2021b). As of January 2023, SECURE-PSORIASIS remained active (Coronavirus and Psoriasis Reporting Registry 2022) (Table 9.1).

Hidradenitis Suppurativa (HS)-COVID

The global HS-COVID-19 registry was launched on April 5th, 2020. The objective of this patient- and provider-facing registry was to help identify factors affecting COVID-19 outcomes in patients with HS. As of June 2022, this registry collected 448 cases (Global Hidradenitis Suppurative COVID-19 Registry 2022). Data from this registry demonstrated that immunosuppressive systemic biologics are not associated with greater severity of COVID-19 symptoms or increased need for COVID-19 treatment (Naik et al. 2020; Naik et al. 2022). As of January 2023, HS-COVID remained active, with plans to compare HS outcomes with other inflammatory conditions. HS-COVID registry also plans to extend data collection to include COVID-19 vaccination data on HS (Alhusayen and Msce 2022) (Table 9.1).

Pediatric Dermatology Research Alliance (PeDRA) Registry

As an international initiative by the Pediatric Dermatology COVID-19 Response Task Force, the PeDRA registry was created on April 12th, 2020. As of March 2021, this provider-facing registry collected data from 467 cases (Freeman et al. 2021). The goal of this registry was to record acral skin changes in pediatric populations in response to a COVID-19 infection. This registry clarified both the short- and long-term courses of acral pernio in COVID-19 (Castelo-Soccio et al. 2021). To date, this registry remains open for new entries, intending to expand to acral manifestations in health conditions beyond COVID-19 (Siegel 2020).

Registry Collaboration

Collaboration between registries within dermatology and beyond was common, which allowed to share patient information and generate larger integrated datasets. AAD/ILDS was known to collaborate with PsoProtect, SECURE-Alopecia, and SECURE-AD with plans of presenting comparative reports in the future (Freeman et al. 2021; Freeman et al. 2020c).

The Impact of COVID-19 on Dermatology Clinical Practice

The volume of patients seen in dermatology practices decreased during the pandemic, secondary to the regional restrictions. Many practices faced disruptions in their workflow due to the need for dedicated triage in outpatient settings, including COVID-19 symptom screening. The decreased volume of in-person visits during the COVID-19 pandemic significantly accelerated the use of teledermatology. Additionally, as the need for frontline physicians increased with rising global cases, dermatologists have been redeployed to various patient settings. Along with changes in practice layouts, dermatologists were faced with a unique set of challenges specific to the COVID-19 pandemic, including the safety of immunosuppressive and biologic treatments in patients who had contracted COVID-19 (Bhargava et al. 2021).

Practice Volume

The effects of the pandemic resulted in a considerable decrease of patient volumes in both outpatient and hospital settings. The total number of consultations was reduced, and appointments were limited to mainly patients receiving biologic treatments and those with suspected malignancies. One study measuring the impact of COVID-19 infection on dermatology practices revealed that of 678 dermatologists, 96.3% reported a reduction in daily work activity, with 49.3% of responses having a reduction in daily work activity of greater than 75% (Conforti et al. 2021), with other studies reporting decreases in dermatology-based office visits ranging from 30 to 70% globally (Litchman et al. 2021; Gisondi et al. 2020). To offset this reduction in work activity, many dermatologists transitioned to remote methods of patient care delivery, with the vast majority of dermatologists increasing teledermatology visits (Conforti et al. 2021).

Teledermatology

Teledermatology uses telecommunication technology to provide dermatologic care to patients through remote means. Teledermatology has several advantages, including reduced wait times to see a specialist, increased access to dermatology services for patients from rural and remote communities, reduced burdens of travel-associated costs and taking time off work. There are, however, challenges with providing care virtually. For example, full body exams are difficult, and some body parts are challenging to examine, such as hair, mucous membranes, and genitals. Additionally, privacy and confidentiality of patient information are held to a high standard, with an important need to use secure and user-friendly telecommunication platforms for virtual clinics. During the COVID-19 pandemic, the development of available services and technologies was accelerated due to increased demand. Ultimately, teledermatology provided dermatologic care while preventing the spread of COVID-19. It also allowed for care to be extended to those with active COVID or those in quarantine. In a study released in early 2021, an estimated 37.8% of dermatology visits were via teledermatology (Conforti et al. 2021). This utilization was increased with changes to legislation for telehealth and insurance policies allowing for improved reimbursement (Bressler et al. 2020). Teledermatology was also utilized within dermatology research in order to maintain subject participation in clinical trials. Many trials allowed some virtual visits to avoid disruption in the study schedule and avoid discontinuation from the trial.

Treatment Modifications

During the COVID-19 pandemic, there were concerns regarding the safety of medications that have suppressive effects on the immune system. Available data suggested continuing immunosuppressants such as azathioprine, cyclosporine, methotrexate, and mycophenolate with careful monitoring during an ongoing COVID-19 infection (Galimberti et al. 2020). There were also recommendations to discontinue oral Janus kinase (JAK) inhibitors and prednisone (Galimberti et al. 2020). Literature regarding systemic biologics and COVID-19 was limited early during the pandemic. The AAD guidelines on COVID-19 and biologic recommended to hold biologic therapy in patients diagnosed with COVID-19 and resume once the infection had resolved. Patients with no-to-mild respiratory symptoms and no close contact with a confirmed COVID-19 case could continue to receive biologic therapy. Later in the pandemic, the safety and efficacy of immunosuppressant medication use in patients receiving the COVID-19 vaccine were questioned (Wack et al. 2021). A study published in March 2022 demonstrated that immunocompromised patients showed improved seroconversion by the second COVID-19 vaccination dose (Lee et al. 2022). Further studies of immunosuppressants and immunomodulators are needed to conclude their relative risk in use for patients with COVID-19 and with COVID-19 vaccination.

The Impact of COVID-19 on Research

Research regarding COVID-19 is a topic of international interest, with numerous journals calling for the submission of relevant manuscripts (Brown and Horton 2020). This international academic response led to the creation of a COVID-19 resource center for patients and physicians with free information in English and Mandarin on the novel coronavirus COVID-19 in January 2020 (Elsevier 2020).

Along with a shift to COVID-19-focused studies, there was a decrease in non-COVID-19-related work. A meta-analysis of over 20,000 publications from high-impact journals found that two primary strategies were taken by journals: (1) decreased non-COVID-19 works while integrating COVID-19-related publications or (2) increased COVID-19 related publications while maintaining the number of non-COVID-19 related works. This study found that COVID-19-related publications accounted for 25.9% of total publications in 2020, with an 18% decrease in non-COVID-19 publications (Raynaud et al. 2021). Another study estimated that 10–20% of all biomedical investigations were related to COVID-19 (Harper et al. 2020). During 2020, there was also an increase in the number of authors on published works. For example, case reports had a median of nine authors on COVID-19 compared to four authors non-COVID-19-related publications, suggesting an increased collaboration in research activities internationally (Raynaud et al. 2021).

The increase in research activities has raised concerns regarding the rigidity of the new evidence. While thousands of new publications, news reports, and opinion pieces emerged, the availability of scientifically robust data remained limited (Weiner et al. 2020).

The Impact of COVID-19 on Dermatology-Specific Research

Topics of interest in dermatology research during the pandemic include cutaneous manifestations of COVID-19, the effects of COVID-19 on existing dermatologic conditions, and the safety of immunosuppressants and immunomodulators in patients with COVID-19 or vaccination. Following a search on MEDLINE and Embase Ovid as of January 1st, 2023, using a combination of keywords of "COVID-19" and "Dermatology" between 2019 and 2022, there has been a significant increase in COVID-19-related publications throughout the pandemic. There was a 192.6% increase in such publications from 2019 to 2020 and a 64.1% increase from 2020 to 2021, with 3000 publications in 2021 alone. This trend continued through 2021,

Table 9.2 Number of COVID-19 related publications from 2019 to 2022

Year	Number of COVID-19 related dermatology publications[a]	% Change from the previous year
2019	37	NA
2020	1967	192.6% increase
2021	3824	64.1% increase
2022	3813	0.3% decrease

[a]All searches performed in MEDLINE and Embase Ovid databases on January 1st, 2023, using a combination of keywords "COVID-19" and "Dermatology". *NA* not applicable

finally seeing a slowdown in 2022 with a mere 0.3% decrease in COVID-19 and dermatology-related publications (Ovid 2022) (Table 9.2).

Multiple studies reported on the incidence of COVID-19 in patients receiving biologic therapy (Poddighe and Kovzel 2021; Abduelmula et al. 2022; Lytvyn et al. 2022; Jones et al. 2021). These studies concluded that no increase in COVID-19 incidence or severity was noted on biologic therapies. Furthermore, these studies suggest that discontinuing treatment due to concerns of a COVID-19 infection is not supported as it may reduce efficacy outcomes and cause flares of dermatologic disease (Georgakopoulos et al. 2020). Further studies on COVID-19 and dermatology publications worldwide are needed to conclude the effects of the pandemic on dermatology research.

Regarding the direct effects of the COVID-19 pandemic on dermatology clinical trials, several recommendations have been provided to optimize the continuation and recruitment of patients to clinical trials effectively. These measures included assessing the patient's fitness for the trials, plans to minimize infection risks, and a contingency plan for ongoing developments regarding the virus (Sheriff et al. 2021). For ongoing trials and registries, quick adaptation in the collection of data was required to ensure continued success. For example, PURE, an international psoriasis registry allowed flexibility in the visit schedule, addition of virtual visits, and modification of the data collection forms to record type of visit and COVID-19-related AEs (Lynde et al. 2022). A report examining dermatology clinical trials between April 2019 and May 2020 observed an increase in the withdrawal, termination, and suspension of dermatology clinical trials in this period (Desai et al. 2021). This study observed over 1000 active, recruiting and enrolling by invitation trials for dermatologic conditions. An estimated 9.1% (92/1010) of these trials had been suspended, withdrawn, or terminated, with over half occurring from March to May of 2020. Among these affected trials, it was reported that 56% had been suspended due to COVID-19. The majority of these trials were either in phase 2 or 3 (Desai et al. 2021).

Conclusion

The COVID-19 pandemic has affected many aspects of dermatology practice, including decreased patient visit volumes, implementation of teledermatology, creation of the COVID-19 dermatology registries, and the rapid acceleration of COVID-19-related research. Ongoing clinical trials required adaptation to continue to collect data and minimize discontinuation, as well as allowing virtual visits and updated AE collection to include COVID-19 specific events. While the rates of COVID-19 have declined and society is slowly returning to pre-pandemic practices, the changes during COVID-19 will leave a lasting impact on dermatology. Teledermatology became integrated into many practices and will likely remain to some degree going forward. The adaptability and organization of the international dermatology community have been remarkable, and lessons learned from this pandemic will have a lasting impact on how medicine is practiced.

Funding Sources None.

Conflicts of Interest Dr. Abrahim Abduelmula has no relevant disclosures.

Dr. Yuliya Lytvyn has no relevant disclosures.

Dr. Khalad Maliyar has no relevant disclosures.

Dr. Muskaan Sachdeva has no relevant disclosures.

Dr. Jorge R. Georgakopoulos has no relevant disclosures.

Dr. Asfandyar Mufti has no relevant disclosures.

Dr. Melinda J. Gooderham has been an investigator, speaker, consultant, or advisory board member for AbbVie, Amgen, Akros, Arcutis, AnaptysBio, Aristea, Bausch Health, Boehringer Ingelheim, BMS, Celgene, Dermira, Dermavant, Galderma, GSK, Eli Lilly, Incyte, Janssen, Kyowa Kirin, Leo Pharma, Medimmune, Meiji, Merck, Moonlake, Nimbus, Novartis, Pfizer, Regeneron, Reistone, Roche, Sanofi Genzyme, Sun Pharma, UCB, and Ventyx.

Dr. Jensen Yeung has been an advisor, consultant, speaker, and/or investigator for AbbVie, Allergan,

Amgen, Astellas, Boehringer Ingelheim, Celgene, Centocor, Coherus, Dermira, Eli Lilly, Forward,

Galderma, GSK, Janssen, LEO Pharma, Medimmune, Merck, Novartis, Pfizer, Regeneron, Roche,

Sanofi Genzyme, Sun Pharma, Takeda, UCB, Valeant, and Xenon.

References

Abduelmula A, Georgakopoulos JR, Mufti A, et al. Incidence of COVID-19 in patients with chronic idiopathic urticaria and asthma on omalizumab: a multicentre retrospective cohort study. J Cutan Med Surg. 2022;26(3):319–20. https://doi.org/10.1177/12034754211049707.

Alhusayen R, Msce M. Global Hidradenitis Suppurative COVID-19 Registry. https://hscovid.ucsf.edu/. Accessed 31 Dec 2022.

Bhargava S, Negbenebor N, Sadoughifar R, Ahmad S, Kroumpouzos G. Global impact on dermatology practice due to the COVID-19 pandemic. Clin Dermatol. 2021;39(3):479–87. https://doi.org/10.1016/j.clindermatol.2021.01.017.

Bressler MY, Siegel DM, Markowitz O. Virtual dermatology: a COVID-19 update. Cutis. 2020;105(4):163–4; E2.

Brown A, Horton R. A planetary health perspective on COVID-19: a call for papers. Lancet. 2020;395(10230):1099. https://doi.org/10.1016/S0140-6736(20)30742-X.

Brumage D. Home. PsoProtect. 2016. https://psoprotect.org/. Accessed 31 Dec 2022.

Brumage D. PsoProtect Me Registry: current data. PsoProtect Me. 2020. https://psoprotectme.org/current-data/. Accessed 31 Dec 2022.

Castelo-Soccio L, Lara-Corrales I, Paller AS, et al. Acral changes in pediatric patients during COVID 19 pandemic: registry report from the COVID 19 response task force of the Society of Pediatric Dermatology (SPD) and Pediatric Dermatology Research Alliance (PeDRA). Pediatr Dermatol. 2021;38(2):364–70. https://doi.org/10.1111/pde.14566.

Conforti C, Lallas A, Argenziano G, et al. Impact of the COVID-19 pandemic on dermatology practice worldwide: results of a survey promoted by the International Dermoscopy Society (IDS). Dermatol Pract Concept. 2021;11(1):e2021153. https://doi.org/10.5826/dpc.1101a153.

Coronavirus and Psoriasis Reporting Registry. Wake Forest University School of Medicine. https://school.wakehealth.edu/departments/dermatology/secure-psoriasis. Accessed 31 Dec 2022.

COVID-19 Data Explorer. Our world in data. https://ourworldindata.org/explorers/coronavirus-data-explorer. Accessed 31 Dec 2022.

COVID-19 Dermatology Registry. Aad.org. https://www.aad.org/member/practice/coronavirus/registry. Accessed 31 Dec 2022.

Desai S, Manjaly P, Lee KJ, Li SJ, Manjaly C, Mostaghimi A. The impact of COVID-19 on dermatology clinical trials. J Invest Dermatol. 2021;141(3):676–8. https://doi.org/10.1016/j.jid.2020.06.032.

Elsevier. Novel coronavirus information center. Elsevier Connect; 2020. https://www.elsevier.com/connect/coronavirus-information-center. Accessed 31 Dec 2022.

Freeman EE, McMahon DE, Fitzgerald ME, et al. The American Academy of Dermatology COVID-19 registry: crowdsourcing dermatology in the age of COVID-19. J Am Acad Dermatol. 2020a;83(2):509–10. https://doi.org/10.1016/j.jaad.2020.04.045.

Freeman EE, McMahon DE, Lipoff JB, et al. The spectrum of COVID-19-associated dermatologic manifestations: an international registry of 716 patients from 31 countries. J Am Acad Dermatol. 2020b;83(4):1118–29. https://doi.org/10.1016/j.jaad.2020.06.1016.

Freeman EE, McMahon DE, Hruza GJ, et al. International collaboration and rapid harmonization across dermatologic COVID-19 registries. J Am Acad Dermatol. 2020c;83(3):e261–6. https://doi.org/10.1016/j.jaad.2020.06.050.

Freeman EE, Chamberlin GC, McMahon DE, et al. Dermatology COVID-19 registries: updates and future directions. Dermatol Clin. 2021;39(4):575–85. https://doi.org/10.1016/j.det.2021.05.013.

Freeman EE, Galvan Casas C, Prasad S, et al. The American Academy of Dermatology and International League of Dermatological Societies Monkeypox Registry: expanding the COVID-19 registry to emerging infections. J Am Acad Dermatol. 2022;87(6):1278–80. https://doi.org/10.1016/j.jaad.2022.08.053.

Galimberti F, McBride J, Cronin M, et al. Evidence-based best practice advice for patients treated with systemic immunosuppressants in relation to COVID-19. Clin Dermatol. 2020;38(6):775–80. https://doi.org/10.1016/j.clindermatol.2020.05.003.

Georgakopoulos JR, Mufti A, Vender R, Yeung J. Treatment discontinuation and rate of disease transmission in psoriasis patients receiving biologic therapy during the COVID-19 pandemic: a Canadian multicenter retrospective study. J Am Acad Dermatol. 2020;83(4):1212–4. https://doi.org/10.1016/j.jaad.2020.07.021.

Gisondi P, Piaserico S, Conti A, Naldi L. Dermatologists and SARS-CoV-2: the impact of the pandemic on daily practice. J Eur Acad Dermatol Venereol. 2020;34(6):1196–201. https://doi.org/10.1111/jdv.16515.

Global Hidradenitis Suppurative COVID-19 Registry. Dissemination of findings. https://hscovid.ucsf.edu/dissemination-findings. Accessed 31 Dec 2022.

Harper L, Kalfa N, Beckers GMA, et al. The impact of COVID-19 on research. J Pediatr Urol. 2020;16(5):715–6. https://doi.org/10.1016/j.jpurol.2020.07.002.

Jones ME, Kohn AH, Pourali SP, et al. The use of biologics during the COVID-19 pandemic. Dermatol Clin. 2021;39(4):545–53. https://doi.org/10.1016/j.det.2021.05.010.

Lee ARYB, Wong SY, Chai LYA, et al. Efficacy of covid-19 vaccines in immunocompromised patients: systematic review and meta-analysis. BMJ. 2022;376:e068632. https://doi.org/10.1136/bmj-2021-068632.

Litchman GH, Marson JW, Rigel DS. The continuing impact of COVID-19 on dermatology practice: office workflow, economics, and future implications. J Am Acad Dermatol. 2021;84(2):576–9. https://doi.org/10.1016/j.jaad.2020.08.131.

Lopez S, Vakharia P, Vandergriff T, Freeman EE, Vasquez R. Pernio after COVID-19 vaccination. Br J Dermatol. 2021;185(2):445–7. https://doi.org/10.1111/bjd.20404.

Lynde C, Papp K, Beecker J, Albrecht L, Delorme I, Dei-Cas I, Vieira A, Rihakova L, Gooderham M. 35158 Adaptations in the PURE registry in response to the COVID 19 pandemic: the impact of well-designed modifications in real-world data collection in a psoriasis registry. J Am Acad Dermatol. 2022;87:AB135. https://doi.org/10.1016/j.jaad.2022.06.573.

Lytvyn Y, Georgakopoulos JR, Mufti A, et al. Incidence and prognosis of COVID-19 in patients with psoriasis on apremilast: a multicentre retrospective cohort study. J Eur Acad Dermatol Venereol. 2022;36(2):e94–5. https://doi.org/10.1111/jdv.17749.

Mahil SK, Yates M, Langan SM, et al. Risk-mitigating behaviours in people with inflammatory skin and joint disease during the COVID-19 pandemic differ by treatment type: a cross-sectional patient survey. Br J Dermatol. 2021a;185(1):80–90. https://doi.org/10.1111/bjd.19755.

Mahil SK, Dand N, Mason KJ. Factors associated with adverse COVID-19 outcomes in patients with psoriasis-insights from a global registry-based study. J Allergy Clin Immunol. 2021b;147(1):60–71. https://doi.org/10.1016/j.jaci.2020.10.00.

McMahon DE, Amerson E, Rosenbach M, et al. Cutaneous reactions reported after Moderna and Pfizer COVID-19 vaccination: a registry-based study of 414 cases. J Am Acad Dermatol. 2021;85(1):46–55. https://doi.org/10.1016/j.jaad.2021.03.092.

Naik HB, Alhusayen R, Frew J, et al. Global Hidradenitis Suppurativa COVID-19 Registry: a registry to inform data-driven management practices. Br J Dermatol. 2020;183(4):780–1. https://doi.org/10.1111/bjd.19345.

Naik HB, Alhusayen R, Frew J, et al. Biologic therapy is not associated with increased COVID-19 severity in patients with hidradenitis suppurativa: initial findings from the Global Hidradenitis Suppurativa COVID-19 Registry. J Am Acad Dermatol. 2022;86(1):249–52. https://doi.org/10.1016/j.jaad.2021.09.016.

Ovid: Welcome to Ovid. Ovid.com. https://ovidsp.dc2.ovid.com/ovid-a/ovidweb.cgi. Accessed 31 Dec 2022.

Poddighe D, Kovzel E. Impact of anti-type 2 inflammation biologic therapy on COVID-19 clinical course and outcome. J Inflamm Res. 2021;14:6845–53. https://doi.org/10.2147/JIR.S345665.

Raynaud M, Goutaudier V, Louis K, et al. Impact of the COVID-19 pandemic on publication dynamics and non-COVID-19 research production. BMC Med Res Methodol. 2021;21(1):255. https://doi.org/10.1186/s12874-021-01404-9.

SECURE-AD Patient Survey. Secure Derm. 2020. https://secure-derm.com/secure-pad/. Accessed 31 Dec 2022.

SECURE-Alopecia Registry. Secure Derm. 2020. https://secure-derm.com/secure-alopecia/. Accessed 31 Dec 2022.

Sheriff T, Dickenson-Panas H, Murrell DF. Conducting dermatology clinical trials during the COVID-19 pandemic. Clin Dermatol. 2021;39(1):104–6. https://doi.org/10.1016/j.clindermatol.2020.12.019.

Siegel M. COVID-19 web resources for PeDRA members. 2020. Pedraresearch.org. https://pedra-research.org/2020/04/06/covid-19-websites-for-pedra-members. Accessed 31 Dec 2022.

Singh H, Kaur H, Singh K, Sen CK. Cutaneous manifestations of COVID-19: a systematic review. Adv Wound Care (New Rochelle). 2021;10(2):51–80. https://doi.org/10.1089/wound.2020.1309.

Wack S, Patton T, Ferris LK. COVID-19 vaccine safety and efficacy in patients with immune-mediated inflammatory disease: review of available evidence. J Am Acad Dermatol. 2021;85(5):1274–84. https://doi.org/10.1016/j.jaad.2021.07.054.

Weiner DL, Balasubramaniam V, Shah SI, Javier JR, Pediatric Policy Council. COVID-19 impact on research, lessons learned from COVID-19 research, implications for pediatric research. Pediatr Res. 2020;88(2):148–50. https://doi.org/10.1038/s41390-020-1006-3.

Impact of COVID-19 on Dermatology Medical Education

10

Katherine L. Perlman, Rachel M. Reardon, and Steven T. Chen

Introduction

The COVID-19 pandemic caused significant changes to the medical education system as students, trainees, institutions, and societies tried to navigate the unprecedented events. Medical education curricula and policies were forced to adapt to follow public health regulations and keep students, faculty, and patients healthy. Like other specialties, dermatology medical education was drastically impacted by the pandemic. This chapter aims to assess the impact of the COVID-19 pandemic on medical education in dermatology.

Learning Objectives

- Provide an overview of the impacts of the COVID-19 pandemic on medical education in dermatology.
- Evaluate the influence of the transition to virtual learning formats on medical students preparing for and applying to dermatology residencies.
- Assess the challenges and adaptations experienced in dermatology residency training programs in response to the COVID-19 pandemic.

Medical Student Dermatology Education

General Changes

Due to public health regulations, medical students had disruptions in clinical rotations, away rotations, United States Medical Licensing Examinations (USMLE), and grading policies (Samimi et al. 2021; Adusumilli et al. 2021). Schools adapted to pandemic-related changes by reducing in-person clinical activities and transitioning to virtual formats. Schools quickly adopted web-based resources such as Zoom or Webex to hold virtual didactics, virtual grand rounds, and virtual patient visits for students (Oki et al. 2021; Lipner et al. 2021). Medical school dermatology curricula were similarly impacted by the abrupt switch to virtual learning. Some programs utilized online learning tools such as the American Academy of Dermatology (AAD) Basic Dermatology Curriculum, VisualDx, and *The New England Journal of Medicine* (NEJM) Photo Challenge to supplement students' derma-

K. L. Perlman
Department of Dermatology, Massachusetts General Hospital, Boston, MA, USA

University of Illinois College of Medicine, Chicago, IL, USA
e-mail: KPERLMAN@mgh.harvard.edu

R. M. Reardon · S. T. Chen (✉)
Department of Dermatology, Massachusetts General Hospital, Boston, MA, USA

Harvard Medical School, Boston, MA, USA
e-mail: RMREARDON@mgh.harvard.edu; STCHEN@MGB.ORG

© The Author(s), under exclusive license to Springer Nature Switzerland AG 2023
H. H. Oon, C. L. Goh (eds.), *COVID-19 in Dermatology*, Updates in Clinical Dermatology,
https://doi.org/10.1007/978-3-031-45586-5_10

tology curriculum (Bell et al. 2021). Many medical schools also suspended or cancelled clinical rotations for medical students (Samimi et al. 2021; Ladha et al. 2021; Jones et al. 2021). The sudden cancellation of both clinical and non-clinical opportunities significantly affected medical students. Students now had decreased opportunities for longitudinal service, advocacy, and research, which impacted their specialty choice and ability to obtain strong letters of recommendation for their residency applications (Samimi et al. 2021).

Some medical students in states with particularly high numbers of COVID-19 cases, such as New York, chose to graduate early in order to bolster the hospital workforce (American Medical Association 2022). States granted early graduates temporary medical licenses that allowed them to work in a COVID-19 service capacity until they acquired their trainee licenses (American Medical Association 2022; AAMC 2022). Early graduates worked as interns before starting their own residency programs later that year in July. Though they were able to contribute to pandemic relief efforts, early graduation impacted the usual training timeline and transition between medical school graduation and working as a resident physician.

Away Rotations

Away rotations are important for students applying into competitive specialties such as dermatology, as they allow students to have advanced clinical experiences, meet new dermatology mentors, and learn about resident life at different institutions (Adusumilli et al. 2021; Stewart et al. 2020). Away rotations are similarly important for residency programs, as the dermatology trainees and faculty are able to work with students applying to their program and can evaluate a candidate's fit in a more longitudinal manner than applications and interview days will allow (Adusumilli et al. 2021; Stewart et al. 2020). During the early phases of the pandemic, most away rotations were cancelled, including those available in dermatology (Adusumilli et al.

2021). To address this issue, some dermatology residency programs created virtual visiting clinical rotations and research rotations for students (Adusumilli et al. 2021; Bell et al. 2021). These virtual rotations allowed students to interact with dermatology residents and faculty and attend virtual educational activities including journal club, grand rounds, resident didactics, and clinicopathologic conferences (Adusumilli et al. 2021). Students were also able to participate in telemedicine consults and patient visits (Bell et al. 2021). While this allowed students to work with dermatology teams at other institutions and see more dermatology cases, virtual rotations could not fully replicate a traditional away rotation experience. Compared to in-person away rotations, virtual rotations reduced students' ability to obtain letters of recommendation and engage in research opportunities (Adusumilli et al. 2021).

Teledermatology

In 2020, the Association of American Medical Colleges (AAMC) released guidelines recommending that medical students should not participate in clinical activities until there was an adequate supply of personal protective equipment (PPE), space for social distancing, and COVID-19 testing (Whelan et al. 2020). Consequently, medical students were removed from clinical settings in order to follow social distancing guidelines and reduce unnecessary COVID-19 exposures (Jones et al. 2021). To address this reduction of in-person clinical experience, medical schools turned to teledermatology to deliver patient care and education.

Since dermatology is a highly visual specialty, online platforms may be useful for dermatology medical education (Lam and Doiron 2021). Many medical schools utilized asynchronous and/or synchronous telehealth, which allowed students to study cases, form differential diagnoses, write clinical notes, and discuss skin exam findings (Ladha et al. 2021; Su et al. 2020; Ashrafzadeh et al. 2021). Medical students were also able to participate in virtual patient visits and consults (Bell et al. 2021).

The shift from in-person teaching to teledermatology was very useful for social distancing, as students were able to complete their work remotely. Teledermatology also put an increased reliance on accurate verbal descriptions of dermatology pathologies (Lam and Doiron 2021). Medical students were able to practice asking pertinent questions and improving other aspects of communication, due to the inability for an in-person exam (Lam and Doiron 2021). Teledermatology could also reach a larger pool of learners and preceptors, as anyone with internet connection could join these sessions (Lam and Doiron 2021). While teledermatology has unique benefits, there are also significant limitations. Students are unable to observe or assist in procedures that are commonly done in dermatology, such as biopsies and cryotherapy (Lipner et al. 2021; Ashrafzadeh et al. 2021). Similarly, students were unable to perform full body skin exams (FBSE) which is a commonly used and very important skill for dermatology trainees. Dermatology pathologies often require tactile exams for accurate diagnosis and management, which cannot be done through virtual formats (Lam and Doiron 2021). Since students were working with patients virtually, they also had more limited opportunities for practicing nonverbal communication skills, bedside manner, and other aspects of interpersonal professionalism (Lam and Doiron 2021).

Mentorship

With the decreased in-person opportunities for medical student education, pandemic-related changes created new challenges for medical students searching for dermatology mentors (Jones et al. 2021). Typically, students identified mentors who worked at their home dermatology program or who worked in their geographical regions (Fernandez et al. 2021). The shift to virtual dermatology education reduced students' ability to develop relationships with local dermatologists, and this impact was worse for students who did not have a home dermatology program.

During the pandemic, there was an increase in virtual opportunities for mentorship in dermatology (Fernandez et al. 2021). Students could meet with their mentors over platforms such as Zoom to discuss their residency applications and conduct remote research (Jones et al. 2021). Before the pandemic, minority students reported limited access to mentorship and cited this as a major barrier for applying to dermatology residencies (Fernandez et al. 2021; Soliman et al. 2019). Virtual mentorship allowed students who may have limited mentorship at their home institution to find mentors in dermatology (Fernandez et al. 2021). While virtual opportunities have increased access to mentors, there may still exist a shortage of mentorship for certain medical students.

Dermatology Residency Applicants

Fourth-year medical students applying into dermatology faced significant changes to the application cycle, including in interviews, application schedules, decreased clinical opportunities, and unique considerations while crafting their applications.

Dermatology Residency Applications

Dermatology is one of the most competitive medical specialties to match into, and the pandemic only increased applicants' stress (National Resident Matching Program 2020; Yeh et al. 2022). Dermatology applicants typically have the highest number of publications, research, and volunteer experiences across all specialties (Rosman et al. 2020). COVID-19 restrictions significantly impacted volunteer opportunities, research projects, and clinical rotations – many of which were cancelled (Rosman et al. 2020). Further compounding application stress, in 2020, the Association of American Medical Colleges (AAMC) delayed the opening of the Electronic Residency Application Service (ERAS) by 5 weeks, which significantly compressed the timeline for application review by dermatology residency programs (Samimi et al. 2021).

Application Sessions

Because of the unprecedented changes in the residency application cycle, application education sessions were held to address applicant concerns (Samimi et al. 2021). Organizations such as the Dermatology Interest Group Association (DIGA) and many dermatology residency programs hosted national webinars for dermatology applicants (Samimi et al. 2021; Bell et al. 2021). A majority of members of the Association of Professors of Dermatology (APD) reported holding application-focused educational sessions for medical students during the pandemic, with a large reported increase in session number from before the pandemic (Bell et al. 2021). Webinars allowed dermatology applicants to speak with dermatology residency program directors, faculty, and residents to learn more about residency programs and have their application concerns addressed (Samimi et al. 2021; Brumfiel et al. 2021). While these extra sessions allowed students to speak with dermatology residency programs, the addition of these webinars may have also contributed to increased student stress due to the time commitment of attending sessions for each program.

Dermatology Residency Programs

The pandemic also caused significant changes to dermatology residency programs and the typical application process. In the spring of 2020, the APD released statements encouraging programs to limit in-person away rotations to applicants without a home dermatology program, create virtual away experiences, perform holistic application review, consider COVID-related changes to applications, and have virtual interviews (Samimi et al. 2021; Rosman et al. 2020). Holistic application review aimed to shift the emphasis away from standardized metrics to focus more on an applicant's overall strengths and contributions to their communities, including leadership and service experiences (Samimi

et al. 2021). Residency programs also turned to social media to showcase their programs and provide virtual mentorship and outreach opportunities (Samimi et al. 2021; Zheng et al. 2021). After May 2020, there was an increase in official dermatology residency program social media accounts on Instagram, Twitter, and Facebook (Harp et al. 2021). Programs shared educational topics, information on residency life, and more to engage with applicants on these virtual platforms.

Dermatology Resident and Fellow Education

General Changes

Like changes seen in medical school curricula, many dermatology residency and fellowship educational experiences also transitioned to virtual formats. Dermatology training programs turned to virtual conferences, didactics, virtual pathology sessions, collaborative teaching from other programs, and online lectures to continue education during the pandemic (Jones et al. 2021; Gehret et al. 2022). Virtual teaching allowed for increased exposure to guest lectures, as programs were able to invite speakers to teach from across the country. While there was an increased ability for guest lectures, trainees lost opportunities for peer-to-peer teaching and for rotating between different hospitals (Gehret et al. 2022; Mufti et al. 2020). The transition to online education also caused residents to have decreased patient volumes and in-person clinical visits, which resulted in less clinical dermatology experience than trainees had prior to the pandemic (Samimi et al. 2021; Jones et al. 2021; Mufti et al. 2020; Sattler et al. 2021). Additionally, some dermatology residents were redeployed to other clinical teams to help with COVID-19 patients in overloaded departments and, consequently, spent less time in dermatology training and education (Samimi et al. 2021; Mufti et al. 2020; Sattler et al. 2021; Oldenburg and Marsch 2020).

Teledermatology

Teledermatology was widely used by most, if not all, dermatology training programs (Samimi et al. 2021; Jones et al. 2021). Programs used teledermatology such as e-visits and e-consults using store-and-forward technology and live video virtual visits (Samimi et al. 2021). In 2020, the Centers for Medicare and Medicaid Services (CMS) lifted restrictions on teledermatology, allowing physicians to practice across state lines during the pandemic (American Academy of Dermatology n.d.). Consequently, teledermatology expanded into most areas of dermatology practice including inpatient consults, outpatient visits, and dermatopathology (Loh et al. 2022).

Teledermatology has many benefits for dermatology trainees. First, teledermatology can be used for inpatient dermatology as well as outpatient care (Trinidad et al. 2020). After CMS eased teledermatology restrictions, dermatology trainees had the unique opportunity to virtually work with patients across the country (Farr et al. 2021). This expansion not only increased access to dermatologic care for patients but also allowed dermatology residents and fellows to have experience with a more diverse patient population and a wider variety of dermatological conditions (Jones et al. 2021). Further, virtual consults allowed for high patient caseloads in a low-stress learning environment (Loh et al. 2022; Zakaria et al. 2021). Implementation of teledermatology in the inpatient setting allowed for the conservation of PPE and decreased unnecessary COVID-19 exposures for the dermatology clinicians while still allowing trainees to work with inpatient dermatology cases (Samimi et al. 2021; Trinidad et al. 2020). While there were benefits of teledermatology during the pandemic, there are also important limitations to these methods of providing patient care. First, use of teledermatology for patient visits may be difficult as skin lesions may not be accurately displayed and there may be technology issues and internet bandwidth limitations (Jones et al. 2021). Programs must also check all patient images used are for Protected Health Information (PHI) and ensure all platforms used are Health Insurance Portability and Accountability Act (HIPAA) compliant and secure (Samimi et al. 2021). Additionally, similar to the challenges faced by medical students, dermatology residents and fellows had fewer opportunities to hone their nonverbal communication and bedside manner/professionalism skills than their predecessors.

Procedural Education

Dermatology residents across the United States reported that pandemic-related changes had the most negative impact on dermatology procedural education, surgical dermatology, and cosmetic dermatology education (Gehret et al. 2022). During the pandemic, dermatology departments postponed and/or cancelled many elective outpatient procedural or surgical visits out of concern for both patients and providers (Samimi et al. 2021; Jones et al. 2021; Mufti et al. 2020; Pollock et al. 2021). Dermatology residents are at risk for COVID-19 infection because of procedures and evaluations around the nose and mouth, which requires patients to unmask while in close proximity to clinicians for prolonged periods of time (Samimi et al. 2021; Sattler et al. 2021; Pollock et al. 2021). These changes caused a significant overall decrease in procedural volume for dermatology trainees, which created concern for the procedural education during the pandemic (Samimi et al. 2021; Pollock et al. 2021). Procedural education is necessary knowledge for dermatology residents and fellows, as the Accreditation Council for Graduate Medical Education (ACGME) and the American Society for Dermatologic Surgery (ASDS) require trainees to demonstrate proficiency in common dermatology procedures for board certification (Pollock et al. 2021).

Some dermatology programs addressed these issues with procedural education by creating virtual experiences with home procedural kits and virtual oversight for residents (Samimi et al.

2021; Tassavor et al. 2021). The ASDS also created virtual procedural videos for trainees to help trainees meet the number of cases required for ACGME requirements (Pollock et al. 2021). However, these virtual experiences could not fully replicate the in-person procedural education done before the pandemic.

Dermatopathology Education

While the pandemic caused many negative changes to dermatology trainee education, dermatopathology education was more readily adaptable. A survey of US dermatology residents reported that pandemic changes had the least negative impact on dermatopathology education, and 30% of respondents said it had a positive impact (Gehret et al. 2022). Prior to the pandemic, dermatopathology was taught in-person in the pathology department (Wolner et al. 2022; Blum et al. 2021). This style of teaching was limited by space constraints and available microscopes (Wolner et al. 2022; Blum et al. 2021). During the pandemic, dermatology programs transitioned dermatopathology didactics, sign-out, and consensus conferences to online platforms such as virtual microscopy (Samimi et al. 2021; Jones et al. 2021; Blum et al. 2021). Using this method, dermatopathologists utilized light microscopy that was simultaneously shown virtually so the dermatology team could attend dermatopathology sign-out remotely and in real time (Blum et al. 2021; Mahmood 2021). Dermatology trainees also utilized online educational tools for dermatopathology such as the Clearpath app, myDermPath app, PathPresenter, DermpathPRO, and Dermpedia (Mahmood 2021). Use of virtual microscopy and virtual educational tools allowed dermatology residents and fellows to continue their dermatopathology education during the pandemic.

Board Certification

In March 2020, the ACGME cancelled all site visits and adjusted program requirements in response to the COVID-19 pandemic. The ACGME issued a modified framework for how graduate medical education (GME) can effectively operate during the pandemic, which included three stages defined along a continuum: "business as usual," increased clinical demands, and pandemic emergency status (Samimi et al. 2021; Accreditation Council for Graduate Medical Education n.d.-a). The ACGME also began to allow sponsoring institutions and programs to request Emergency Categorization in order to adapt GME and board certification requirements in response to local COVID-related educational disruptions (Accreditation Council for Graduate Medical Education n.d.-b). The American Board of Dermatology (ABD) similarly adapted their certification requirements during the pandemic, allowing residents in mandated COVID-19 quarantine to count their time as contributing to clinical education requirements if they were able to complete structured remote academic activities during quarantine (American Board of Dermatology 2023).

Dermatology trainees faced further obstacles when large conferences, such as the AAD Annual Meeting, were cancelled. These cancellations caused challenges for dermatology residents and fellows who previously used educational sessions at these conferences for high-yield dermatology board review (Samimi et al. 2021). Dermatology board exams were also delayed and transitioned to a virtual format (Samimi et al. 2021; Sattler et al. 2021). Additionally, decreased procedural volumes for dermatology trainees created concern for trainees' ability to meet ACGME case log minimums (Samimi et al. 2021; Pollock et al. 2021). To address these concerns, dermatology programs held virtual board reviews, paid for residents to access question banks, and hosted webinars to address certification concerns (Samimi et al. 2021; Adusumilli et al. 2020). Still, dermatology residents expressed concern about passing the board examination and meeting certification requirements (Adusumilli et al. 2020).

Research and Future Employment

Dermatology trainees' research opportunities and future employment were also impacted by the COVID-19 pandemic. Since national dermatology conferences were cancelled, trainees lost key networking and socializing opportunities. Conferences are usually crucial events for networking and time with potential employers, research partners, and training programs (Sattler et al. 2021). Further, dermatology residents and fellows applying for jobs had fewer chances to assess programs in person (Sattler et al. 2021). Trainees had to rely on virtual tours and Zoom sessions with program faculty to learn about employment opportunities. Some institutions and dermatology practices implemented hiring freezes, which increased trainees' stress about jobs (Sattler et al. 2021). Among surveyed third-year dermatology residents, a majority reported high levels of anxiety regarding employment and how pandemic-related educational changes will be perceived by future employers (Adusumilli et al. 2020).

Research opportunities were also negatively impacted during the pandemic. During early phases of the pandemic, many non-essential research projects were halted (Sattler et al. 2021). Trainees, consequently, had fewer opportunities to practice research and work with mentors in the field. Further, removal of childcare resources during the pandemic compounded with the disproportionate burden of childcare on women widened the gender gap seen in academia (Sattler et al. 2021). Throughout the pandemic, journal submissions from women declined, whereas submissions from men increased (Sattler et al. 2021). This is a significant change as research productivity and publications are important factors for academic hires and promotions. Female dermatology trainees may have been negatively impacted by the pandemic more significantly than male trainees.

Dermatology Societies

Prior to the COVID-19 pandemic, most dermatology society meetings were held in person. During the pandemic, they were either delayed, cancelled, or made completely virtual (Samimi et al. 2021; Loh et al. 2022). Many societies chose to use virtual formats in order to continue providing education, networking, and research education during the pandemic. Dermatology societies also created new virtual education sessions to help dermatology trainees address educational gaps created by the pandemic (Jones et al. 2021; Pollock et al. 2021). For example, the Medical Dermatology Society (MDS) and the Society of Dermatology Hospitalists (SDH) released guidance on how to manage dermatology patients taking immunosuppressive therapy during the COVID-19 pandemic (Zahedi Niaki et al. 2020). The AAD released Dialogues in Dermatology podcasts centered on pandemic-specific discussions. The Women's Dermatology Society (WDS) curated Resident Education Series Events through Zoom for dermatology residents and fellows. WDS also waived membership fees for 6 months so more trainees could take advantage of these learning opportunities. The ASDS hosted webinars on topics specific to COVID-19, monthly surgical journal clubs, virtual didactics, virtual procedural videos, and live learning sessions on social media platforms during the pandemic (Pollock et al. 2021). Overall, dermatology societies aimed to continue providing opportunities while following public health recommendations and ensuring safety for dermatology trainees.

Conclusion

Since the early stages of the COVID-19 pandemic, dermatology medical education has rapidly and drastically changed. Virtual education was widely implemented, which allowed students and trainees to learn remotely without increased risk of COVID-19 exposure. Dermatology programs utilized teledermatology more often to deliver patient care and allow students and trainees to safely participate in patient care. Pandemic-related changes also caused significant stress for dermatology residency applicants, who worried how the pandemic negatively impacted their applications and their ability to network with dermatology residency programs. Dermatology residents and fellows were similarly negatively impacted by reductions in patient caseload, procedural experience, and concerns regarding meeting certification requirements.

It has become clear that COVID-19 is here to stay for the time being and the healthcare system will continue to grapple with the potential for frequent labor shortages and educational interruptions due to COVID-19 infections and mandatory quarantines (Assistant Secretary for Planning and Evaluation 2022; COVID is here to stay 2022). In order to lessen the impact on medical education and dermatology training, teledermatology and other virtual learning methods may continue to be utilized to allow for continued education.

References

AAMC. "Itching to get back in": Medical students graduate early to join the fight. https://www.aamc.org/news-insights/itching-get-back-medical-students-graduate-early-join-fight. Accessed 7 Dec 2022.

Accreditation Council for Graduate Medical Education. Three Stages of GME During the COVID-19 Pandemic [Internet]. https://www.acgme.org/covid-19/-Archived-Three-Stages-of-GME-During-the--COVID-19-Pandemic/#:~:text=Stage%201%20%E2%80%93%20%E2%80%9Cbusiness%20as%20usual,focus%20only%20on%20patient%20care.

Accreditation Council for Graduate Medical Education. Sponsoring Institution Emergency Categorization [Internet]. https://www.acgme.org/covid-19/sponsoring-institution-emergency-categorization/.

Adusumilli NC, Eleryan M, Tanner S, Friedman AJ. Third-year dermatology resident anxiety in the era of COVID-19. J Am Acad Dermatol. 2020;83(3):969–71.

Adusumilli NC, Kalen J, Hausmann K, Friedman AJ. Dermatology applicant perspectives of a virtual visiting rotation in the era of COVID-19. J Am Acad Dermatol. 2021;84(6):1699–701.

American Academy of Dermatology. Teledermatology during the COVID-19 pandemic [Internet]. https://www.aad.org/member/practice/telederm/toolkit

American Board of Dermatology. Impact of COVID-19 on Dermatology Resident Education [Internet]. 2023. https://www.abderm.org/public/announcements/impact-of-covid-19-on-dermatology-resident-education.

American Medical Association. COVID-19 and early medical school graduation: a primer for M4s. https://www.ama-assn.org/medical-students/medical-student-health/covid-19-and-early-medical-school-graduation-primer-m4s. Accessed 6 Dec 2022.

Ashrafzadeh S, Imadojemu SE, Vleugels RA, Buzney EA. Strategies for effective medical student education in dermatology during the COVID-19 pandemic. J Am Acad Dermatol. 2021;84(1):e33–4.

Assistant Secretary for Planning and Evaluation. Impact of the COVID-19 Pandemic on the Hospital and Outpatient Clinical Workforce [Internet]. Department of Health and Human Services; 2022. p. 1–27. https://aspe.hhs.gov/sites/default/files/documents/9cc72124abd9ea25d58a22c7692dccb6/aspe-covid-workforce-report.pdf.

Bell KA, Porter C, Woods AD, Akkurt ZM, Feldman SR. Impact of the COVID-19 pandemic on dermatology departments' support of medical students: a survey study. Dermatol Online J. 2021;27(7). https://escholarship.org/uc/item/7x57v28j. Accessed 21 Sep 2022.

Blum AE, Murphy GF, Lee JJ. Digital dermatopathology: the time is now. J Cutan Pathol. 2021;48(4):469–71.

Brumfiel CM, Jefferson IS, Wu AG, Strunck JL, Veerabagu S, Lin K, et al. A national webinar for dermatology applicants during the COVID-19 pandemic. J Am Acad Dermatol. 2021;84(2):574–6.

COVID is here to stay: Countries must decide how to adapt. Nature. 2022;601(7892):165.

Farr MA, Duvic M, Joshi TP. Teledermatology during COVID-19: an updated review. Am J Clin Dermatol. 2021;22(4):467–75.

Fernandez JM, Behbahani S, Marsch AF. A guide for medical students and trainees to find virtual mentorship in the COVID era and beyond. J Am Acad Dermatol. 2021;84(5):e245–8.

Gehret NL, Brooks BE, Vance TM, Wambier CG, Libby TJ. Impact of the COVID-19 pandemic on dermatology residency education in the United States: a cross-sectional survey. JAAD Int. 2022;8:134–5.

Harp T, Szeto MD, Presley CL, Meckley AL, Geist R, Anderson J, et al. Usage and engagement with Instagram by dermatology residency programs during the COVID-19 pandemic compared with twitter and Facebook. J Am Acad Dermatol. 2021;85(5):e313–5.

Jones VA, Clark KA, Puyana C, Tsoukas MM. Rescuing medical education in times of COVID-19. Clin Dermatol. 2021;39(1):33–40.

Ladha MA, Lui H, Carroll J, Doiron P, Kirshen C, Wong A, et al. Medical student and resident dermatology education in Canada during the COVID-19 pandemic. J Cutan Med Surg. 2021;25(4):437–42.

Lam M, Doiron PR. The use of Teledermatology in medical education. Med Sci Educ. 2021;32(1):243–6.

Lipner SR, Shukla S, Stewart CR, Behbahani S. Reconceptualizing dermatology patient care and education during the COVID-19 pandemic and beyond. Int J Womens Dermatol. 2021;7(5 Part B):856–7.

Loh CH, Ong FLL, Oh CC. Teledermatology for medical education in the COVID-19 pandemic context: a systematic review. JAAD Int. 2022;6:114–8.

Mahmood MN. Dermatopathology resident training and education during the COVID-19 pandemic: challenges faced and lessons learned. Clin Dermatol. 2021;39(5):907–10.

Mufti A, Maliyar K, Sachdeva M, Doiron P. Modifications to dermatology residency education during the COVID-19 pandemic. J Am Acad Dermatol. 2020;83(3):e235–6.

National Resident Matching Program. The Match. National Resident Matching Program. Results and Data: 2020 Main Residency Match; 2020. p. 1–128.

Oki O, Shah S, Scrivens L, Guckian J. COVID-19: challenges and solutions for the future of UK dermatology undergraduate curriculum delivery. Clin Exp Dermatol. 2021;46(1):171–3.

Oldenburg R, Marsch A. Optimizing teledermatology visits for dermatology resident education during the COVID-19 pandemic. J Am Acad Dermatol. 2020;82(6):e229.

Pollock SE, Nathan NR, Nassim JS, Shadi Kourosh A, Mariwalla K, Tsao SS. The show must go on: dermatologic procedural education in the era of COVID-19. Int J Womens Dermatol. 2021;7(2):224–7.

Rosman IS, Schadt CR, Samimi SS, Rosenbach M. Approaching the dermatology residency application process during a pandemic. J Am Acad Dermatol. 2020;83(5):e351–2.

Samimi S, Choi J, Rosman IS, Rosenbach M. Impact of COVID-19 on dermatology residency. Dermatol Clin. 2021;39(4):609–18.

Sattler SS, Kraus CN, Wu JJ. How the COVID-19 pandemic is affecting graduating dermatology residents and fellows. Dermatol Online J. 2021;27(3):18. https://escholarship.org/uc/item/92c9v9dj. Accessed 21 Sep 2022.

Soliman YS, Rzepecki AK, Guzman AK, Williams RF, Cohen SR, Ciocon D, et al. Understanding perceived barriers of minority medical students pursuing a career in dermatology. JAMA Dermatol. 2019;155(2):252–4.

Stewart CR, Chernoff KA, Wildman HF, Lipner SR. Recommendations for medical student preparedness and equity for dermatology residency applications during the COVID-19 pandemic. J Am Acad Dermatol. 2020;83(3):e225–6.

Su MY, Lilly E, Yu J, Das S. Asynchronous teledermatology in medical education: lessons from the COVID-19 pandemic. J Am Acad Dermatol. 2020;83(3):e267–8.

Tassavor M, Shah A, Hashim P, Torbeck R. Flipped classroom curriculum for dermatologic surgery during COVID-19: a prospective cohort study. J Am Acad Dermatol. 2021;85(5):e297–8.

Trinidad J, Kroshinsky D, Kaffenberger BH, Rojek NW. Telemedicine for inpatient dermatology consultations in response to the COVID-19 pandemic. J Am Acad Dermatol. 2020;83(1):e69–71.

Whelan A, Prescott J, Young G, Catanese VM, McKinney R. Guidance on Medical Students' participation in direct in-person patient contact activities. 2020. https://www.aam c.org/system/files/2020-08/meded-August-14-Guidance-on-Medical-Students-on-Clinical-Rotations.pdf.

Wolner ZJ, Nguyen H, Kong HE, Perricone AJ, Stoff BK, Cheeley JT. Virtual clinicopathologic correlation rounds for inpatient consult skin biopsies during the COVID-19 pandemic: a quality improvement study. J Cutan Pathol. 2022;49(1):107–9.

Yeh C, Desai AD, Wilson BN, Elkattawy O, Shah R, Behbahani S, et al. Cross-sectional analysis of scholarly work and mentor relationships in matched dermatology residency applicants. J Am Acad Dermatol. 2022;86(6):1437–9.

Zahedi Niaki O, Anadkat MJ, Chen ST, Fox LP, Harp J, Micheletti RG, et al. Navigating immunosuppression in a pandemic: a guide for the dermatologist from the COVID task force of the Medical Dermatology Society and Society of Dermatology Hospitalists. J Am Acad Dermatol. 2020;83(4):1150–9.

Zakaria A, Maurer T, Amerson E. Impact of Teledermatology program on dermatology resident experience and education. Telemed E-Health. 2021;27(9):1062–7.

Zheng DX, Mulligan KM, Scott JF. #DermTwitter and digital mentorship in the COVID-19 era. J Am Acad Dermatol. 2021;85(1):e17–8.

Management of Immunosuppressed Dermatology Patients During COVID-19

11

James P. Pham and John W. Frew

Many early dermatological guidelines provided guidelines regarding the management of immunosuppressed patients during the era of COVID-19 (Niaki et al. 2020; Price et al. 2020; Schwartz et al. 2020; Fahmy et al. 2020; Lebwohl et al. 2020). These suggestions were largely based on extrapolations of pre-clinical data (Price et al. 2020) or incidence rates of other upper respiratory viruses reported in pivotal trials (Lebwohl et al. 2020). For example, Price et al. suggest antimetabolites (methotrexate, mycophenolate mofetil, azathioprine, etc.), calcineurin inhibitors (tacrolimus or cyclosporine) and glucocorticoids may impair T cells to a greater degree than biologics, and cessation in active infection can be considered (Price et al. 2020).

However, understanding of COVID-19 pathophysiology has evolved substantially since the publication of these initial guidelines. Therefore, 3 years on from the onset of the pandemic, it is necessary to re-examine these initial recommendations with the benefit of clinical outcome datasets and improved knowledge of the immunobiology of SARS-CoV2 infection and thus the possible interactions with immunosuppressive medications. This chapter will summarise updates in COVID-19 pathophysiology relevant for the clinical dermatologist, as well as present four scenarios which may be encountered in daily practice—with suggestions for how to manage immunosuppression in each scenario. A dynamic approach to practise guidelines reflecting updates in knowledge will be essential in providing safe and evidence-based patient care in the ongoing pandemic especially for the immunosuppressed.

COVID-19 Pathophysiology

Research into COVID-19 quickly demonstrated that it is a distinct disease from influenza and other coronaviruses to which it was initially compared. The majority of patients infected with SARS-CoV-2 will develop respiratory involvement—80% mild-to-moderate (no oxygen requirement), 15% severe (needing oxygen support) and 5% critical (acute respiratory distress syndrome, multi-organ failure) (Osuchowski et al. 2021). However, it has been shown that, unlike other respiratory viruses, multiple organ systems may be infected by SARS-CoV-2,

J. P. Pham
School of Clinical Medicine, UNSW Medicine and Health, Sydney, NSW, Australia

J. W. Frew (✉)
School of Clinical Medicine, UNSW Medicine and Health, Sydney, NSW, Australia

Department of Dermatology, Liverpool Hospital, Liverpool, NSW, Australia

Laboratory of Translational Cutaneous Medicine, Ingham Institute for Applied Medical Research, Liverpool, NSW, Australia
e-mail: john.frew@unsw.edu.au

© The Author(s), under exclusive license to Springer Nature Switzerland AG 2023
H. H. Oon, C. L. Goh (eds.), *COVID-19 in Dermatology*, Updates in Clinical Dermatology,
https://doi.org/10.1007/978-3-031-45586-5_11

including intestinal epithelial cells (Stanifer et al. 2020), myocardial cells (Bearse et al. 2021) and the brain (Serrano et al. 2021), particularly in severe disseminated COVID-19.

Figure 11.1 summarises the effects of COVID-19 infection on the immune system, including the 'cytokine storm' that characterises severe disease. Figure 11.2 details the targets of immunosuppressants commonly used in dermatology and their effects on T cells.

Interestingly, contrary to early guidelines suggesting avoidance of immunosuppression to prevent infection or reduce complications in confirmed infections (both scenarios discussed in detail in later sections), clinical data have highlighted the efficacy of immunomodulatory drugs in reducing adverse outcomes in COVID-19. For example, dexamethasone has been shown to reduce mortality in COVID-19 patients requiring oxygen support with a hazard ratio of 0.64–0.82 (Horby et al. 2021). Similarly, improved survival outcomes have been demonstrated with the addition of the IL-6 inhibitor tocilizumab (Stone et al. 2020), the Janus kinase inhibitor baricitinib (Kalil et al. 2021) and the IL-1 receptor antagonist anakinra (Huet et al. 2020) to standard of care in patients with severe COVID-19.

Therefore, rather than a blanket approach of avoiding or ceasing certain immunosuppressive medications to minimise COVID-19 complications, dermatologists should consider the specific clinical contexts and medications in their practice. Ongoing research into the immunobiology of COVID-19 infection is vital in guiding this

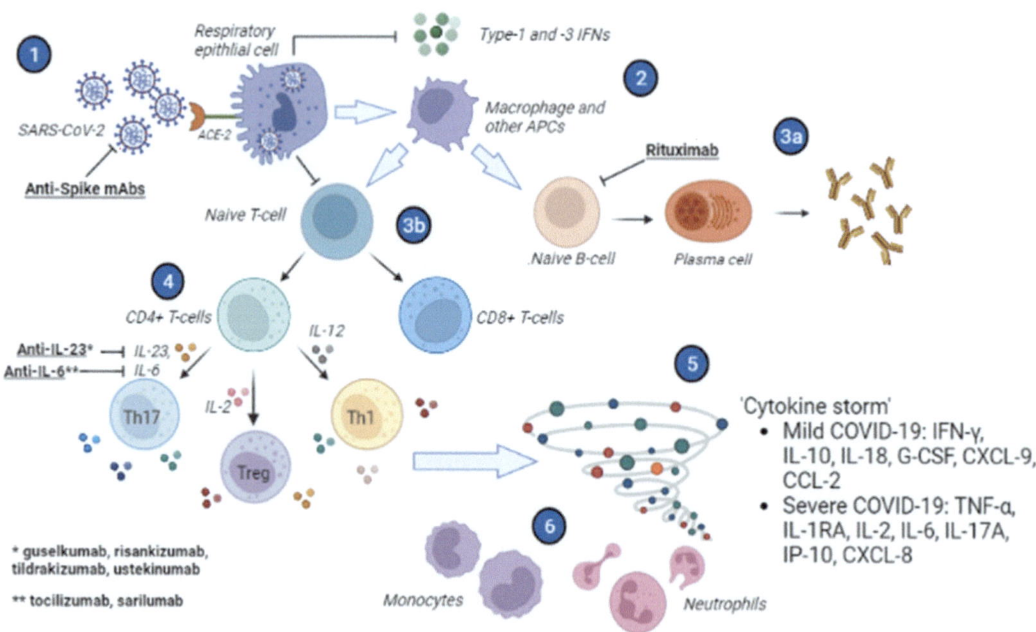

Fig. 11.1 Schematic summarising the immunobiology of COVID-19 infection: (1) SARS-CoV-2 virus infecting the respiratory epithelium via ACE-2 receptors, enabling replication by suppressing Type-1 and Type-3 IFN and T-cell responses (the latter contributing to lymphopenia in severe disease) (Blanco-Melo et al. 2020; Shen et al. 2022; Cizmecioglu et al. 2021); (2) presentation of viral antigens by APCs leading to the differentiation of (3a) naïve B cells to plasma cells secreting anti-SARS-CoV-2 antibodies (Cox and Brokstad 2020) and (3b) naïve T cells to activated SARS-CoV-2-specific CD4+ and CD8+ effector cells (Cox and Brokstad 2020); (4) further subtype differentiation of CD4+ T cells, with a skew towards Th17/Th1 over Treg cells in severe disease (Meckiff et al. 2020); (5) 'cytokine storm' characterising mild-to-severe infection (Blanco-Melo et al. 2020; Zhang et al. 2020; Del Valle et al. 2020; Wang et al. 2020), resulting in (6) the overactivation of innate immune pathways (monocytes and neutrophils) which can precipitate a hyperinflammatory state, multi-organ failure and death (Vanderbeke et al. 2021). Relevant targets of immunosuppressive/immunomodulatory medications used in dermatology as well as for the treatment of COVID-19 itself are also included in the diagram

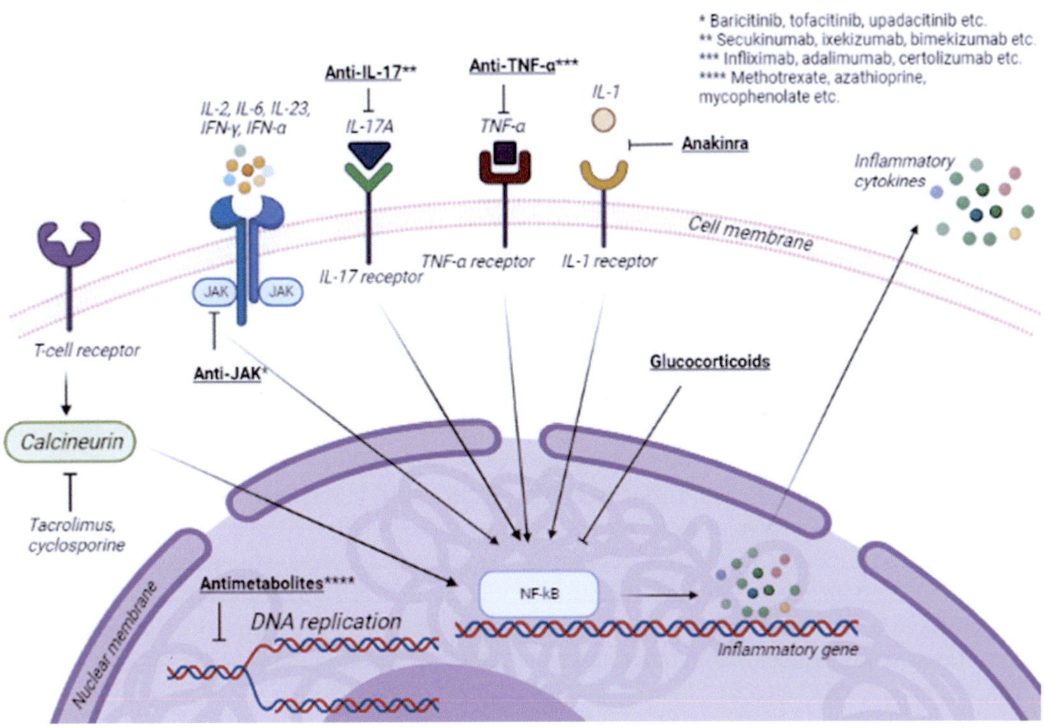

Fig. 11.2 Schematic summarising common immunosuppressants utilised in dermatology and their targets within a representative T cell. These include monoclonal antibodies targeting interleukin (*IL*)-17; tumour necrosis factor (*TNF*)-α; Janus kinase (*JAK*) inhibitors blocking the signalling of cytokines such as IL-2, IL-6, IL-23, interferon (*IFN*)-α and IFN-Υ; glucocorticoids inhibiting nuclear factor (*NF*)-κβ; calcineurin inhibitors inhibiting cytokine transcription (via the nuclear factor of activated T cells [*NFAT*] pathway); and antimetabolites inhibiting DNA replication

practice, as much of the data to date have been from patients with severe disease and therefore the potential for immunosuppressants to modulate mild-to-moderate infection is largely unknown. However, based on the available evidence, four clinical scenarios where dermatologists may require modification of immunosuppression are presented herein.

Scenario 1: Minimising Infection and Transmission

At the time of writing (December 2022), many countries have eased public lockdown orders due to socioeconomic ramifications and improvements in COVID-19 mortality with effective vaccination and antiviral strategies. However, this has resulted in significant increases in infection rates worldwide—with over 190,000 new daily infections reported presently worldwide (WHO Coronavirus (COVID-19) Dashboard 2022). This may pose a concern for dermatologists in regard to the vulnerability of their patients to contracting COVID-19 due to potential increased susceptibility to infection by SARS-CoV-2 and possible increased risk of associated complications (the latter discussed below). Guidelines from the American Academy of Dermatology (AAD) do not currently support stopping immunosuppressive drugs in patients who have not tested positive for COVID-19 (American Academy of Dermatology 2022).

It is unclear if dermatology patients treated with immunosuppressants are at an increased risk of COVID-19. One case-control study from the Lombardia region of Italy during a 'red-zone' declaration identified that psoriasis patients treated with biologics (22% anti-TNF-α, 45% anti-IL-17, 20% anti-IL-12/23, 5% anti-IL-23) were more likely to test positive to SARS-CoV-2 than the general population, with an unadjusted odds ratio of 3.43 (Damiani et al. 2020). Notably, however, this study did not account for the high comorbidity burden in the psoriasis cohort which may have contributed to COVID-19 infection, such as 20% being active smokers and 18% being obese. Of note, none of the 17 psoriasis patients who contracted COVID-19 in this cohort developed severe disease or died.

It has been suggested that ACE-2 receptors on keratinocytes may allow for transcutaneous infection by SARS-CoV-2, with findings of increased ACE-2 expression in skin lesions in active COVID-19 (Sun et al. 2020; Colmenero et al. 2020). Certain dermatological conditions may predispose patients to cutaneous SARS-CoV-2 tropism, rather than the immunosuppressive treatments for them. For example, transcriptomic analysis of lesional skin and blood from patients with psoriasis identified significantly higher ACE-2 levels than controls (Tembhre et al. 2021). Similar upregulated ACE-2 expression patterns have been observed in lesional and perilesional skin in hidradenitis suppurativa and pyoderma gangrenosum (Flora and Frew 2022). However, correlation between cutaneous ACE-2 expression and COVID-19 infection risk has not been demonstrated. Interestingly, IL-17 inhibitors have shown to decrease ACE-2 expression in psoriatic skin (Xu et al. 2021; Krueger et al. 2021). This is theorised to decrease SARS-CoV-2 infection risk by decreasing ACE-2 on other epithelial tissues (e.g. alveolar cells) (Krueger et al. 2021); however, this has not been proven.

However, there are some considerations for dermatologists managing immunosuppressed patients from a public health perspective. Firstly, nosocomial COVID-19 infection of patients and clinicians in a healthcare setting is high, estimated to be up to 60% (Abbas et al. 2021). Therefore, dermatologists can consider strategies to reduce hospital exposure and patient-clinician or patient-patient interactions to lower transmission risk. For example, in patients requiring treatment with a TNF-α inhibitor, subcutaneous medications such as adalimumab may be preferred over intravenous options such as infliximab as they do not require administration in an infusion centre, with similar efficacy for conditions such as HS (Prens et al. 2021). In cases where there are limited alternatives to intravenous therapy, such as rituximab for AIBD, patient visits may be spaced out as able with appropriate social distancing and personal protective equipment use. Similar approaches have been recommended for phototherapy during the pandemic (Lim et al. 2020).

Secondly, in immunosuppressed patients with possible COVID-19 exposures, dermatologists may be able to liaise with infectious disease specialists to discuss the appropriateness of post-exposure prophylaxis. These include monoclonal antibody combinations targeting the SARS-CoV-2 Spike protein such as bamlanivimab-etesevimab or tixagevimab-cilgavimab (Evusheld®), which were shown to reduce COVID-19 infection in high-risk groups (Cohen et al. 2021; Marovich et al. 2020; Levin et al. 2022). In the USA, the Food and Drug Administration authorises bamlanivimab-etesevimab for post-exposure prophylaxis in patients who are not vaccinated, or who are unlikely to mount sufficient antiviral responses due to immunosuppression (discussed further below), at the discretion of their treating physicians (U.S. Food and Drug Administration 2022). As the pattern of circulating variants varies over time, these monoclonal antibodies may have absent or reduced activity against new dominant subvariants, and alternative drugs may need to be used. Monoclonal antibodies may therefore be considered on a case-by-case basis to mitigate the community spread of COVID-19, with immunosuppressed patients informed to notify the relevant physicians (infectious diseases, emergency medicine) or their treating dermatologist in case of high-risk exposure.

In summary, the following recommendations regarding the management of immunosuppressed dermatology patients who have not tested posi-

Table 11.1 Recommendations to mitigate infection and community spread

Recommendation	GRADE
Immunosuppressant use should continue, with limited evidence their use increases the risk of COVID-19 infection	D
Insufficient evidence that targeting ACE-2 (e.g. via IL-17 inhibition) reduces the risk of COVID-19 infection	D
Consider alternative modes of delivery of medication to reduce nosocomial transmission	D
Consider post-exposure prophylaxis with anti-spike antibodies in heavily immunosuppressed patients[a]	B

[a]Dependent on susceptibility of prevailing variants

tive for COVID-19 are made, with corresponding GRADE levels of evidence (Siemieniuk and Guyatt 2021) (Table 11.1):

Scenario 2: Active Infection

Another scenario dermatologists are likely to face is the management of immunosuppressed dermatology patients who test positive to COVID-19. A large, propensity-matched analysis of over 1.16 million people in the USA with immune-mediated inflammatory disorders infected with COVID-19 found a slightly increased risk of critical care unit admission or death, hazard ratio (HR) 1.15 (95%CI 1.11–1.18) (MacKenna et al. 2022). Of the 769,816 patients with inflammatory skin disease (90% psoriasis), this HR was 1.12 (95%CI 1.04–1.21). Use of 'standard immunosuppressants' (defined as methotrexate, mycophenolate, cyclosporine, azathioprine, etc.) versus biologics (used in 90.5 and 9.5% of patients, respectively) was not associated with significantly different risk in adverse COVID-19 outcomes in this cohort. However, it was unclear whether the increased mortality risk in this study was due to immunosuppressant use or the underlying inflammatory disorders themselves.

In another propensity-matched analysis of 12,841 long-term immunosuppressed patients admitted to hospital with COVID-19, there was no significant increase in mortality risk (HR 0.97, 95%CI 0.91–1.02), and there was a slight reduction in mechanical ventilation requirements (HR 0.89, 95%CI 0.83–0.96) (Andersen et al. 2022). However, on subgroup analysis of individual drugs, a history of rituximab use for rheumatological conditions was associated with an increased mortality risk (HR 1.72, 95%CR 1.10–2.69). The impact of immunosuppression on COVID-19 severity should also be considered in the context of available data for specific inflammatory skin disorders. For example, in a matched database analysis of 5574 dermatomyositis patients with COVID-19, lower mortality was observed (HR 0.76, 95%CI 0.60–0.97) (Pakhchanian et al. 2022). Among patients with dermatomyositis, a 1-year history of DMARD or corticosteroid use was associated with an increased risk of severe COVID-19 (HR 2.25, 95%CI 1.15–4.39). However, this sub-analysis did not adjust for dermatomyositis severity or the presence of interstitial lung disease (also an independent risk factor for severe COVID-19, HR 1.64, 95%CI 1.02–2.64) as confounders.

A similar database analysis in HS identified no significant difference in mortality or severe COVID-19 compared to controls and no increased risk for complications with TNF-α inhibitor use in patients with HS (Raiker et al. 2021). Furthermore, in an international registry-based study of psoriasis patients infected with SARS-CoV-2, hospitalisation was increased in patients receiving non-biologic treatment versus biologics (HR 2.84, 95%CI 1.31–6.18) (Mahil et al. 2021). However, this study was limited by patient-reported data and the potential for unadjusted confounders, such as self-isolation compliance (significantly lower in patients receiving non-biologic treatments).

Therefore, there is insufficient evidence to recommend ceasing regular immunosuppressants and especially biologics for dermatological disorders in cases of active infection, as suggested by the AAD (American Academy of Dermatology 2022). In some cases, this may even be to the detriment of patients, as breaks in treatment dosing may precipitate the formation of anti-drug antibodies and therefore reduced efficacy on restarting (Norden et al. 2022; Reich et al. 2018; Hsu and Armstrong 2013).

However, special attention should be paid for patients who have been treated with rituximab, such as for autoimmune bullous disorders (AIBD), cutaneous lupus or dermatomyositis. Patients with pemphigus may be particularly vulnerable to COVID-19, with pneumonia and respiratory sepsis representing the most common cause of death in the pre-pandemic era (Schmidt et al. 2019). B-cell depletion with rituximab was theorised to predispose to severe COVID-19 via hypogammaglobulinaemia (Mehta et al. 2020), with uncontrolled studies and case reports suggesting poor outcomes in patients treated for multiple sclerosis, haematological malignancies and rheumatic disorders (Esmaeili et al. 2021; Levavi et al. 2021). Therefore, in patients who have received rituximab in the preceding year who develop COVID-19, anti-spike monoclonal antibodies against SARS-CoV-2 should be considered even in mild or early infection to mitigate the effects of hypogammaglobulinaemia (Gupta et al. 2021; Dougan et al. 2021). Maintenance rituximab infusions should also be postponed until after acute infection, particularly given the risk of exposure at infusion centres, although this must be balanced against the risk of flaring underlying inflammatory skin disorders, particularly AIBD.

Another aspect regarding the management of immunosuppressed patients to consider is the potential for prolonged infectious periods in this population. Cohort studies suggest patients receiving immunosuppressive medications, including corticosteroids, are more likely to remain infectious beyond 3 weeks (Li et al. 2021; Campioli et al. 2020). A case report of a renal transplant patient receiving prednisolone, tacrolimus and mycophenolate identified a prolonged infectious period (confirmed by serial PCR testing) of 63 days (Man et al. 2020). However, this phenomenon has not been validated in a dermatology-specific setting, and therefore, generalisability is unclear. Rather than 5-day isolation as suggested by authorities (Tanne 2021), for the purposes of reducing community transmis-

Table 11.2 Recommendations in case of active COVID-19 infection

Recommendation	GRADE
Limited evidence to recommend ceasing immunosuppressants in acute infection, particularly biologics	D
Inflammatory skin disorders and associated comorbidities may themselves predispose to severe COVID-19	D
Patients treated with rituximab warrant careful follow-up and consideration of anti-spike antibody therapies	C
Consider counselling heavily immunosuppressed patients (e.g. multiple agents, conventional non-selective) on the potential for extended infectious periods	D

sion, dermatologists may consider counselling immunosuppressed patients (particularly those on multiple or conventional non-selective agents) who test positive to remain isolated until no longer symptomatic or until PCR testing is negative, as appropriate.

In summary, the following recommendations regarding the management of immunosuppressed dermatology patients who have tested positive for COVID-19 are made (Table 11.2):

Scenario 3: Vaccination

The development of effective vaccines against SARS-CoV-2 has been essential in combating the COVID-19 pandemic. Four COVID-19 vaccine classes currently exist—inactivated virus vaccines (e.g. Sinopharm's Covilo), mRNA vaccines (e.g. Pfizer-BioNTech's BNT162b2), adenoviral vector vaccines (e.g. Johnson & Johnson-Janssen's Ad26.COV2.S) and adjuvanted protein vaccines (e.g. Novavax's Nuvaxovid) (Barouch 2022). A meta-analysis of 51 controlled studies estimated these vaccines were effective in preventing severe infection and death by 89 and 99%, respectively (Zheng et al. 2022). COVID-19 vaccines are engineered to induce both cellular and humoral immune memory against SARS-CoV-2 spike proteins, generating robust neutralising T_H1/CD8+ T-cell and antibody responses, respectively (Sahin et al. 2020; Swanson et al. 2021).

However, the ability to develop such immune memory may be impaired by immunosuppressive medications. A non-randomised cohort study demonstrated lower anti-SARS-CoV-2 antibody generation and responses, as well as spike-specific IFN-γ-mediated CD4+ cellular immunity following mRNA vaccination in people receiving immunosuppressive therapies compared to controls (Collier et al. 2022). On multivariate analysis, this was particularly prominent in patients receiving corticosteroids, antimetabolites, calcineurin inhibitors and combination therapy. This may translate to reduced clinical efficacy of vaccines in this cohort—with one national cohort study in Israel reporting immunocompromised patients represented 40% of breakthrough infections (Brosh-Nissimov et al. 2021). In a similar real-world US study, immunosuppressed people comprised 44% of breakthrough infections, with a vaccine effectiveness of only 63% in a case-control sub-analysis (versus 91% in non-immunosuppressed people) (Tenforde et al. 2022).

The potential for immunosuppressive medications to suppressive anti-SARS-CoV-2 immune memory differ between classes of agents. In a cohort of patients with inflammatory bowel disease, anti-spike antibodies were lower in those receiving infliximab, tofacitinib or infliximab-thiopurine combination compared to healthy controls (Alexander et al. 2022). A similar study including patients with inflammatory skin disorders identified reduced seroconversion following the first vaccination (mRNA or adenoviral vector) in patients receiving non-biologic immunosuppressants compared to biologics, HR 0.29 (Al-Janabi et al. 2022). This effect remained significant on multivariate analysis for methotrexate (HR 0.097), prednisolone (HR 0.04) and methotrexate-based combinations (HR 0.025–0.052). However, after the second dose, only 1.6% of patients did not seroconvert, with the only significant risk factor being exposure to rituximab (HR 0.001).

As rituximab depletes CD20+ B and plasma cells, it is well established as a contributor to vaccine inefficacy (Eisenberg et al. 2013; Van Assen et al. 2010). In a case-control study of 96 anti-CD20-treated patients, only 14% developed both cellular and humoral immunity after the second mRNA vaccination, compared to 75% of controls (Moor et al. 2021). On multivariate analysis, longer time since anti-CD20 dosing (>7.6 months) and higher peripheral B-cell count (>27 cells per μL) were predictive of humoral response. In another small study of five rituximab-treated patients, reduced neutralising antibody titres following mRNA vaccination was observed (Bonelli et al. 2021). Interestingly, despite this, all rituximab-treated patients were able to generate IFN-γ responses to SARS-CoV-2 peptides similar to controls, suggesting preserved cellular immunity. A third booster vaccination may improve efficacy in rituximab-treated patients—with 100% generating cellular CD4/CD8+ immune responses in one cohort, although only 16% developed neutralising antibodies (Jyssum et al. 2022).

Booster vaccination should also be considered in other patients receiving immunosuppressive therapies, particularly with evidence of failed seroconversion. In a randomised trial of 46 immunosuppressed patients who failed to seroconvert after 2 doses of an mRNA vaccine, seroconversion was higher after a third mRNA booster rather than an adenoviral vector booster (63 vs. 18%, $p = 0.006$) (Mrak et al. 2022). However, there were no differences in T-cell responses between patients who received an mRNA or adenoviral boosters, although these were diminished relative to healthy controls. While this suggests that immunosuppressed patients may benefit from boosters, the majority (76%) were on combination therapy, mostly for solid organ transplants (80%), and so whether this applies to the dermatology patient population is unclear. It should be noted that booster vaccines are also recommended in the general, non-immunosuppressed, population due to waning antibody responses (approximately 6–8 months between classes) and emergence of new SARS-CoV-2 variants for which T-cell immune memory is more significant in defending against (Barouch 2022).

Dermatologists may also consider counselling their patients on the potential for COVID-19 vaccines themselves to exacerbate underlying

Table 11.3 Recommendations regarding COVID-19 vaccination

Recommendation	GRADE
All patients regardless of immunosuppression should be counselled on the benefits of COVID-19 vaccination	A
Timing of vaccination should be considered in patients receiving anti-CD20 treatment, with greater efficacy when vaccines are administered later after anti-CD20	C
Booster vaccination should be counselled in patients, particularly in immunosuppressed patients	B
Dermatologists should discuss the risk of COVID-19 vaccines flaring underlying dermatoses, for shared decision-making	D

inflammatory skin disorders. While supportive data is largely limited to case series and cohort studies (Damiani et al. 2021; Sotiriou et al. 2021), a national data-linkage study showed no increased risk of psoriasis or eczema exacerbations post-COVID-19 vaccines (Adams et al. 2022). Regardless, concerns regarding potential flaring of inflammatory skin conditions may lead to patient hesitancy towards vaccination. Shared decision-making between dermatologists and patients is essential in improving compliance to recommended vaccine schedules for personal and community protection while also mitigating harms from any cutaneous flares that may result.

In summary, the following recommendations regarding the management of immunosuppressed dermatology patients regarding COVID-19 vaccination are made (Table 11.3):

Scenario 4: Clinical Trials

Clinical trials are an essential method of testing new drugs for safety and efficacy prior to broader patient access, in dermatology and medicine as a whole. As a consequence of the COVID-19 pandemic and associated public health measures including lockdowns, clinical trials were significantly disrupted worldwide (van Dorn 2020). These disruptions included closure of laboratories, diversion of funding towards COVID-19-related research, conference cancellations and the inability to conduct face-to-face safety and monitoring visits. An analysis of the US National Library of Medicine's ClinicalTrials.Gov in early 2020 identified 1052 suspended clinical trials, 905 of which (86%) listed the COVID-19 pandemic as the reason (Asaad et al. 2020). Dermatological clinical trials were similarly affected early in the pandemic, with 9% of those registered on ClinicalTrials.Gov terminated in early 2020, affecting 7141 patients (Desai et al. 2021). Common conditions for which trials were suspended included atopic dermatitis ($n = 7$), psoriasis ($n = 7$) and HS ($n = 5$).

While many trials have since resumed since the easing of COVID-19 lockdowns, dermatologists should consider the ongoing pandemic in their approach towards future clinical research. Guidelines have been published regarding the safe conduct of dermatology clinical trials during the pandemic (Collier et al. 2020; Sheriff et al. 2021), recommending the use of telehealth follow-up, appropriate sanitation and physical distancing measures and carefully assessing the risks and benefits of trial participation and continuation. However, careful attention regarding trials of immunosuppressive medications is also warranted.

Many 'first-in-class' immunosuppressive agents in dermatology have largely unknown risk profiles. These new agents may carry increased risk of infection, demonstrated in a randomised phase 2 trial of the IL-36 inhibitor spesolimab in pustular psoriasis with a 17% infection rate compared to 6% with placebo (Bachelez et al. 2021). In a similar phase 2 trial in atopic dermatitis, 9% of patients receiving spesolimab developed upper respiratory tract infections compared to none in the placebo control group (Bissonnette et al. 2022). Future, particularly early-phase, trials should consider and assess the potential for immunosuppressive medications to worsen COVID-19 outcomes in their pre-clinical research and establish plans with institutional review boards for if a trial participant is infected with SARS-CoV-2. This may include informing the patient to immediately notify their trial coordinator and treating physician to decide whether or not to continue or withhold the immunosuppressive medication.

During periods of acute rise in community infections with easing of public lockdowns, dermatologists should also carefully consider whether it is safe for patients to continue on trial, particularly for immunosuppressive medications. Patients may also rely on clinical trials for access to medications that they otherwise may not be able to afford (Torre and Shahriari 2017), and continuing an effective drug may be to their benefit. Furthermore, suspension of clinical trials may also delay regulatory approval which relies on their data (Drugs. U.S. Food and Drug Administration 2022). Dermatologists who conduct clinical research should therefore weigh the potential harms of enrolling and continuing patients on immunosuppressive drugs (non-maleficence) with the benefits of continuing the trials (beneficence). This is likely to be a dynamic process that reflects updated knowledge regarding the adverse events of each medication and the current state of the COVID-19 pandemic and public health orders.

In summary, the following recommendations regarding the management of immunosuppressed dermatology patients regarding clinical trials are made (Table 11.4):

Table 11.4 Recommendations regarding clinical trials

Recommendation	GRADE
Clinical trials may be safely continued with appropriate safety measures and use of telehealth to minimise exposure	D
Patients receiving immunosuppressive trial drugs should be informed to notify their treating physician that they are on a trial if they develop COVID-19	D
Institutional review boards should also consider the possibility of patients becoming infected with COVID-19, in balancing the risks and benefits of the trials	D
Patients should also know to inform the trial investigators promptly if they develop COVID-19, to decide whether it is necessary to withhold or suspend the trial drug(s)	D

Conclusion

The COVID-19 pandemic has resulted in monumental changes to the world as a whole, and the medical community has been no exception. Dermatologists caring for immunosuppressed patients have had to balance the risks of immunosuppression in case of SARS-CoV-2 infection with the benefits of controlling inflammatory skin disorders. Suggestions made in this chapter (regarding mitigating infection risk, active COVID-19, vaccination and clinical trials in dermatology) are based on the available data to date and may be subject to change based on future research to best optimise patient care. The data presentation and the proposed management strategies may enable dermatologists to lead evidence-based discussions with patients regarding the management of their risk profiles in the ongoing pandemic climate.

Funding Disclosures Nil relevant disclosures.

Conflicts of Interest JWF has conducted advisory work for Janssen, Boehringer Ingelheim, Pfizer, Kyowa Kirin, LEO Pharma, Regeneron, ChemoCentryx, AbbVie and UCB; participated in trials for Pfizer, UCB, Boehringer Ingelheim, Eli Lilly and CSL; and received research support from Ortho Dermatologics and Sun Pharma.

References

Abbas M, Robalo Nunes T, Martischang R, et al. Nosocomial transmission and outbreaks of coronavirus disease 2019: the need to protect both patients and healthcare workers. Antimicrob Resist Infect Control. 2021;10:1–13.

Adams L, Nakafero G, Grainge MJ, et al. Is vaccination against Covid-19 associated with psoriasis or eczema flare? Self-controlled case series analysis using data from the clinical practice research datalink (aurum). Br J Dermatol. 2022;188:297.

Alexander JL, Kennedy NA, Ibraheim H, et al. COVID-19 vaccine-induced antibody responses in immunosuppressed patients with inflammatory bowel disease (VIP): a multicentre, prospective, case-control study. Lancet Gastroenterol Hepatol. 2022;7:342–52.

Al-Janabi A, Ra A, Littlewood Z, et al. The effect of immunomodulators on seroconversion to BNT162b2 and AZD1222 vaccines in patients with immune-mediated inflammatory diseases: a prospective cohort study. Br J Dermatol. 2022;188:ljac109.

American Academy of Dermatology. Guidance on the use of immunosuppressive agents. https://www.aad.org/member/practice/coronavirus/clinical-guidance/biologics. Accessed 14 Dec 2022.

Andersen KM, Bates BA, Rashidi ES, et al. Long-term use of immunosuppressive medicines and in-hospital COVID-19 outcomes: a retrospective cohort study using data from the national COVID cohort collaborative. Lancet Rheumatol. 2022;4:e33–41.

Asaad M, Habibullah NK, Butler CE. The impact of COVID-19 on clinical trials. Ann Surg. 2020;272:e222–e3.

Bachelez H, Choon S-E, Marrakchi S, et al. Trial of spesolimab for generalized pustular psoriasis. N Engl J Med. 2021;385:2431–40.

Barouch DH. Covid-19 vaccines—immunity, variants, boosters. N Engl J Med. 2022;387:1011–20.

Bearse M, Hung YP, Krauson AJ, et al. Factors associated with myocardial SARS-CoV-2 infection, myocarditis, and cardiac inflammation in patients with COVID-19. Mod Pathol. 2021;34:1345–57.

Bissonnette R, Abramovits W, Saint-Cyr Proulx É, et al. Spesolimab, an anti-interleukin-36 receptor antibody, in patients with moderate-to-severe atopic dermatitis: results from a multicenter, randomized, double-blind, placebo-controlled, phase IIa study. J Eur Acad Dermatol Venereol. 2022;37:549.

Blanco-Melo D, Nilsson-Payant BE, Liu W-C, et al. Imbalanced host response to SARS-CoV-2 drives development of COVID-19. Cell. 2020;181:1036–45.

Bonelli MM, Mrak D, Perkmann T, Haslacher H, Aletaha D. SARS-CoV-2 vaccination in rituximab-treated patients: evidence for impaired humoral but inducible cellular immune response. Ann Rheum Dis. 2021;80:1355–6.

Brosh-Nissimov T, Orenbuch-Harroch E, Chowers M, et al. BNT162b2 vaccine breakthrough: clinical characteristics of 152 fully vaccinated hospitalized COVID-19 patients in Israel. Clin Microbiol Infect. 2021;27:1652–7.

Campioli CC, Cevallos EC, Assi M, Patel R, Binnicker MJ, O'Horo JC. Clinical predictors and timing of cessation of viral RNA shedding in patients with COVID-19. J Clin Virol. 2020;130:104577.

Cizmecioglu A, Akay Cizmecioglu H, Goktepe MH, et al. Apoptosis-induced T-cell lymphopenia is related to COVID-19 severity. J Med Virol. 2021;93:2867–74.

Cohen MS, Nirula A, Mulligan MJ, et al. Effect of bamlanivimab vs placebo on incidence of COVID-19 among residents and staff of skilled nursing and assisted living facilities: a randomized clinical trial. JAMA. 2021;326:46–55.

Collier EK, Hsiao JL, Shi VY. Conducting clinical trials during the COVID-19 pandemic. J Dermatol Treat. 2020;31:330–2.

Collier AY, Yu J, McMahan K, et al. Coronavirus Disease 2019 Messenger RNA vaccine immunogenicity in immunosuppressed individuals. J Infect Dis. 2022;225:1124–8.

Colmenero I, Santonja C, Alonso-Riaño M, et al. SARS-CoV-2 endothelial infection causes COVID-19 chilblains: histopathological, immunohistochemical and ultrastructural study of seven paediatric cases. Br J Dermatol. 2020;183:729–37.

Cox RJ, Brokstad KA. Not just antibodies: B cells and T cells mediate immunity to COVID-19. Nat Rev Immunol. 2020;20:581–2.

Damiani G, Pacifico A, Bragazzi NL, Malagoli P. Biologics increase the risk of SARS-CoV-2 infection and hospitalization, but not ICU admission and death: real-life data from a large cohort during red-zone declaration. Dermatol Ther. 2020;33:e13475.

Damiani G, Pacifico A, Pelloni F, Iorizzo M. The first dose of COVID-19 vaccine may trigger pemphigus and bullous pemphigoid flares: is the second dose therefore contraindicated? J Eur Acad Dermatol Venereol. 2021;35:e645.

Del Valle DM, Kim-Schulze S, Huang H-H, et al. An inflammatory cytokine signature predicts COVID-19 severity and survival. Nat Med. 2020;26:1636–43.

Desai S, Manjaly P, Lee KJ, Li SJ, Manjaly C, Mostaghimi A. The impact of COVID-19 on dermatology clinical trials. J Invest Dermatol. 2021;141:676.

Dougan M, Nirula A, Azizad M, et al. Bamlanivimab plus etesevimab in mild or moderate Covid-19. N Engl J Med. 2021;385:1382–92.

Drugs. U.S. Food and Drug Administration. Development & approval process. https://www.fda.gov/drugs/development-approval-process-drugs. Accessed 14 Dec 2022.

Eisenberg RA, Jawad AF, Boyer J, et al. Rituximab-treated patients have a poor response to influenza vaccination. J Clin Immunol. 2013;33:388–96.

Esmaeili S, Abbasi MH, Abolmaali M, et al. Rituximab and risk of COVID-19 infection and its severity in patients with MS and NMOSD. BMC Neurol. 2021;21:183.

Fahmy DH, El-Amawy HS, El-Samongy MA, et al. COVID-19 and dermatology: a comprehensive guide for dermatologists. J Eur Acad Dermatol Venereol. 2020;34:1388–94.

Flora A, Frew JW. Angiotensin-converting enzyme 2 expression is elevated in tissue of hidradenitis suppurativa and pyoderma gangrenosum and demonstrates a different pattern of expression to psoriasis vulgaris. J Eur Acad Dermatol Venereol. 2022;37:e372.

Gupta A, Gonzalez-Rojas Y, Juarez E, et al. Early treatment for Covid-19 with SARS-CoV-2 neutralizing antibody sotrovimab. N Engl J Med. 2021;385:1941–50.

Horby P, Lim WS, Emberson JR, et al. Dexamethasone in hospitalized patients with Covid-19. N Engl J Med. 2021;384:693–704.

Hsu L, Armstrong AW. Anti-drug antibodies in psoriasis: a critical evaluation of clinical significance and impact on treatment response. Expert Rev Clin Immunol. 2013;9:949–58.

Huet T, Beaussier H, Voisin O, et al. Anakinra for severe forms of COVID-19: a cohort study. Lancet Rheumatol. 2020;2:e393–400.

Jyssum I, Kared H, Tran TT, et al. Humoral and cellular immune responses to two and three doses of SARS-

CoV-2 vaccines in rituximab-treated patients with rheumatoid arthritis: a prospective, cohort study. Lancet Rheumatol. 2022;4:e177–e87.

Kalil AC, Patterson TF, Mehta AK, et al. Baricitinib plus remdesivir for hospitalized adults with Covid-19. N Engl J Med. 2021;384:795–807.

Krueger JG, Murrell DF, Garcet S, et al. Secukinumab lowers expression of ACE2 in affected skin of patients with psoriasis. J Allergy Clin Immunol. 2021;147:1107–9.

Lebwohl M, Rivera-Oyola R, Murrell DF. Should biologics for psoriasis be interrupted in the era of COVID-19? J Am Acad Dermatol. 2020;82:1217–8.

Levavi H, Lancman G, Gabrilove J. Impact of rituximab on COVID-19 outcomes. Ann Hematol. 2021;100:2805–12.

Levin MJ, Ustianowski A, De Wit S, et al. Intramuscular AZD7442 (Tixagevimab-Cilgavimab) for prevention of Covid-19. N Engl J Med. 2022;386:2188–200.

Li TZ, Cao ZH, Chen Y, et al. Duration of SARS-CoV-2 RNA shedding and factors associated with prolonged viral shedding in patients with COVID-19. J Med Virol. 2021;93:506–12.

Lim HW, Feldman SR, Van Voorhees AS, Gelfand JM. Recommendations for phototherapy during the COVID-19 pandemic. J Am Acad Dermatol. 2020;83:287–8.

MacKenna B, Kennedy NA, Mehrkar A, et al. Risk of severe COVID-19 outcomes associated with immune-mediated inflammatory diseases and immune-modifying therapies: a nationwide cohort study in the OpenSAFELY platform. Lancet Rheumatol. 2022;4:e490–506.

Mahil SK, Dand N, Mason KJ, et al. Factors associated with adverse COVID-19 outcomes in patients with psoriasis—insights from a global registry–based study. J Allergy Clin Immunol. 2021;147:60–71.

Man Z, Jing Z, Huibo S, Bin L, Fanjun Z. Viral shedding prolongation in a kidney transplant patient with COVID-19 pneumonia. Am J Transplant. 2020;20:2626–7.

Marovich M, Mascola JR, Cohen MS. Monoclonal antibodies for prevention and treatment of COVID-19. JAMA. 2020;324:131–2.

Meckiff BJ, Ramírez-Suástegui C, Fajardo V, et al. Imbalance of regulatory and cytotoxic SARS-CoV-2-reactive CD4+ T cells in COVID-19. Cell. 2020;183:1340–53.e16.

Mehta P, Porter JC, Chambers RC, Isenberg DA, Reddy V. B-cell depletion with rituximab in the COVID-19 pandemic: where do we stand? Lancet Rheumatol. 2020;2:e589–e90.

Moor MB, Suter-Riniker F, Horn MP, et al. Humoral and cellular responses to mRNA vaccines against SARS-CoV-2 in patients with a history of CD20 B-cell-depleting therapy (RituxiVac): an investigator-initiated, single-centre, open-label study. Lancet Rheumatol. 2021;3:e789–e97.

Mrak D, Sieghart D, Simader E, et al. Heterologous vector versus homologous mRNA COVID-19 booster vaccination in non-seroconverted immunosuppressed patients: a randomized controlled trial. Nat Commun. 2022;13:5362.

Niaki OZ, Anadkat MJ, Chen ST, et al. Navigating immunosuppression in a pandemic: a guide for the dermatologist from the COVID task force of the Medical Dermatology Society and Society of Dermatology Hospitalists. J Am Acad Dermatol. 2020;83:1150–9.

Norden A, Moon JY, Javadi SS, Munawar L, Maul JT, Wu JJ. Anti-drug antibodies of IL-23 inhibitors for psoriasis: a systematic review. J Eur Acad Dermatol Venereol. 2022;36:1171.

Osuchowski MF, Winkler MS, Skirecki T, et al. The COVID-19 puzzle: deciphering pathophysiology and phenotypes of a new disease entity. Lancet Respir Med. 2021;9:622–42.

Pakhchanian H, Khan H, Raiker R, et al. COVID-19 outcomes in patients with dermatomyositis: a registry-based cohort analysis. Semin Arthritis Rheum. 2022;56:152034.

Prens LM, Bouwman K, Aarts P, et al. Adalimumab and infliximab survival in patients with hidradenitis suppurativa: a daily practice cohort study. Br J Dermatol. 2021;185:177–84.

Price KN, Frew JW, Hsiao JL, Shi VY. COVID-19 and immunomodulator/immunosuppressant use in dermatology. J Am Acad Dermatol. 2020;82:e173–e5.

Raiker R, Pakhchanian H, Pham J, Phan K. Coronavirus disease 2019 complications in patients with hidradenitis suppurativa: a multicenter analysis. J Dermatol. 2021;48:1619–21.

Reich K, Jackson K, Ball S, et al. Ixekizumab pharmacokinetics, anti-drug antibodies, and efficacy through 60 weeks of treatment of moderate to severe plaque psoriasis. J Investig Dermatol. 2018;138:2168–73.

Sahin U, Muik A, Derhovanessian E, et al. COVID-19 vaccine BNT162b1 elicits human antibody and TH1 T cell responses. Nature. 2020;586:594–9.

Schmidt E, Kasperkiewicz M, Joly P. Pemphigus. Lancet. 2019;394:882–94.

Schwartz RA, Pradhan S, Murrell DF, et al. COVID-19 and immunosuppressive therapy in dermatology. Dermatol Ther. 2020;33:e14140.

Serrano GE, Walker JE, Arce R, et al. Mapping of SARS-CoV-2 brain invasion and histopathology in COVID-19 disease. Medrxiv; 2021.

Shen X-R, Geng R, Li Q, et al. ACE2-independent infection of T lymphocytes by SARS-CoV-2. Signal Transduct Target Ther. 2022;7:1–11.

Sheriff T, Dickenson-Panas H, Murrell DF. Conducting dermatology clinical trials during the COVID-19 pandemic. Clin Dermatol. 2021;39:104–6.

Siemieniuk R, Guyatt G. What is GRADE? BMJ Best Practice. 2021.

Sotiriou E, Tsentemeidou A, Bakirtzi K, Lallas A, Ioannides D, Vakirlis E. Psoriasis exacerbation after COVID-19 vaccination: a report of 14 cases from a single centre. J Eur Acad Dermatol Venereol. 2021;35:e857.

Stanifer ML, Kee C, Cortese M, et al. Critical role of type III interferon in controlling SARS-CoV-2 infection in human intestinal epithelial cells. Cell Rep. 2020;32:107863.

Stone JH, Frigault MJ, Serling-Boyd NJ, et al. Efficacy of tocilizumab in patients hospitalized with Covid-19. N Engl J Med. 2020;383:2333–44.

Sun Y, Zhou R, Zhang H, et al. Skin is a potential host of SARS-CoV-2: a clinical, single-cell transcriptome-profiling and histologic study. J Am Acad Dermatol. 2020;83:1755–7.

Swanson PA, Padilla M, Hoyland W, et al. AZD1222/ChAdOx1 nCoV-19 vaccination induces a polyfunctional spike protein–specific TH1 response with a diverse TCR repertoire. Sci Transl Med. 2021;13:eabj7211.

Tanne JH. Covid-19: CDC shortens isolation period as US cases hit record high. British Medical Journal Publishing Group; 2021.

Tembhre MK, Parihar AS, Sharma VK, et al. Enhanced expression of angiotensin-converting enzyme 2 in psoriatic skin and its upregulation in keratinocytes by interferon-γ: implication of inflammatory milieu in skin tropism of SARS-CoV-2. Br J Dermatol. 2021;184:577–9.

Tenforde MW, Patel MM, Ginde AA, et al. Effectiveness of severe acute respiratory syndrome coronavirus 2 messenger RNA vaccines for preventing coronavirus Disease 2019 hospitalizations in the United States. Clin Infect Dis. 2022;74:1515–24.

Torre K, Shahriari M. Clinical trials in dermatology. Int J Womens Dermatol. 2017;3:180–3.

U.S. Food and Drug Administration. Fact Sheet for Health Care Providers Emergency Use Authorisation (EUA) of Bamlanivimab and Etesevimab. https://www.fda.gov/media/145802/download. Accessed 14 Dec 2022.

Van Assen S, Holvast A, Benne CA, et al. Humoral responses after influenza vaccination are severely reduced in patients with rheumatoid arthritis treated with rituximab. Arthritis Rheum. 2010;62:75–81.

van Dorn A. COVID-19 and readjusting clinical trials. Lancet. 2020;396:523–4.

Vanderbeke L, Van Mol P, Van Herck Y, et al. Monocyte-driven atypical cytokine storm and aberrant neutrophil activation as key mediators of COVID-19 disease severity. Nat Commun. 2021;12:4117.

Wang J, Jiang M, Chen X, Montaner LJ. Cytokine storm and leukocyte changes in mild versus severe SARS-CoV-2 infection: review of 3939 COVID-19 patients in China and emerging pathogenesis and therapy concepts. J Leukoc Biol. 2020;108:17–41.

WHO Coronavirus (COVID-19) Dashboard. World Health Organization. https://covid19.who.int/. Accessed 13 Dec 2022.

Xu Q, Chen L, Li X, Zheng J. If skin is a potential host of SARS-CoV-2, IL-17 antibody could reduce the risk of COVID-19. J Am Acad Dermatol. 2021;84:e173.

Zhang X, Tan Y, Ling Y, et al. Viral and host factors related to the clinical outcome of COVID-19. Nature. 2020;583:437–40.

Zheng C, Shao W, Chen X, Zhang B, Wang G, Zhang W. Real-world effectiveness of COVID-19 vaccines: a literature review and meta-analysis. Int J Infect Dis. 2022;114:252–60.

Therapeutic Considerations of COVID-19 on Aesthetic Dermatology, Dermatosurgery and Skin Cancer

Danica Xie and John R. Sullivan

Introduction

Dermatological consultation, procedures and post-procedure care should be performed in a way that minimises the risk of COVID-19 transmission without compromising on safety measures or the quality of care provided. Individual clinicians' therapeutic preferences and cosmetic practices vary, so this chapter will include general considerations around COVID-19 and aesthetic dermatology, dermatosurgery and skin cancer. Since 2020, vaccine rollouts and improved COVID-19 testing worldwide continue to change the landscape of safe practice recommendations. This has provided clinics with a good opportunity to review their infection control, including droplet and electrosurgical and laser plume precautions.

There are three accepted modes of viral transmission: direct contact with contaminated surfaces (fomites), larger respiratory droplets and small micro-droplets known as aerosols. Droplets spread remains the main infection concern with SARS-CoV-2 which can be enhanced by speaking.

Aerosol-generating procedures have been identified to be of risk to healthcare workers (HCWs). Examples include nebulised therapy and airway suctioning. Generally, dermatology procedures do not generate aerosols; however, persistent and/or severe coughing and screaming (children) can also generate aerosols. The risk of transmission can be increased with the prolonged, close proximity involved in performing procedures near the nose or mouth. Asymptomatic (and symptomatic) patients and staff capable of transmitting the virus will continue to attend dermatologic procedures, necessitating a level of standard and close patient contact precautions. Measures should continue to minimise the risk of patients with suspected or confirmed SARS-CoV-2 infection attending the practice for consultation, treatment or follow-up.

General precautions in distancing during history-taking and consent processes remain advised, maintaining greater than 1 m distance where possible and incorporating the benefits of universal mask wearing (Chu et al. 2020). When in close proximity such as examination and treatments, attention should be directed to appropriate personal protective equipment and careful patient preparation.

Further, it is important to consider evolution in the COVID-19 pandemic including case surges that may be seasonal or related to new strains. Variation in community prevalence, second and subsequent infections, impact of vaccination

D. Xie · J. R. Sullivan (✉)
Dermatology Department, The Sutherland Hospital, Sydney, NSW, Australia

Faculty of Medicine, University of New South Wales, Sydney, NSW, Australia
e-mail: jrsullivan@kdaa.com.au

© The Author(s), under exclusive license to Springer Nature Switzerland AG 2023
H. H. Oon, C. L. Goh (eds.), *COVID-19 in Dermatology*, Updates in Clinical Dermatology,
https://doi.org/10.1007/978-3-031-45586-5_12

including bivalent COVID-19 mRNA vaccines, access to anti-viral medications and other factors all need to be taken into account in the provision of dermatological care. The aim of this chapter is to provide guidance; however, recommendations are not proscriptive.

Dermatology care should normally include the following precautions to protect and minimise infections for patients and staff in the context of local government regulations and requirements along with hospital policies.

This chapter focuses on several procedural dermatology areas. The impact of SARS-CoV-2 overlaps but also differs for aesthetic dermatology, dermatosurgery or skin cancer. Important differences include the generally elective nature of aesthetic dermatology. Many aesthetic dermatology procedures however are performed also for therapeutic indications and can have psychological benefits.

Whilst the priority of a preventative 'field cancerisation' treatment is similarly not as medically time sensitive, the timely management of skin cancer remains important. The SARS-CoV-2 pandemic saw a 32% decrease in melanoma diagnosis in Australia, with a similar delay in diagnosis in other cancers which may be quick to metastasise (Boniface and Tapia-Rico 2022; Roseleur et al. 2021). This likely varied between countries due to differences in their pandemic management strategies, such as the duration and nature of lockdowns. High-risk SARS-CoV-2 individuals, such as solid organ transplant patients, are particularly vulnerable to delaying scheduled skin cancer screening (Mokos and Bašić-Jukić 2021). The increased utilisation of audio-visual participation has also assisted multidisciplinary team involvement in patient care where appropriate (Abi Rafeh et al. 2021). Deferment of elective treatment also has significant health implications and should be limited.

COVID infection including 'long COVID' should also be considered, with its range of physical and psychological symptoms. This can include anxiety, depression, posttraumatic stress disorder and cognitive symptoms (Crook et al. 2021; Luo et al. 2020). 'Long COVID' should be considered, for example, for aesthetic dermatology treatments. This could include opting for botulinum toxin A (BoNT-A) over a greater morbidity and downtime-associated procedure such as an aggressive laser resurfacing treatment in a mentally fragile patient.

The safety of individual staff at higher risk of severe SARS-CoV-2 infection needs to be also considered. Pregnancy, for example, appears to worsen the clinical course of COVID-19, and infection appears to increase maternal and neonatal morbidity (risk of preterm birth, preeclampsia) and mortality (Villar et al. 2021).

In summary, patient-centred care should aim to do no harm, and this is particularly important for patients in vulnerable or high-risk COVID-19 settings.

Infection Control

Despite the enormous published literature in regard to COVID-19 including its transmission, the level of evidence for precautions to prevent infection in clinical areas remains low level or grade. Lessons from the COVID-19 pandemic however have provided impetus for clinicians and providers to review infection control and occupational health and safety precautions including respiratory protection precautions regarding the safety and quality of the air both staff and patients breathe.

The importance of aseptic precautions including skin asepsis should be guided by our traditional infective concerns including common pathogens from *Staph aureus* to biofilms for procedures involving implants such as hyaluronic acid fillers and skin threads.

The risk of SARS-CoV-2 transmission via contaminated surfaces (fomites) emphasises the importance of clean, uncluttered, disinfected work areas along with antisepsis. This is key for performing procedural dermatology services safely.

Review of ventilation of indoor work areas including clinical spaces should be done. The monitoring of carbon dioxide (CO_2) levels in clinical and work areas over the course of a working day can be useful. CO_2 levels rise in occupied spaces that are inadequately ventilated. Consideration should also be given to using portable high-efficiency particulate air (HEPA) filtration systems (Lindsley et al. 2021). Some portable air filters also contain carbon filters which may have additional benefits for electrosurgery and ablative laser plume.

Fortunately, good clinical practice precautions and facility design also appear to provide benefits to reduce COVID-19 transmission from appropriate handwashing, skin cleaning and antisepsis through to eye protection and air management.

Viral Infectivity and Dermatological Procedures

Human-to-human spread of SARS-CoV-2 is common via droplets and aerosols, where the virus can survive for several hours (Doremalen et al. 2020). Many dermatological procedures are focused on the face, where the nose, mouth and mucosal surfaces represent areas of high SARS-CoV-2 exposure. There is a theoretical increased risk of transmission with aerosol-generating procedures. These are not commonly utilised in dermatology; however, dermatologic laser and electrosurgery can generate smoke or plumes. Such plumes have been reported to contain HPV DNA in the plume, including those generated by the CO_2 laser treatment of respiratory tract papillomas and plantar warts (Garden et al. 1988; Kashima et al. 1991). Further, SARS-CoV-2 can remain infective on porous fomites (e.g. cotton gown, paper, gloves) for a few hours or on nonporous surfaces (e.g. stainless steel, plastic) for 4 days with complete decay at 9 days (Aboubakr et al. 2021).

Regular handwashing before and after patient contact, including after removal of PPE, is recommended to reduce the risk of COVID-19 transmission (Narla et al. 2021). In addition to possible fomite transmission, the survival time of SARS-CoV-2 on the human skin is approximately 9 h (Hirose et al. 2021). Washing hands with soap and water for at least 20 s removes 99.7% bacteria based on a study done for the food industry (Jensen et al. 2015). Alcohol-based hand sanitisers containing at least 60% alcohol can be used; however, they may not be as effective when hands are visibly soiled. Latex and nitrite gloves are preferable to vinyl, to minimise the risk of viral exposure (Rego and Roley 1999; Rundle et al. 2020). Generally, it is advisable to avoid touching the eyes, nose and mouth.

Personal Protective Precautions (Table 12.1)

Masks Minimise Droplet Transmission

Patients and healthcare providers are recommended to use masks to reduce the risk of transmitting COVID-19. In asymptomatic individuals, thousands of oral fluid droplets of inhalable par-

Table 12.1 Guidance for personal protective equipment (PPE) according to different levels of precautions in the aesthetic and surgical dermatology setting

Level of precautions[a]	Examples in aesthetic and surgical dermatology	Suggested PPE
Standard	Routine consultation Reception or waiting room	Precautions to vary with community COVID-19 transmission
Close patient contact	Full skin examination Cryotherapy Photodynamic therapy Chemical peels BoNT-A Dermal fillers	Consider droplet or airborne transmission precautions Surgical or N95 masks Eye shields or wrap-around glasses or combined mask/upper face shield
Laser and electrosurgical plumes	Laser procedures Monopolar or bipolar cautery	N95/P2 masks Eye shields or wrap-around protective (including laser[b]) glasses
Aerosol-generating procedures (uncommon in dermatology)	Medical gases aerosolised by a mask Surgical procedures requiring general anaesthetic Screaming child	N95/P2 masks Eye shields or wrap-around glasses Face shield Protective gown

[a]Will vary with the level of community transmission and healthcare worker risk
[b]Appropriate laser safety glass choice should be based on laser (or light) hazard requirements

ticle size (<5 µm diameter) are produced when speaking, potentially transmitting pre-symptomatic SARS-CoV-2 (Anfinrud et al. 2020). High viral loads of SARS-CoV-2 have been detected in oral fluids of COVID-19 patients with and without symptoms (Chan et al. 2020). Further, a recent small study demonstrated that SARS-CoV-2 and SARS-CoV-2 remained viable and infectious in aerosols for at least 3 h ($n = 2$) (Van Doremalen et al. 2020). A laser rated or N95 mask should also be considered for any PM2.5 (particulate matter) (≤2.5 µm)-generating procedures in dermatology including laser, electrocautery and cryotherapy with high levels of PM2.5 reported to be associated with an increase in respiratory disease and infection (Mermiri et al. 2022).

Dermatology Procedures Near the Face Pose a Transmission Risk

In dermatology, physician and staff masking is particularly important for procedures near the nose and mouth (Narla et al. 2021). Healthcare professionals that manage patient with diseases of the aerodigestive tract (including dentists, head and neck surgeons, otolaryngologists, respiratory physicians, gastroenterologists and speech therapists) or ophthalmologists are most susceptible to become infected (risk ratio 2.13) (Kowalski et al. 2020). Aside from the possible spread from respiratory secretions in these specialties, there is also a strong association between proximity of the exposed individual and the risk of infection, with an absolute risk of 12.8% with shorter distance (<1 m) vs. 2.6% with further distance (≥1 m) (risk difference −10.2%, 95% CI −11.5 to −7.5) (Chu et al. 2020).

Surgical Masks vs. Respirator Masks

There is no high-quality evidence on whether N95 respirators are better than surgical masks for healthcare worker protection from SARS-CoV-2 (Iannone et al. 2020). For SARS-CoV-2, respiratory aqueous droplets are the main infection risk concern rather than individual viral particles and are filtered by surgical masks. The facial seal has been shown to be important in the effectiveness of masks for filtering the air we breathe and

exhale. N95 have become a good laser and mask for performing head and neck procedures as they traditionally provide a better face seal (Li et al. 2021). However, it should be noted the fit and protection provided are reduced in those with more facial hair (Sandaradura et al. 2020). If wearing N95 masks, clinicians should undergo fit-testing with an appropriate mask.

When it comes to electrosurgical and laser plumes, seal and fit are likely similarly important. Electrosurgical and laser plumes generate smaller particles such as PM2.5, carcinogens and ultra-fine particles (UFP) (<0.1 µm) that are inhalable and can be deposited in the alveoli (Brace et al. 2014). Smaller particles carry chemical (and PM) risks, whilst large particles have been demonstrated to exhibit infectivity potential (Mowbray et al. 2013).

There are no studies on the effect on COVID-19 transmission between standard surgical masks and N95 masks in dermatology or aesthetic dermatology procedures or during other minor dermatosurgery procedures in a clinic setting. Bartoszko and colleagues (Bartoszko et al. 2020) performed a systemic review and meta-analysis on the efficacy of surgical masks and N95 respirators for preventing COVID-19 in healthcare workers. Low certainty evidence suggests that both masks offer similar protection against viruses including coronavirus in non-aerosol-generating procedures. In another systematic review and meta-analysis including composite data for SARS-CoV-2, severe acute respiratory syndrome (SARS) and Middle East respiratory syndrome (MERS), Chu et al. found that face masks could result in a large reduction in risk of infection ($n = 2647$; aOR 0.15, 95% CI 0.07 to 0.34, RD −14.3%, −15.9 to −10.7), with stronger associations with N95 or similar respirators compared with disposable surgical masks (Chu et al. 2020). Further, this interaction was also seen when adjusting for aerosol-generating procedures ($p = 0.048$).

Other Protective Precautions

Eye protection is recommended during laser and dermatologic surgery to protect from eye injury and infection transmission. Evidence reinforces its value also regarding COVID-19 transmission (Narla et al. 2021). A recent systematic review and meta-analysis of composite data for SARS-CoV-2, SARS and MERS found that eye protection was associated with less infection ($n = 3713$; aOR 0.22, 95% CI 0.12 to 0·39, RD −10.6%, 95% CI −12.5 to −7.7) (Chu et al. 2020). Most laser and light protection glasses are wrap-around in design, similar to surgical safety protective eyewear. The wearing of corrective glasses can generally be accommodated by selective appropriate laser glasses and safety eyewear. Some advocate for an additional face shield for high-risk patients, staff and procedures.

As SARS-CoV-2 can remain infective on cotton for a few hours, clinicians may choose to wear disposable gowns on top of work scrubs and may change out of these on leaving work (Ren et al. 2020).

Equipment Care

Cleaning and disinfection of surfaces and medical equipment is an important aspect of infection control. Equipment including dermatoscopes and energy-based devices should be cleaned with detergent and then disinfected. Both 70–90% alcohol and sodium hypochlorite 0.05–0.1% are recommended disinfectants (World Health Organization 2020); however, it is important to follow manufacturer recommendations of compatible products with many other disinfectants shown to have activity against pathogens including COVID-19 (Kampf et al. 2020; World Health Organization 2020). It is important to note that bleach is often damaging to surfaces and medical equipment such as lasers and medical devices. Always check with the manufacturer regarding suitable products.

Existing recommendations are based on a significant reduction of coronavirus activity on surfaces within 30 s to 1 min exposure time. Low-touch or minimally contaminated surfaces such as laser touch screens should also be disinfected between patients. Single-use patient eye protection should be considered. It is otherwise important to ensure re-useable patient eye protec-

tion or equipment should be cleaned and disinfected between patients. This should take into account agents used and eye risks such as seen with chlorhexidine. Again, 70–80% alcohol remains a safe choice.

Patient Preparation and Antisepsis

To reduce patient time spent in the practice including waiting areas, some practices advocate for patient self-application of anaesthetic creams prior to arrival. Patients should remove creams or cosmetic products and wash areas being treated for at least 20 s prior to skin antisepsis.

Commonly used skin antisepsis agents can also protect against SARS-CoV-2. These are chosen based on procedure, patient and balance of risks. Skin antisepsis should be chosen to cover and protect against known pathogen and treatment risks.

Appropriate skin antisepsis remains important for patient safety for dermatologic surgery and aesthetic dermatology including dermal fillers and skin threads.

There remains no evidence to show that ablative laser procedures increase the risk of contracting COVID-19. Laser (and electrosurgical) plumes however have been shown to contain viruses (HPV), bacteria and deoxyribonucleic acid along with carbon particles and toxic gases. Skin antisepsis should be considered to reduce some of these risks; this would not however eliminate the risk of aerosolised blood and blood-borne pathogens or those found in other secretions when treating near or on mucosal areas.

Dwell time is the duration of time disinfectants' need to remain wet on surfaces to properly disinfect. Alcohol (isopropyl- or ethyl-) with or without chlorhexidine 0.05–0.1% or povidone-iodine are fast acting and have proven to inactivate SARS-CoV-2 with dwell times between 15 and 30 s (Bidra et al. 2020). Specific points for different agents are listed below:

Hand rubs:

- Ethanol and 2-propanol of >30% (vol/vol) are sufficient for the complete viral inactivation of

SARS-CoV-2 in 30 s (Kratzel et al. 2020). However, ethanol 70% which is a commercially available concentration can completely inactivate SARS-CoV-2 at 30 s of contact (Bidra et al. 2020).

In regard to disinfecting surfaces and equipment, it is important to both clean and then disinfect. Some agents have been designed to do both.

Any disinfectant product should meet the criteria for use against SARS-CoV-2 such as WHO standards or the Environmental Protection Agency (EPA).

Surface disinfectants:

- Sodium hypochlorite 0.1% and 0.05% can inactivate SARS-CoV-2 in less than 1 min (Kampf et al. 2020).
- Hydrogen peroxide 0.5% is effective against human coronavirus (HCoV) within 1 min of exposure time (Kampf et al. 2020). However, studies of the in vitro effectiveness of hydrogen peroxide 1.5% against SARS-CoV-2 demonstrate minimal effectiveness (Davies et al. 2021).

Laser treatment is one area where there is significant variation in current practice, and COVID-19 provides a good opportunity to review these practices. For ablative laser procedures, it is common to utilise an antiseptic. However, consider chromophore and avoid povidone-iodine (a competing chromophore) for lasers in the visible spectrum.

Aerosol-Generating Procedures

Laser and electrosurgical plumes contain PM2.5 particles along with potential carcinogens (Mowbray et al. 2013). Positive association between air pollutants and the transmission and severity of COVID-19 serves as a reminder as to the importance of effective electrosurgical and laser plume management for staff and patient health (Wu et al. 2020; Domingo and Rovira 2020; Marquès and Domingo 2022).

Wearing correctly fitted N95 and using a smoke evacuator are recommended. Guidance includes holding the tip of the smoke evacuator handpiece within 2.5 cm of the site of laser skin interaction.

Aesthetic Dermatology

Laser Plumes

There remains no good evidence that laser and electrosurgical plumes are a source of COVID infection. Plume management aims to address other infective and health risks.

Smoke evacuator systems for managing electrosurgical and laser plumes now commonly include ULPA filters, which are designed to also filter out individual viral particles such as HPV. Some include HEPA filters which filter out most viral particles but not individual viral particles. Carbon filters are also now usually included (for filtering carcinogens).

Air-Cooling and Cryocooling Systems During Laser Procedures

Cooling devices are utilised for both patient safety and comfort during laser and light procedures. Air handling appears important in SARS-CoV-2 transmission. The virus favours cool environments as demonstrated by outbreaks in abattoir and meat processing facilities. Cryocoolers may also dissipate the virus.

There is insufficient study to provide guidance, but it is prudent for staff to wear eye and respiratory protection whilst cooling systems are in use. Antisepsis of skin areas being treated and patient wearing of a mask where appropriate and practical could also be considered.

Patients routinely should be provided eye protection for other safety reasons, but masks are not always practical with many laser treatments frequently addressing head and neck concerns.

Chemical Peels

Many laser- and energy-based treatments along with stronger chemical peels lead to breaks in the skin barrier and thus an impaired skin barrier.

Although risk has not been demonstrated that skin provides a clinically significant source of infection, it has not been studied as to whether broken inflamed skin puts a patient at an increased risk of infection via the skin by infected droplets. The theoretical risk can stem from *ACE2* receptors being found on keratinocytes of the human skin, a key receptor of the SARS-CoV-2 spike protein.

Dermatosurgery

Electrosurgical Treatments (Cautery)

Having portable HEPA air filters has been shown to reduce and clear airborne COVID-19, and many also include carbon filters, ionisers or ultraviolet light to remove viral particles (see section "Laser Plumes").

When using electrosurgery, consideration should be given to using a smoke evacuator and N95 mask for other infection control and respiratory health reasons. This may have benefits in reducing aerosolised tissue particles or blood. Electrosurgery using bipolar also produces less electrosurgical plume compared to monopolar (hyfrecation). Bipolar electrosurgery could be considered where a smoke evacuator and N95 masks are not available.

Medical Gases Aerosolised Via a Mask

COVID-19 considerations around analgesia delivery in surgical procedures include the aerosolisation of nitrous oxide. Free-flow mask delivery carries a greater potential aerosol generation versus demand delivery systems. Demand delivery also has greater safety in limiting dosing.

In paediatric procedures, consider a screaming child as an aerosol risk (potentially enhanced by a free-flow nitrous mask). Age can limit use of demand delivery systems.

Skin Cancer

Cryotherapy

There is no proven additional transmission risk of cryotherapy but often performed around the sites of increased theoretical transmission, such as the nose and mouth. See section "Air-Cooling and Cryocooling".

Photodynamic Therapy

Some people utilise water spraying, fan and cooling for laser treatments, which carry a risk relating to improper air handling or droplet protection.

Non-Aerosol- and Laser Plume-Generating Procedures

Adverse Reactions to Hyaluronic Acid Filler Following SARS-CoV-2 Infection

There are several reports of reactions to cosmetic procedures in the context of SARS-CoV-2 infection or vaccination (Munavalli et al. 2022). Rowland-Warmann (Rowland-Warmann 2021) reports a patient who presented with delayed-type hypersensitivity reaction to hyaluronic dermal filler after a severe SARS-CoV-2 infection. This presented as induration, erythema, tenderness and swelling around the radix 3 weeks post confirmed SARS-CoV-2 infection, where HA dermal filler was placed for a non-surgical rhinoplasty 4 months prior. Similarly, another patient experienced sudden swelling in the periocular area 3 weeks after SARS-CoV-2 had HA dermal filler placed for facial rejuvenation 10 months prior (Shome et al. 2021).

COVID Vaccine-Related Adverse Effects

Dermal filler reactions (swelling, erythema, tenderness, lip angioedema) have been reported post-Moderna COVID-19 vaccine in areas that had previously undergone dermal filler placement (n = 3/15,184) (Food and Drug Administration (FDA) Center for Biologics Evaluation and Research (CBER) 2020). Filler placement ranged from 2 weeks to 6 months prior to vaccination. These rare adverse events often resolved without treatment; however, oral steroids and hyaluronidase have been utilised to manage this uncommon occurrence.

Additionally, a rare interaction between BoNT-A and COVID-19 vaccination has been reported in two patients (Guo et al. 2021). Both patients developed generalised facial swelling and flu-like symptoms within 12 h of BoNT-A administration, which was 2 weeks and 2 months post-Sinovac (Vero Cell COVID) vaccination, respectively. Given that both patients had previous BoNT-A treatment which were uneventful, the possibility of allergy to BoNT-A was less likely. Neither patients had respiratory compromise and were managed with oral steroids and antihistamines in the emergency department.

Other Clinic and Patient Factors

Patient Flow

Patients vary in their susceptibility to severe disease. Patient flow and safety precautions need to take into consideration these more vulnerable patients. In aesthetic dermatology practice, the elective nature and importance of patient experience have always made patient scheduling and designing waiting areas to provide patients with their own space an important consideration. Fomite risks should lead to a review of plush finishing in treatment (and waiting) areas such as fur-like throws and cushions on treatment couches in some cosmetic practices and decorative items that make cleaning and disinfecting harder. Safety should be prioritised over a cosmetic sense of luxury where they may compromise infection control. It is important to emphasise that these are medical treatments and designing cosmetic treatment rooms with infection control and health and safety can be prioritised without compromising patient comfort.

The COVID-19 pandemic provided impetus for keeping patient waiting times and the duration of attendance to a minimum. Consideration should be given where practical to working between multiple rooms allowing time for cleaning of rooms and equipment between patients and reducing time spent in common waiting areas. Socially distanced chairs in the waiting room can also minimise risk of transmission.

Although cosmetic injectables and laser or light treatments may be performed at the same patient visit, consideration should be given to avoiding scheduling multiple procedures during the same patient visit. This is particularly if it involves prolonged period of patient contact including the use of multiple rooms, the involvement of multiple staff members and a greater range of medical equipment.

Although carers and support people remain important in many circumstances, discouraging attendance of relatives and friends remains prudent unless indicated or needed.

The SARS-CoV-2 pandemic also enhanced our telemedicine options. This should continue to be utilised for the enhanced follow-up of patients after procedures for complications and to reduce the need for clinic attendance.

Vaccination

Levels of vaccination and recency of vaccination vary between countries, along with the effectiveness of vaccines. Recency of infection and boosters including those designed to include more recent strains all alter infection risks. Vaccination has been shown to reduce the risk of developing more severe disease and death. The risk of infection still persists but can be minimised with opportunistic counselling of unvaccinated patients. All healthcare workers including support staff and admin should be encouraged to receive vaccination according to government protocol (Narla et al. 2021).

Sedation and General Anaesthetic

Most of our procedures are performed on an awake patient and utilise local anaesthetic and analgesia rather than sedation. This carries less risk for the patient should they unknowingly be infected with SARS-CoV-2. Sedation and general anaesthetic are however utilised and need to factor in SARS-CoV-2 and follow local guidance. This may be utilised for skin cancer surgery, ablative laser and field photodynamic therapy. These include the recommendation to avoid elective surgery within 7 weeks of infection unless the benefits of doing so exceed the risk of waiting (El-Boghdadly et al. 2022). The risk of infection for staff also requires special consideration in regard to non-urgent or 'elective' surgery within 10 days of a patient diagnosis of SARS-CoV-2 infection.

Increased perioperative risks including mortality are seen throughout the 6 weeks after asymptomatic SARS-CoV-2 infection with previous variants. Other factors beyond timing are also important including the severity of infection and assessment of increased anaesthetic risk. It is also preferable that patients have had three vaccine doses where possible. Depending on population risk, screening and testing for SARS-CoV-2 infection should be considered in patients where general anaesthetic is planned.

Training

The SARS-CoV-2 pandemic has reduced training opportunities for junior staff and others wanting to upskill. Continued training is essential as highlighted by the ongoing pressures on the healthcare system several years after the pandemic was declared. The value of training of junior dermatology staff along with that of practice nurses assisting with laser treatments and surgical procedures should not be neglected. With ongoing COVID-19 concerns, it is important to make sure patient, staff and trainee numbers are kept appropriate regarding social distancing and facility limitations. It remains important to adhere to local requirements; small group and peer learning may also improve the patient experience when done well. Small group peer training also improves collegial connection, contributes to

well-being and reduces professional stress, all of which remain important for healthcare worker health.

Conclusion

In 2020, healthcare workers constituted a substantial proportion of all COVID-19 infections in Australia, and data suggests that the majority of HCWs acquired it at the workplace. COVID precautions in the dermatology medical setting however appear to have worked well. For many dermatologists, the workplace has not been the main source of reported COVID-19 infections but rather, family, friends, conferences and travel.

It is important to have a safe working environment. The SARS-CoV-2 pandemic has led to a review of workflow, the precautions taken, infection control and use of personal protective equipment. This has helped reinforce good infection control across aesthetic dermatology, dermatosurgery and skin cancer procedures. Therein lies a benefit beyond COVID-19 era for optimal outcomes for both patients and practices.

Precautions utilised will evolve over time including as the level of community of transmission varies and new knowledge. A standard level of precautions will likely persist. Where there is close patient contact, including many aesthetic dermatology, dermatology surgery and skin cancer treatments, droplet or airborne transmission precautions should be considered. With the increased availability of N95 masks, these should now be routinely utilised for procedures involving significant laser and electrosurgical plumes.

The SARS-CoV-2 pandemic has led to several positive changes and an improvement in awareness of infection control measures. This has included handwashing before and after patient contact, good respiratory hygiene and the increased availability and use of alcohol-based hand sanitisers. The increased use of properly fitted N95 masks for procedures involving electrosurgical and laser plumes and the use of smoke evacuators have benefits for clinicians beyond their reduction in risk of SARS-CoV-2 transmission.

References

Abi Rafeh J, Cattelan L, Zargham H, Jafarian F. Growing role of telemedicine in dermatology: a practical, timely application for skin cancer screening in organ transplant recipients. J Cutan Med Surg. 2021;25(1):104–5.

Aboubakr HA, Sharafeldin TA, Goyal SM. Stability of SARS-CoV-2 and other coronaviruses in the environment and on common touch surfaces and the influence of climatic conditions: a review. Transbound Emerg Dis. 2021;68(2):296–312.

Anfinrud P, Stadnytskyi V, Bax CE, Bax A. Visualizing speech-generated oral fluid droplets with laser light scattering. N Engl J Med. 2020;382(21):2061–3.

Bartoszko JJ, Farooqi MAM, Alhazzani W, Loeb M. Medical masks vs N95 respirators for preventing COVID-19 in healthcare workers: a systematic review and meta-analysis of randomized trials. Influenza Other Resp Viruses. 2020;14(4):365–73.

Bidra AS, Pelletier JS, Westover JB, Frank S, Brown SM, Tessema B. Rapid in-vitro inactivation of severe acute respiratory syndrome coronavirus 2 (SARS-CoV-2) using povidone-iodine oral antiseptic rinse. J Prosthodont. 2020;29(6):529–33.

Boniface D, Tapia-Rico G. Oncology during the COVID-19 pandemic: a lockdown perspective. Curr Oncol Rep. 2022;1-17:1219.

Brace MD, Stevens E, Taylor SM, Butt S, Sun Z, Hu L, et al. 'The air that we breathe': assessment of laser and electrosurgical dissection devices on operating theater air quality. J Otolaryngol Head Neck Surg. 2014;43(1):1–9.

Chan JF-W, Yip CC-Y, To KKW, Tang TH-C, Wong SC-Y, Leung K-H, et al. Improved molecular diagnosis of COVID-19 by the novel, highly sensitive and specific COVID-19-RdRp/Hel real-time reverse transcription-PCR assay validated in vitro and with clinical specimens. J Clin Microbiol. 2020;58(5):e00310–20.

Chu DK, Akl EA, Duda S, Solo K, Yaacoub S, Schünemann HJ, et al. Physical distancing, face masks, and eye protection to prevent person-to-person transmission of SARS-CoV-2 and COVID-19: a systematic review and meta-analysis. Lancet. 2020;395(10242):1973–87.

Crook H, Raza S, Nowell J, Young M, Edison P. Long covid—Mechanisms, risk factors, and management. BMJ. 2021;374:n1648.

Davies K, Buczkowski H, Welch SR, Green N, Mawer D, Woodford N, et al. Effective in vitro inactivation of SARS-CoV-2 by commercially available mouthwashes. J Gen Virol. 2021;102(4):001578.

Domingo JL, Rovira J. Effects of air pollutants on the transmission and severity of respiratory viral infections. Environ Res. 2020;187:109650.

Doremalen N, Bushmaker T, Morris DH, Holbrook MG, Gamble A, Brandi NW, Tamin A, Harcourt JL, Thornburg NJ, Gerber SI, Lloyd-Smith JO, de Wit E, Munster VJ. Aerosol and surface stability of SARS-CoV-2 as compared with SARS-CoV-1. N Engl J Med. 2020;382:1564–7.

El-Boghdadly K, Cook T, Goodacre T, Kua J, Denmark S, McNally S, et al. Timing of elective surgery and risk assessment after SARS-CoV-2 infection: an update: a multidisciplinary consensus statement on behalf of the Association of Anaesthetists, Centre for Perioperative Care, Federation of Surgical Specialty Associations, Royal College of Anaesthetists, Royal College of Surgeons of England. Anaesthesia. 2022;77(5):580–7.

Food and Drug Administration (FDA) Center for Biologics Evaluation and Research (CBER). In: Zhang R, editor. 163rd Vaccines and Related Biological Products Advisory Committee (VRBPAC) Meeting; 2020.

Garden JM, O'Banion MK, Shelnitz LS, Pinski KS, Bakus AD, Reichmann M, et al. Papillomavirus in the vapor of carbon dioxide laser-treated verrucae. JAMA. 1988;259(8):1199–202.

Guo X, Li T, Wang Y, Jin X. Sub-acute hypersensitive reaction to botulinum toxin type a following Covid-19 vaccination: case report and literature review. Medicine. 2021;100(49):e27787.

Hirose R, Ikegaya H, Naito Y, Watanabe N, Yoshida T, Bandou R, et al. Survival of severe acute respiratory syndrome coronavirus 2 (SARS-CoV-2) and influenza virus on human skin: importance of hand hygiene in coronavirus disease 2019 (COVID-19). Clin Infect Dis. 2021;73(11):e4329–e35.

Iannone P, Castellini G, Coclite D, Napoletano A, Fauci AJ, Iacorossi L, et al. The need of health policy perspective to protect healthcare workers during COVID-19 pandemic. A GRADE rapid review on the N95 respirators effectiveness. PLoS One. 2020;15(6):e0234025.

Jensen DA, Danyluk MD, Harris LJ, Schaffner DW. Quantifying the effect of hand wash duration, soap use, ground beef debris, and drying methods on the removal of Enterobacter aerogenes on hands. J Food Prot. 2015;78(4):685–90.

Kampf G, Todt D, Pfaender S, Steinmann E. Persistence of coronaviruses on inanimate surfaces and their inactivation with biocidal agents. J Hosp Infect. 2020;104(3):246–51.

Kashima HK, Kessis T, Mounts P, Shah K. Polymerase chain reaction identification of human papillomavirus DNA in CO2 laser plume from recurrent respiratory papillomatosis. Otolaryngol Head Neck Surg. 1991;104(2):191–5.

Kowalski LP, Sanabria A, Ridge JA, Ng WT, de Bree R, Rinaldo A, et al. COVID-19 pandemic: effects and evidence-based recommendations for otolaryngology and head and neck surgery practice. Head Neck. 2020;42(6):1259–67.

Kratzel A, Todt D, V'kovski P, Steiner S, Gultom M, Thao TTN, et al. Inactivation of severe acute respiratory syndrome coronavirus 2 by WHO-recommended hand rub formulations and alcohols. Emerg Infect Dis. 2020;26(7):1592.

Li Y, Liang M, Gao L, Ahmed MA, Uy JP, Cheng C, et al. Face masks to prevent transmission of COVID-19: a systematic review and meta-analysis. Am J Infect Control. 2021;49(7):900–6.

Lindsley WG, Derk RC, Coyle JP, Martin SB Jr, Mead KR, Blachere FM, et al. Efficacy of portable air cleaners and masking for reducing indoor exposure to simulated exhaled SARS-CoV-2 aerosols—United States, 2021. Morb Mortal Wkly Rep. 2021;70(27):972.

Luo M, Guo L, Yu M, Jiang W, Wang H. The psychological and mental impact of coronavirus disease 2019 (COVID-19) on medical staff and general public—a systematic review and meta-analysis. Psychiatry Res. 2020;291:113190.

Marquès M, Domingo JL. Positive association between outdoor air pollution and the incidence and severity of COVID-19. A review of the recent scientific evidences. Environ Res. 2022;203:111930.

Mermiri M, Mavrovounis G, Kanellopoulos N, Papageorgiou K, Spanos M, Kalantzis G, et al. Effect of PM2.5 levels on ED visits for respiratory causes in a Greek semi-urban area. J Pers Med. 2022;12(11):1849.

Mokos M, Bašić-Jukić N. Diagnostic delays for non-melanoma skin cancers in renal transplant recipients during the COVID-19 pandemic: what is hiding behind the mask? Acta Dermatovenerol Croat. 2021;29(2):111–3.

Mowbray N, Ansell J, Warren N, Wall P, Torkington J. Is surgical smoke harmful to theater staff? A systematic review. Surg Endosc. 2013;27(9):3100–7.

Munavalli GG, Guthridge R, Knutsen-Larson S, Brodsky A, Matthew E, Landau M. COVID-19/SARS-CoV-2 virus spike protein-related delayed inflammatory reaction to hyaluronic acid dermal fillers: a challenging clinical conundrum in diagnosis and treatment. Arch Dermatol Res. 2022;314(1):1–15.

Narla S, Alam M, Ozog MDM, Bertucci V, Chan HHL, Goldman MP, et al. (2021). American Society of Dermatologic Surgery Association (ASDSA) and American Society for Laser Medicine & Surgery (ASLMS) guidance for cosmetic dermatology practices during COVID-19.

Rego A, Roley L. In-use barrier integrity of gloves: latex and nitrile superior to vinyl. Am J Infect Control. 1999;27(5):405–10.

Ren S-Y, Wang W-B, Hao Y-G, Zhang H-R, Wang Z-C, Chen Y-L, et al. Stability and infectivity of coronaviruses in inanimate environments. World J Clin Cases. 2020;8(8):1391.

Roseleur J, Gonzalez-Chica D, Emery J, Stocks N. Skin checks and skin cancer diagnosis in Australian general practice before and during the COVID-19 pandemic, 2011–2020. Br J Dermatol. 2021;185(4):853–5.

Rowland-Warmann M. Hypersensitivity reaction to hyaluronic acid dermal filler following novel coronavirus infection—a case report. J Cosmet Dermatol. 2021;20(5):1557–62.

Rundle CW, Presley CL, Militello M, Barber C, Powell DL, Jacob SE, et al. Hand hygiene during COVID-19: recommendations from the American Contact Dermatitis Society. J Am Acad Dermatol. 2020;83(6):1730–7.

Sandaradura I, Goeman E, Pontivivo G, Fine E, Gray H, Kerr S, et al. A close shave? Performance of P2/N95 respirators in healthcare workers with facial hair: results of the BEARDS (BEnchmarking adequate respiratory DefenceS) study. J Hosp Infect. 2020;104(4):529–33.

Shome D, Doshi K, Vadera S, Kapoor R. Delayed hypersensitivity reaction to hyaluronic acid dermal filler post-COVID-19 viral infection. J Cosmet Dermatol. 2021;20(5):1549.

Van Doremalen N, Bushmaker T, Morris DH, Holbrook MG, Gamble A, Williamson BN, et al. Aerosol and surface stability of SARS-CoV-2 as compared with SARS-CoV-1. N Engl J Med. 2020;382(16):1564–7.

Villar J, Ariff S, Gunier RB, Thiruvengadam R, Rauch S, Kholin A, et al. Maternal and neonatal morbidity and mortality among pregnant women with and without COVID-19 infection: the INTERCOVID multinational cohort study. JAMA Pediatr. 2021;175(8):817–26.

World Health Organization. Cleaning and disinfection of environmental surfaces in the context of COVID-19: interim guidance. Geneva: World Health Organization; 2020.

Wu X, Nethery RC, Sabath MB, Braun D, Dominici F. Air pollution and COVID-19 mortality in the United States: strengths and limitations of an ecological regression analysis. Sci Adv. 2020;6(45):eabd4049.

Psychological Aspects, Psychodermatology, and Vaccine Hesitancy During the COVID-19 Pandemic

Woo Chiao Tay, Anthony Bewley, Julia-Tatjana Maul, and Hazel H. Oon

Abbreviations

AAD	American Academy of Dermatology
AD	Atopic dermatitis
AIBD	Autoimmune bullous diseases
BDD	Body dysmorphic disorder
BFRB	Body-focused repetitive behaviors
DLQI	Dermatology Life Quality Index
HCW	Healthcare workers
IES-R	Impact of Event Scale-Revised
IL	Interleukins
ILDS	International League of Dermatological Societies
MMR	Measles, mumps, and rubella
mRNA	Messenger RNA
OR	Odds ratio
PGWB	Psychological General Well-Being Index
PPE	Personal protective equipment
PTSD	Post-traumatic stress disorder
SAGE	Strategic Advisory Group of Experts on Immunization
TE	Telogen effluvium
TNF	Tumor necrosis factor
WHO	World Health Organization

W. C. Tay (✉) · H. H. Oon
National Skin Centre, Singapore, Singapore
e-mail: derm@hazeloon.com

A. Bewley
Department of Dermatology, Barts Health NHS Trust and Queen Mary University, London, UK
e-mail: anthony.bewley@nhs.net

J.-T. Maul
Department of Dermatology and Venereology, University Hospital of Zurich, Zurich, Switzerland

Faculty of Medicine, University of Zurich, Zurich, Switzerland
e-mail: Julia-Tatjana.Maul@usz.ch

Introduction

The COVID-19 pandemic has impacted the lifestyle of almost every person globally. Not only has the virus caused physical illness in those who were infected, it has also affected their mental health, including those who were not infected (Chernyshov et al. 2020; Xiong et al. 2020; Stamu-O'Brien et al. 2020; Jones et al. 2021; Gilsbach et al. 2021). The long drawn nature of this pandemic offered little respite, prolonging its detrimental mental health effect (Xiong et al. 2020; Manchia et al. 2022).

Psychodermatology became increasingly relevant in this pandemic. The psychological effects of the pandemic, such as fear, stress, and isolation, had a significant impact on skin health; it is essential to understand the interconnection between mental health and the skin (Pendlebury et al. 2022; Ferreira et al. 2021).

One of the biggest challenges in fighting the pandemic has been the development and distribution of vaccines. While there are several vaccine

© The Author(s), under exclusive license to Springer Nature Switzerland AG 2023
H. H. Oon, C. L. Goh (eds.), *COVID-19 in Dermatology*, Updates in Clinical Dermatology,
https://doi.org/10.1007/978-3-031-45586-5_13

options available, some dermatology patients have been hesitant to get vaccinated and complete booster doses. Patients were concerned about the vaccine's safety and efficacy and whether the vaccine would worsen existing dermatoses (Prabani et al. 2022; Pires 2022).

Psychological Aspects

Many countries engaged mass lockdowns and mandatory social isolation policies as means to control the spread of the virus. The rapidly evolving situation of the pandemic had also led to multiple policy changes to the global, public, and private economy, resulting in fears and uncertainties on the ground.

There are several ongoing research projects reviewing the psychological repercussions of the COVID-19 pandemic (Nicola et al. 2020; Holmes et al. 2020). Studies indicated that individuals who had contracted COVID-19 experienced increased risk of developing mental health issues (Hossain et al. 2020a). A systematic review reported that quarantine and isolation caused mental health problems such as depression, anxiety disorders, mood disorders, and PTSD (Hossain et al. 2020b). A Lancet review showed 73% and 57% of participants had low mood and increased irritability during the quarantine, respectively (Brooks et al. 2020).

Psychological Impact on Patients with Dermatoses

Even before the COVID-19 pandemic, studies had shown that major natural disasters and economy crisis led to an increase in rates of psychological distress and disorders (Chaves et al. 2018). Beaglehole et al. in a systemic review and meta-analysis published in 2018 reported that there were increased rates of depression, anxiety disorders, substance abuse, suicidal tendencies, and PTSD following natural disasters and post-disaster response (Beaglehole et al. 2018). The COVID-19 pandemic was more drawn out than

the severe acute respiratory syndrome (SARS) of 2003. Long periods of solitary confinement in custodial care, mandatory masking up, and quarantine for illness had adverse mental health effects (Stickley and Koyanagi 2016). Mental health, quality of life, and well-being were all known to be affected by quarantines. Physical distance, social distance, and diverse security measures had hindered social connections and diminished empathy for others (Saladino et al. 2020; Luchetti et al. 2020).

Patients with Psoriasis and Connective Tissue Disorders

There are global efforts to collect data from dermatological patients who contracted COVID-19. PsoProtect (Psoriasis Registry for Outcomes, Therapy and Epidemiology of COVID-19 Infection) is an international registry for HCW to report outcomes of COVID-19 in individuals with psoriasis. Psoriasis patients receiving biologics self-reported high rates of social and self-isolation compared to those receiving non-biologic systemic therapies (Mahil et al. 2021a). Compared to conventional systemics, COVID-19 infection rates were lower in the psoriasis biologic cohort who received TNF, IL-17, and IL-23 inhibitors.

Results from PsoProtectMe were analyzed with another online self-reported survey RMD (Rheumatology Register CORE-UK) for rheumatic and musculoskeletal diseases (UK only), and it demonstrated that 60.8% of patients adopted "shielding" or risk-mitigating measures such as social distancing, staying home, and quarantining (Mahil et al. 2021b). Shielding was linked to the use of targeted therapy (biologics, Janus kinase inhibitors), risk factors for severe COVID-19 disease (male, obesity, comorbidity burden), and presence of depression/anxiety. The impact of rigorous shielding practices and attendant social isolation in individuals with more baseline depression, anxiety, and disease burden from chronic skin diseases such as psoriasis and lupus remains to be determined. Patients were also afraid that dermatological therapies, especially the immunosuppressants, could lead to an increased risk and complications of COVID-19 infections.

Thirty-six percent of patients with psoriasis in online questionnaire conducted in India had a feeling of depression during the lockdown (Narang et al. 2022). There were others who complained of altered sleep pattern and affected daily routines, e.g., eating habits, physical activity, and earnings and commuting.

Some patients with psoriasis felt that they were more susceptible to contracting COVID-19 infection because of the pre-existing skin condition (Narang et al. 2022). This finding was similar in Taiwan, where 94.3% of the 423 COVID-19-naïve psoriasis patients reported feeling vulnerable to the COVID-19 threat, especially seen in patients with prolonged psoriasis treatment history (Chiu et al. 2021).

Psoriasis patients also reported their fears of transmitting COVID-19 virus to their family members in the event of infection. Other common concerns cited by psoriasis patients during the COVID-19 pandemic included disrupted access to medication for psoriasis treatment during the pandemic and fear of catching the virus at the hospital when attending dermatology outpatient clinics (Chiu et al. 2021).

A cross-sectional study using an online questionnaire in India found that 35.9% of patients reported worsening of psoriasis during the lockdown. This could have been partly caused by difficulties in accessing investigations and procuring medication; and some patients with psoriasis had either lessened or halted all forms of physical exertion. This in turn led to them feeling depressed (49.2%) and stressed (20%) (Narang et al. 2022).

Rates of treatment non-adherence were higher in psoriasis patients receiving biologics. Patients who chose to discontinue biologics treatment for psoriasis experienced significant worsening of disease control in Italy (Pirro et al. 2022). Dermatologists themselves were also more cautious in the use of biologics and immunosuppressive drugs for the treatment of psoriasis during the pandemic (El-Komy et al. 2021).

Other Dermatoses

The psychological impact of COVID-19 on patients with other dermatoses has been investigated as well. The cancellation of elective operations, rescheduling of outpatient appointments, and delays in treatment led to increased pain and psychosocial distress levels in the patients affected (Knebel et al. 2021; Moreno et al. 2021; Misery et al. 2021).

Face masks caused a worsening of existing dermatological facial diseases, leading to itchiness, redness, and discomforts, especially in patients with acne rosacea and contact dermatitis (İnan Doğan and Kaya 2021).

In a self-reported questionnaire conducted in a skin cancer unit in Italy, there was a significant increase in the Impact of Event Scale-Revised (IES-R) negative responses from 23.6 (±15.6) to 28.3 (±17.2) between patients who visited the center before and after March 2020 (Borsari et al. 2022). Some patients elected to postpone necessary medical consultations to avoid visiting healthcare facilities.

In France, patients with chronic immune-mediated inflammatory diseases (including patients with atopic dermatitis and psoriasis) saw the quarantine as a stressful experience, and it had negatively impacted their work environment and medical conditions. They displayed a greater range of negative emotions to the lockdown: anxiety, distress, work disruption, self-isolation, and fear of infection (Nasseh et al. 2022).

Patients with chronic inflammatory skin conditions reported feeling stigmatized and worsening self-esteem. These negative feelings of shame and guilt increased the tendency toward suicidal ideation (Marasca et al. 2020).

Postponing immunosuppressive therapies during the COVID-19 pandemic in patients with autoimmune blistering dermatosis, e.g., pemphigus, was also associated with higher rates of psychiatric morbidity and impaired quality of life (Elmas et al. 2020).

The psychological impact of long COVID, or post-COVID syndrome, cannot be ignored as well. Even patients with mild symptoms during the acute infection commonly developed fatigue and cognitive impairment post-COVID (Ceban et al. 2022; van Kessel et al. 2022). This had a significant impact on their skin health as well. In a collaboration by the International League of Dermatological Societies (ILDS) and the American Academy of Dermatology (AAD), a crowdsourced international registry for COVID-19 dermatological manifestations was created in April 2020 (Freeman et al. 2020). Chronic psychological stress in long COVID has been postulated to be contributory toward both existing dermatoses and the development of other cutaneous manifestations of pernio, papulosquamous eruptions, and livedo reticularis (Tammaro et al. 2021; McMahon et al. 2021).

Psychological Impact on Dermatologists and Dermatology Allied Health Professionals

The outbreak of COVID-19 has resulted in the temporary restructuring of medical manpower and workload in many hospitals to conserve resources for the screening and treatment of patients with COVID-19.

Studies have shown that HCW were at a higher risk of developing anxiety, depression, stigmatization, and PTSD during the COVID-19 pandemic (Ferreira et al. 2021; Lou et al. 2022; Huerta-González et al. 2021; Della Monica et al. 2022; Honarmand et al. 2022; Rodríguez and Sánchez 2020). In China, a large cross-sectional survey of HCW across different disciplines in 34 hospitals showed a considerable proportion HCW reporting symptoms of distress (71.5%), depression (50.4%), anxiety (44.6%), and insomnia (34.0%) (Lai et al. 2020).

The impact of the COVID-19 pandemic on dermatology staff cannot be understated too (Richardson et al. 2021). Globally, dermatology research studies were paused, amended, or even discontinued during the lockdown periods in many countries. There was uncertainty about whether basic science work requiring in-person experiments could continue. In Singapore, laboratory and research staff were redeployed to help in COVID testing, administration, and contact tracing. Research may have changed focus to COVID-related projects and retrospective studies to remain viable. Changing infection control measures, quarantine periods, drawing up of vaccine-related protocols for dermatology patients and staff, freezing of annual leave, and inability to travel have resulted in a difficult time for dermatology HCW.

Reduced work hours with attendant pay reduction, leave of absence, and job uncertainty may have led to resignation with career changes, retrenchment, and early retirement for less financially resilient allied health workers, and even dermatologists in private practices faced a severe reduction in clinical load and mounting expenses for PPE.

In Egypt, a cross-sectional study reported that 38% of the dermatologists surveyed had severe or extremely severe depression and 35% had severe or extremely severe anxiety (Elsaie et al. 2021). Female dermatologists living in metropolitan areas and with a shorter professional history exhibited a greater amount of stress symptoms (Elsaie et al. 2021).

Egyptian dermatologists also experienced a surge in stress-induced burnout, due to the increased emotional burden caused by the number of fatalities among patients, lack of control, feelings of responsibility for being unable to do more for their patients, extended working hours, and emotional stress among their support system (Elsaie et al. 2020).

In a French study surveying dermatologists, private practitioners reported that a significant source of stress was the loss of revenue from cancelled and rescheduled appointments (Misery et al. 2021). The number of aesthetic procedures was approximately halved during the pandemic period, and many academic meetings have been cancelled as well (Murrell et al. 2020; Mangini et al. 2022).

Supply Chain Disruption

During the pandemic, a reliable medical supply chain could not be taken for granted. There was a global shortage of PPE for all HCW (Bhargava et al. 2021).

Many pharmaceutical companies rely on overseas manufacturers in their production line. Egger et al. looked at the top 15 most common prescribed generic topical dermatological medications, and 13 of them were at least partially manufactured in China (Egger et al. 2020). Many countries experienced shortage of medications during the pandemic, including IL-17 inhibitor ixekizumab, benzoyl peroxide/clindamycin fixed combination gel, and meladinine solution for soak and bath PUVA. Dermatological staff were pressured to explain the situation to patients and further pressed to prescribe alternative therapies in patients who have been well-controlled on existing medications.

Barbed and jagged edges were reported in a new supply of 30-gauge hypodermic needle used in New Orleans, associated with patients complaining of severe pain during triamcinolone injections for scarring alopecia (Rensch et al. 2022).

Teledermatology

COVID-19 has also challenged the traditional physical model of a doctor-patient face-to-face encounter.

Teledermatology is the practice of dermatology at a distance (Eedy and Wootton 2001). Due to the risks associated with the virus, many dermatologists switched to providing care remotely using teledermatology. The use of teledermatology has increased dramatically since the start of the pandemic and generally been received well by patients (Farr et al. 2021; Loh et al. 2021). First, it allowed patients to avoid coming into contact with other people, which reduces the risk of viral transmission. Second, it conferred more convenience for both patients and doctors, saving time and money for both parties (Ibrahim et al. 2021).

Teledermatology also facilitated the increased utilization of palliative psychodermatological services, and such services can improve quality of life in terminal patients (Hafi et al. 2020).

Marasca et al. introduced psychological consultations through teledermatology for patients suffering from chronic skin condition during the pandemic, with a statistically significant improvement in DLQI at week 4 (Marasca et al. 2022).

Details on other aspects of teledermatology will be covered separately in another chapter in this book.

Psychological Impact on Other HCW

There was an increase of PPE-related irritant dermatosis or pressure injuries seen in HCW (Montero-Vilchez et al. 2021; Kampf et al. 2020; Yu et al. 2021). Cases of occupational hand eczema and face mask dermatitis have been reported (Niesert et al. 2021; Xie et al. 2020; Guertler et al. 2020). This further exacerbated the psychological distress in HCW. Dermatology nurses were deployed to the frontlines to care for patients with COVID-19 infection (Richardson et al. 2021).

For junior doctors, in particular trainees and fellows in dermatology and surgical disciplines, there was also uncertainty regarding the quality of training and maintenance of competency given the reduction of elective procedures and diversion of manpower for service requirements during the pandemic (Wong et al. 2020; Lund et al. 2021; Nagaraj et al. 2021; Friedrich et al. 2021; Hope et al. 2021).

An interview study of pharmacists in Ireland reported many feeling "stressed" during the pandemic (Gleeson et al. 2022). Pharmacists also experienced an increase in workload in the form of home delivery services, provision of patient education virtually, managing medications and stock taking, and poor consumer behavior (Johnston et al. 2022).

Psychodermatology

The concept of psychodermatology was first conceived in the late 1970s and early 1980s, when a group of researchers and clinicians became interested in exploring the connection between mental health and skin conditions. Up to that time, the medical community was primarily focused on managing physical cutaneous disease. However, some clinicians understood the importance of the brain-skin connection, which led to the development of psychodermatology as a sub-specialty. Psychodermatology has grown significantly since its conception, and the field of research has expanded to include a wide variety of skin conditions and mental illnesses.

Ferreira et al. provided a framework of four categories in approaching psychodermatological conditions in COVID-19 era: psychophysiological dermatoses, primary psychopathology focused on the skin, cutaneous sensory disorders, and dermatoses leading to psychosocial comorbidities (Ferreira et al. 2021). Cutaneous sensory disorders are not discussed below as there was little literature specific to COVID-19 at the time of writing.

Psychophysiological Dermatoses

Psychophysiological (or psychosomatic) dermatoses are skin diseases that are triggered or worsened by psychological stress but are not directly affected by it. Many dermatosis, including urticaria, eczema, psoriasis, acne, seborrheic dermatitis, atopic dermatitis, alopecia areata, psychogenic purpura, rosacea, and hyperhidrosis, can be worsened by emotional stress (Ferreira et al. 2021; Steinhoff et al. 2012; Jamerson et al. 2022; Shen et al. 2021; Kuang et al. 2020; Stamu-O'Brien et al. 2021).

The COVID-19 pandemic can cause or worsen dermatoses as a complication of the viral infection itself (covered in other chapters of this book), or it can negatively impact dermatological health through stress. The outbreak of COVID-19 had been a significant stressor for many people and led to an increase in the incidence and severity of these dermatoses (Chernyshov et al. 2020; Ferreira et al. 2021; Brooks et al. 2020).

There was an increase in certain dermatoses during the pandemic, which may have been exacerbated by pandemic-associated stress, rather than the viral infection: telogen effluvium (TE),

psoriasis, eczema, urticaria, seborrheic dermatitis, herpes zoster, and vitiligo (Pendlebury et al. 2022; Mangini et al. 2022). Cases of fragile nail syndrome and contact dermatitis also increased during the pandemic as well (Mangini et al. 2022).

TE can follow COVID-19 infection (Lv et al. 2021; Sharquie and Jabbar 2022; Mieczkowska et al. 2021). However, even in individuals who did not contract the infection, stress from the pandemic situation could have been a trigger for TE. There was a more than 400% increase in incidence of TE in New York City in the months of July–August 2020, even in patients not tested positive for COVID-19 infection (Cline et al. 2021).

In PsoProtectMe, a global cross-sectional survey involving 86 countries, 42.7% of 4043 psoriasis patients reported worsening of psoriasis during the pandemic. Patients with anxiety or depression had an adjusted odds ratio (OR) of 2.01 (95% CI, 1.72–2.34) for worsening psoriasis and increased association (42.8% vs. 32.4%) for non-adherence to treatment during the pandemic (Mahil et al. 2021a, c).

A Chinese questionnaire in 926 patients with psoriasis (only 1 respondent tested positive for COVID-19) reported that outdoor activity restriction and income loss were associated with the exacerbation of psoriasis, stress, and symptoms of anxiety and depression (Kuang et al. 2020).

Primary Cutaneous Psychopathology

In a survey of body-focused repetitive behaviors (BFRB) awareness device users, 67.2% of the 460 respondents reported increased of BFRB symptoms during the COVID-19 pandemic (Pathoulas et al. 2021). Participants with skin picking disorders and hair pulling disorders reported a 2.2- and 1.6-point increase on the modified Skin Picking Scale-Revised and Massachusetts General Hospital Hairpulling Scale, respectively.

The start of the COVID-19 pandemic also saw a significant increase in the total number of self-harm presentations between 2019 and 2020 from an observational study of level 1 trauma center in Birmingham (Henry et al. 2021).

Stressors during COVID-19 social isolation such as longer quarantine duration, infection fears, frustration, boredom, inadequate supplies, inadequate information, financial loss, and stigma could have become triggers for patients with underlying psychological disorder (Stamu-O'Brien et al. 2020; Brooks et al. 2020; Grant and Chamberlain 2020; Prochwicz et al. 2022; Ricketts et al. 2022; Torales et al. 2020).

Dermatoses That Lead to Psychosocial Comorbidities

Most dermatoses can lead to psychosocial complications. Disfiguring skin conditions can contribute to psychosocial distress and comorbidities. These conditions, such as atopic dermatitis, psoriasis, and alopecia areata, can have a large effect on an individual's quality of life (Ferreira et al. 2021; Steinhoff et al. 2012; Jamerson et al. 2022; Shen et al. 2021; Kuang et al. 2020). They can lead to feelings of embarrassment, low self-esteem, and even depression.

The pandemic saw an increase in the utilization of digital platforms such as Zoom (Zoom Technologies, Inc., San Jose, Calif.) for social communications. Long hours of teleconferencing and staring at oneself in a magnified view has led to some individuals having increased awareness of their own physical features and developing "Zoom dysmorphia" – unhappy perceptions on how one views oneself (Ramphul 2021; Gasteratos et al. 2021). On the other hand, a longitudinal study of 319 health club users found no differences in body dysmorphic disorder (BDD) pre- and post-COVID-19 lockdown (Trott et al. 2021). Depending on the individual's lifestyle, some patients might have preferred the lockdown as they were able to stay at home and not forced to socially interact.

The COVID-19 pandemic also had its psychological impact on basic self-cosmetic care (Mościcka et al. 2020). Sixty-six percent of the female medical students surveyed in Nepal reported not taking cosmetic care of their skin, hair, and nail during the pandemic, and consequent negative feelings such as losing self-satisfaction, increased irritability, and feeling stressed were cited (Marahatta et al. 2021).

Future of Psychodermatology and the Role of Dermatologists in the Post-COVID Era

Psychodermatology may be underappreciated (Jafferany et al. 2010; Roberts et al. 2020). Understanding psychodermatology is important for all dermatologists. Dermatologists play a significant role in providing mental health support during the pandemic by helping the patient understand the connection between mental and physical health (Ferreira et al. 2021; Soutou and Tomb 2020).

Dermatologists can partner mental health professionals in psychiatric medicine to set up integrated liaison psychiatry clinics to improve patient care (Magid and Reichenberg 2020). The introduction of dermatology-psychiatry combined clinics is a cost-effective approach to manage patients with co-existing dermatological and psychological conditions. This method prevents erroneous diagnoses, inadequate treatments, unneeded referrals, and the doctor hopping behavior in some patients (Magid and Reichenberg 2020; Roberts et al. 2022). Patel et al. reviewed 20 studies and revealed that patients experienced greater contentment or better results when holistic approaches, involving both pharmacological and non-pharmacological therapies, were employed (Patel and Jafferany 2020).

Dermatologists can also help individuals manage their skin condition and mental well-being by encouraging self-management with online resources and providing referrals to mental health professionals who can support patients with their emotional health (Soutou and Tomb 2020).

Finally, dermatologists play a role in the pandemic by giving advice to patients to achieve good hand hygiene without compromising good skincare (Murrell et al. 2020; Soutou and Tomb 2020).

Vaccine Hesitancy

Even before COVID-19 vaccines, vaccination has been a controversial topic, with different groups holding varying opinions on the matter (Dubé et al. 2013; MacDonald 2015; Jarrett et al. 2015; Xiao and Wong 2020). However, the COVID-19 pandemic has brought this issue of vaccine hesitancy to the forefront.

It is important to understand the reasons behind vaccine hesitancy and the implications it has for public health. Vaccine hesitancy is a complex issue. From understanding cultural and religious beliefs to recognizing the importance of education and communication, we discuss an overview of the key arguments surrounding vaccine hesitancy and steps to overcome it.

Pre-Existing Attitudes Toward Vaccinations

Vaccination is a preventive strategy that has saved millions of lives and is one of the most successful public health interventions in history (Andre et al. 2008). However, this does not mean that everyone is in favor of it (Larson et al. 2014). Vaccine hesitancy is defined as the delay in the acceptance or refusal of vaccination despite the availability of vaccination services (Strategic Advisory Group of Experts 2012).

Vaccines have long been a contentious issue (Dubé et al. 2013; Larson et al. 2014). The infamous 1998 Lancet paper from Wakefield et al. (retracted in 2010) was undoubtedly a catalyst that sparked concerns in many parents that the MMR vaccine was connected to autism. Thimerosal, a mercury-based preservative used in vaccines, has also been a concern for patients (Baker 2008).

The reasons behind vaccine hesitancy are complex. MacDonald and WHO SAGE Working Group on Vaccine Hesitancy summarized these reasons into three main factors: confidence, complacency, and convenience (MacDonald 2015). Some worry about the quality of the production process, potential side effects, and policymakers who decided on them (lack of "confidence").

Others simply do not think they need to get vaccinated ("complacency"). There could be factors beyond "medical reasons" that influence an individual's decision for a vaccine: factors such as a leaning toward natural/alternative remedies, political inclinations, and extreme viewpoints founded on religion can all contribute to the situation. Finally, reduced geographical and financial accessibility may make the vaccine less appealing to some people ("convenience").

Factors Affecting COVID-19 Vaccine Uptake

The COVID-19 pandemic really amplified the discussion of vaccine safety and vaccine hesitancy (Storey 2022).

Concerns About Impact on Skin Health

Localized cutaneous reactions were common after mRNA vaccines, and some patients developed urticarial and morbilliform eruptions. There were infrequent reports of reactivation of herpes zoster, dermatologic filler reactions, and immune thrombocytopenia, mainly occurring in high-risk patient groups (Gronbeck and Grant-Kels 2021).

Individuals with pre-existing dermatological conditions were particularly worried. A questionnaire collected from 707 patients from the International Pemphigus and Pemphigoid Foundation found that only 73.1% of the patients were willing to accept the COVID-19 vaccine. Respondents were concerned that the COVID-19 vaccine could cause a flare or worsening control of their underlying AIBD (Kasperkiewicz et al. 2022).

The data from the global patient-reported PsoProtectMe survey found higher vaccine acceptance rates in patients with psoriasis. In the survey, only a minority of respondents (8%) reported vaccine hesitancy. Young psoriasis patients and patients with negative experiences of healthcare and/or doctors were more likely to be vaccine hesitant. The most common reasons for hesitancy from the survey were concerns regarding the side effects of a new vaccine and if it could lead to psoriasis worsening post-vaccination (Bechman et al. 2022).

Understanding of Vaccines

Some individuals were hesitant to get vaccinated because they were concerned about the way vaccines were developed and tested or of a belief that natural immunity was better than immunity provided by a vaccine (Kricorian et al. 2022; Nazlı et al. 2022; Lockyer et al. 2021). This could stem from a mistrust of the government or pharmaceutical companies or a belief that the vaccine had not been thoroughly tested (Kricorian et al. 2022; Nazlı et al. 2022; Majid et al. 2022). Some were worried about reports that the COVID-19 virus itself was genetically engineered by governments.

Parents of young children also had concerns about the vaccines. A systematic review by Khan et al. looked at 108 studies on vaccine hesitancy and reported that the most common barriers to childhood vaccination were mothers' lower education level, financial instability, low confidence in new vaccines, and unmonitored social media platforms (Khan et al. 2022). The same systemic review, however, also highlighted that measures, e.g., provision of information by healthcare professionals, could improve vaccine uptake (Khan et al. 2022).

Misinformation of Social Media

In this age of booming information technology, the role of social media in the dissemination of medical information (or disinformation) and its impact on an individual's medical choices could not be understated (Chou et al. 2009; Dunn et al. 2015; Wilson and Wiysonge 2020; Larson et al. 2022). Despite the best efforts by various governments in the promotion of the vaccines' safety, there remained a lot of misrepresentations and/or exaggeration of cutaneous adverse events of the vaccine (e.g., COVID arm) on social media (Gronbeck and Grant-Kels 2021). People believed that vaccinations could cause certain diseases or long-lasting health problems (Lee et al. 2022).

The major vehicle exacerbating the anti-vaccine sentiments during this COVID-19 pandemic was undoubtedly the social media infodemic (Hernandez et al. 2021; Knight et al. 2021; Li et al. 2022). The individualized algorithm of social media platforms selects articles and content that panders to the user, setting up echo chambers online and artificially inflating the perceived public concurrence of the misinformation.

Only a small proportion of HCW has stepped out into the digital world in an attempt to correct the misinformation. Other HCW, in fear of retaliation by anonymous online "experts," adopted a less vocal stance on social media, choosing not to actively engage or rectify false information. Hernandez et al. coined this phenomenon "Health Care Provider Social Media Hesitancy" referring to "a public health threat of HCW's nonaction in providing pro-vaccine and scientific information about the vaccine on social media" (Hernandez et al. 2021).

Cultural and Religious Beliefs

There were also individuals who were hesitant to get vaccinated because they have strong cultural or religious beliefs against vaccination (Zimmerman et al. 2022). For example, in some communities or religions, it is believed that vaccinating could cause the spirits of their loved ones to leave the bodies of the people who were vaccinated.

Some believed that the COVID-19 virus were bioweapons developed by the Chinese government (Romer and Jamieson 2020). Other conspiracy theories included "COVID-19 is not real," "(it is) an effort by the government to control society," or that the vaccine contained a chip that would track individuals (Lockyer et al. 2021).

Personal Resistance

Some people might simply be reluctant to get vaccinated because they do not like needles or they don't want to take the time to get vaccinated. Others believed that they were not at risk of contracting the virus and/or believed that even if they did, they had low risk of developing complications (Knight et al. 2021).

Finally, some individuals suffered from "information paralysis," where they became so overwhelmed with the vast amount of information about COVID-19 virus and vaccination that they chose not to make any decisions (Lockyer et al. 2021).

COVID-19 Vaccine Uptake in HCW

HCW are at the forefront of the fight against the virus, and their attitudes toward the vaccine are of particular importance. Estimates of vaccine hesitancy among healthcare workers were similar to the general population (Caiazzo and Witkoski Stimpfel 2022). This was an interesting finding as one would expect HCW to have a greater acceptance toward the vaccine. It is essential to understand the reasons why some HCW remain hesitant toward the COVID-19 vaccine and the implications this has for public health.

HCW, especially those working in acute hospitals with direct contact with patients with COVID-19 and its complications, were generally accepting toward the COVID-19 vaccine. Top reasons cited for vaccine acceptance were to protect their family and friends and to protect themselves given their occupational risk (Koh et al. 2022). HCW who had contracted COVID-19 or have a close friend/family contract COVID-19 were also more likely to accept vaccines (Aw et al. 2022).

On the other hand, some HCW chose not to proceed with the vaccine because of concerns of adverse effects. However, this could be due to selection bias. HCW on the front lines of the pandemic were more likely to see the patients with side effects and complications of the vaccine. This created an impression that overestimated the true incidence of vaccine complications and its side effects.

Educating HCW remains the most important link in overcoming vaccine hesitancy. This cannot be overemphasized. However, HCW, just like members of the public, might be hesitant to get vaccinated due to personal, cultural, or religious beliefs. HCW come from diverse cultural and religious backgrounds, and it becomes very important to recognize and respect the cultural and religious beliefs of HCW (Caiazzo and Witkoski Stimpfel 2022; Koh et al. 2022; Aw et al. 2022; Huang et al. 2022; Navin et al. 2022). Cultural and religious beliefs should be considered when educating HCW about the vaccine.

Overcoming Vaccine Hesitancy

Beyond protecting the vaccinated individual, vaccination is also a public health measure that offers herd immunity, conferring protection to those who could not be vaccinated because of age, contraindications, or other medical reasons.

Trust, or the lack thereof, in medical professionals was a crucial factor in deciding if an individual decides for vaccination (Hernandez et al. 2021). A survey of 2440 adults by Nowak et al. revealed that vaccine hesitancy was greatly associated with individuals with greater trust in friends and family than medical professionals (Nowak et al. 2021).

Many strategies had been put forward to address vaccine hesitancy, though only few had been evaluated for impact (Armitage and Conner 2001; Fisher et al. 2013; Francis et al. 2017). A systemic review by Jarrett et al. looked at 13 studies using social mobilization, mass media, communication-centered training for healthcare personnel, non-monetary incentives, and reminder/recall-based approaches. Results indicated that multicomponent and dialogue-based interventions were the most successful (Jarrett et al. 2015).

In the future, the range of vaccine manufacturers and techniques will become more varied. It is essential to evaluate forthcoming methods (Altmann and Boyton 2022). Dermatologists must not be limited to using only medical and scientific approaches to counter falsehoods stemming from religion, media, or governmental sources but also work in tandem with non-HCW to tackle the damaging misinformation (Knight et al. 2021; Zimmerman et al. 2022).

Conclusion

The psychological aspects of the COVID-19 pandemic were complex and far-reaching. The pandemic had significant impact on mental health, physical health, and social and economic well-being of almost everyone globally. It is important to understand the psychological impact of the pandemic to effectively address the problems it has caused. This is especially true for patients with dermatological conditions, who are at a higher risk of primary or secondary cutaneous complications from the infection.

References

Altmann DM, Boyton RJ. COVID-19 vaccination: the road ahead. Science. 2022;375(6585):1127–32.

Andre F, Booy R, Bock H, Clemens J, Datta S, John T, Lee B, Lolekha S, Peltola H, Ruff T, Santosham M, Schmitt H. Vaccination greatly reduces disease, disability, death and inequity worldwide. Bull World Health Organ. 2008;86(2):140–6.

Armitage CJ, Conner M. Efficacy of the theory of planned behaviour: a meta-analytic review. Br J Soc Psychol. 2001;40(4):471–99.

Aw J, Seah SSY, Seng BJJ, Low LL. COVID-19-related vaccine hesitancy among community hospitals' healthcare workers in Singapore. Vaccine. 2022;10(4):537.

Baker JP. Mercury, vaccines, and autism. Am J Public Health. 2008;98(2):244–53.

Beaglehole B, Mulder RT, Frampton CM, Boden JM, Newton-Howes G, Bell CJ. Psychological distress and psychiatric disorder after natural disasters: systematic review and meta-analysis. Br J Psychiatry. 2018;213(6):716–22.

Bechman K, Cook ES, Dand N, Yiu ZZN, Tsakok T, Meynell F, Coker B, Vincent A, Bachelez H, Barbosa I, Brown MA, Capon F, Contreras CR, De La Cruz C, Di Meglio P, Gisondi P, Jullien D, Kelly J, Lambert J, Lancelot C, Langan SM, Mason KJ, McAteer H, Moorhead L, Naldi L, Norton S, Puig L, Spuls PI, Torres T, Urmston D, Vesty A, Warren RB, Waweru H, Weinman J, Griffiths CEM, Barker JN, Smith CH, Galloway JB, Mahil SK. Vaccine hesitancy and access to psoriasis care during the COVID-19 pandemic: findings from a global patient-reported cross-sectional survey. Br J Dermatol. 2022;187(2):254–6.

Bhargava S, Negbenebor N, Sadoughifar R, Ahmad S, Kroumpouzos G. Global impact on dermatology practice due to the COVID-19 pandemic. Clin Dermatol. 2021;39(3):479–87.

Borsari S, Pampena R, Benati M, Raucci M, Mirra M, Lai M, Lombardi M, Pellacani G, Longo C. Self-reported measure of subjective distress in response to COVID-19 pandemic in patients referred to our skin cancer unit during the first wave. Clin Dermatol. 2022;40(1):93–9.

Brooks SK, Webster RK, Smith LE, Woodland L, Wessely S, Greenberg N, Rubin GJ. The psychological impact of quarantine and how to reduce it: rapid review of the evidence. Lancet. 2020;395(10227):912–20.

Caiazzo V, Witkoski Stimpfel A. Vaccine hesitancy in American healthcare workers during the COVID-19 vaccine roll out: an integrative review. Public Health. 2022;207:94–104.

Ceban F, Ling S, Lui LMW, Lee Y, Gill H, Teopiz KM, Rodrigues NB, Subramaniapillai M, Di Vincenzo JD, Cao B, Lin K, Mansur RB, Ho RC, Rosenblat JD, Miskowiak KW, Vinberg M, Maletic V, McIntyre RS. Fatigue and cognitive impairment in post-COVID-19 syndrome: a systematic review and meta-analysis. Brain Behav Immun. 2022;101:93–135.

Chaves C, Castellanos T, Abrams M, Vazquez C. The impact of economic recessions on depression and individual and social Well-being: the case of Spain (2006–2013). Soc Psychiatry Psychiatr Epidemiol. 2018;53(9):977–86.

Chernyshov PV, Tomas-Aragones L, Augustin M, Svensson A, Bewley A, Poot F, Szepietowski JC, Marron SE, Manolache L, Pustisek N, Suru A, Salavastru CM, Blome C, Salek MS, Abeni D, Sampogna F, Dalgard F, Linder D, Evers AWM, Finlay AY. Position statement of the European Academy of Dermatology and Venereology task force on quality of life and patient oriented outcomes on quality of life issues in dermatologic patients during the COVID-19 pandemic. J Eur Acad Dermatol Venereol. 2020;34(8):1666–71.

Chiu HY, Liao NFC, Lin Y, Huang YH. Perception of the threat, mental health burden, and healthcare-seeking behavior change among psoriasis patients during the COVID-19 pandemic. PloS One. 2021;16(12):1–13.

Chou WS, Hunt YM, Beckjord EB, Moser RP, Hesse BW. Social media use in the United States: implications for health communication. J Med Internet Res. 2009;11(4):e48.

Cline A, Kazemi A, Moy J, Safai B, Marmon S. A surge in the incidence of telogen effluvium in minority predominant communities heavily impacted by COVID-19. J Am Acad Dermatol. 2021;84(3):773–5.

Della Monica A, Ferrara P, Dal Mas F, Cobianchi L, Scannapieco F, Ruta F. The impact of Covid-19 healthcare emergency on the psychological Well-being of health professionals: a review of literature. Annali Di Igiene Medicina Preventiva e Di Comunita. 2022;34(1):27–44.

Dubé E, Laberge C, Guay M, Bramadat P, Roy R, Bettinger JA. Vaccine hesitancy: an overview. Hum Vaccin Immunother. 2013;9(8):1763–73.

Dunn AG, Leask J, Zhou X, Mandl KD, Coiera E. Associations between exposure to and expression of negative opinions about human papillomavirus vaccines on social media: an observational study. J Med Internet Res. 2015;17(6):e144.

Eedy DJ, Wootton R. Teledermatology: a review. Br J Dermatol. 2001;144(4):696–707.

Egger A, Abrouk M, Brodsky M, Kirsner RS. COVID-19 supply chain considerations for prescription drugs in dermatology. J Drugs Dermatol. 2020;19(6):666–7.

El-Komy MHM, Abdelnaby A, El-Kalioby M. How does COVID-19 impact psoriasis practice, prescription patterns, and healthcare delivery for psoriasis patients? A cross-sectional survey study. J Cosmet Dermatol. 2021;20(6):1573–9.

Elmas ÖF, Demirbaş A, Türsen Ü, Atasoy M, Lotti T. Pemphigus and COVID-19: critical overview of management with a focus on treatment choice. Dermatol Ther. 2020;33(6):1–6.

Elsaie ML, Hussein SM, Zaky MS, Hanafy NS, Jafferany M. Therapeutic implications of prevalence and predictor risk factors for burn out syndrome in Egyptian dermatologists: a cross sectional study. Dermatol Ther. 2020;33(6):1–8.

Elsaie ML, Hasan MS, Zaky MS, Hussein SM, Kadah AS, Omar AM. Implication of COVID-19 on the mental health of Egyptian dermatologists: a cross-sectional study. J Cosmet Dermatol. 2021;20(10):3066–73.

Farr MA, Duvic M, Joshi TP. Teledermatology during COVID-19: an updated review. Am J Clin Dermatol. 2021;22(4):467–75.

Ferreira BR, Jafferany M, Misery L. Psychodermatology in the era of COVID-19. J Clin Aesthet Dermatol. 2021;14(3 Suppl 1):S24–7.

Fisher WA, Kohut T, Salisbury CMA, Salvadori MI. Understanding human papillomavirus vaccination intentions: comparative utility of the theory of reasoned action and the theory of planned behavior in vaccine target age women and men. J Sex Med. 2013;10(10):2455–64.

Francis DB, Cates JR, Wagner KPG, Zola T, Fitter JE, Coyne-Beasley T. Communication technologies to improve HPV vaccination initiation and completion: a systematic review. Patient Educ Couns. 2017;100(7):1280–6.

Freeman EE, McMahon DE, Fitzgerald ME, Fox LP, Rosenbach M, Takeshita J, French LE, Thiers BH, Hruza GJ. The American Academy of Dermatology COVID-19 registry: crowdsourcing dermatology in the age of COVID-19. J Am Acad Dermatol. 2020;83(2):509–10.

Friedrich A-KU, DiComo JA, Golshan M. The impact of COVID-19 on breast surgery fellowships. Curr Breast Cancer Rep. 2021;13(4):235–40.

Gasteratos K, Spyropoulou G-A, Suess L. "Zoom dysmorphia": a new diagnosis in the COVID-19 pandemic era? Plast Reconstr Surg. 2021;148(6):1073e–4e.

Gilsbach S, Herpertz-Dahlmann B, Konrad K. Psychological impact of the COVID-19 pandemic on children and adolescents with and without mental disorders. Front Public Health. 2021;9(November):1–8.

Gleeson LL, Ludlow A, Clyne B, Ryan B, Argent R, Barlow J, Mellon L, De Brún A, Pate M, Kirke C, Moriarty F, Flood M. Pharmacist and patient experiences of primary care during the COVID-19 pandemic: an interview study. Explor Res Clin Soc Pharm. 2022;8:100193.

Grant JE, Chamberlain SR. Prevalence of skin picking (excoriation) disorder. J Psychiatr Res. 2020;130:57–60.

Gronbeck C, Grant-Kels JM. Attention all anti-vaccinators: the cutaneous adverse events from the mRNA COVID-19 vaccines are not an excuse to avoid them! Clin Dermatol. 2021;39(4):674–87.

Guertler A, Moellhoff N, Schenck TL, Hagen CS, Kendziora B, Giunta RE, French LE, Reinholz M. Onset of occupational hand eczema among healthcare workers during the SARS-CoV-2 pandemic: comparing a single surgical site with a COVID-19 intensive care unit. Contact Dermatitis. 2020;83(2):108–14.

Hafi B, Uvais NA, Jafferany M, Afra TP, Muhammed RT. Palliative psychodermatology care during COVID-19 pandemic. Dermatol Ther. 2020;33(4):19–20.

Henry N, Parthiban S, Farroha A. The effect of COVID-19 lockdown on the incidence of deliberate self-harm injuries presenting to the emergency room. Int J Psychiatry Med. 2021;56(4):266–77.

Hernandez RG, Hagen L, Walker K, O'Leary H, Lengacher C. The COVID-19 vaccine social media infodemic : healthcare providers' missed dose in addressing misinformation and vaccine hesitancy. Hum Vaccin Immunother. 2021;17(9):2962–4.

Holmes EA, O'Connor RC, Perry VH, Tracey I, Wessely S, Arseneault L, Ballard C, Christensen H, Cohen Silver R, Everall I, Ford T, John A, Kabir T, King K, Madan I, Michie S, Przybylski AK, Shafran R, Sweeney A, Worthman CM, Yardley L, Cowan K, Cope C, Hotopf M, Bullmore E. Multidisciplinary research priorities for the COVID-19 pandemic: a call for action for mental health science. Lancet Psychiatry. 2020;7(6):547–60.

Honarmand K, Yarnell CJ, Young-Ritchie C, Maunder R, Priestap F, Abdalla M, Ball IM, Basmaji J, Bell CM, Jeffs L, Shah S, Chen J, LeBlanc D, Kayitesi J, Eta-Ndu C, Mehta S. Personal, professional, and psychological impact of the COVID-19 pandemic on hospital workers: a cross-sectional survey. PloS One. 2022;17(2 February):1–18.

Hope C, Reilly J-J, Griffiths G, Lund J, Humes D. The impact of COVID-19 on surgical training: a systematic review. Tech Coloproctol. 2021;25(5):505–20.

Hossain MM, Tasnim S, Sultana A, Faizah F, Mazumder H, Zou L, McKyer ELJ, Ahmed HU, Ma P. Epidemiology of mental health problems in COVID-19: a review. F1000Research. 2020a;9:636.

Hossain MM, Sultana A, Purohit N. Mental health outcomes of quarantine and isolation for infection prevention: a systematic umbrella review of the global evidence. Epidemiol Health. 2020b;42:e2020038.

Huang D, Ganti L, Graham EW, Shah D, Aleksandrovskiy I, Al-Bassam M, Fraunfelter F, Falgiani M, Leon L, Lopez-Ortiz C. COVID-19 vaccine hesitancy among healthcare providers. Health Psychol Res. 2022;10(2):34218.

Huerta-González S, Selva-Medrano D, López-Espuela F, Caro-Alonso PÁ, Novo A, Rodríguez-Martín B. The psychological impact of covid-19 on front line nurses: a synthesis of qualitative evidence. Int J Environ Res Public Health. 2021;18(24):12975.

Ibrahim AE, Magdy M, Khalaf EM, Mostafa A, Arafa A. Teledermatology in the time of COVID-19. Int J Clin Pract. 2021;75(12):1–9.

İnan Doğan E, Kaya F. Dermatological findings in patients admitting to dermatology clinic after using face masks during Covid-19 pandemia: a new health problem. Dermatol Ther. 2021;34(3):1–7.

Jafferany M, Vander Stoep A, Dumitrescu A, Hornung RL. The knowledge, awareness, and practice patterns of dermatologists toward psychocutaneous disorders: results of a survey study. Int J Dermatol. 2010;49(7):784–9.

Jamerson TA, Li Q, Sreeskandarajan S, Budunova IV, He Z, Kang J, Gudjonsson JE, Patrick MT, Tsoi LC. Roles played by stress-induced pathways in driving ethnic heterogeneity for inflammatory skin diseases. Front Immunol. 2022;13:845655.

Jarrett C, Wilson R, O'Leary M, Eckersberger E, Larson HJ. Strategies for addressing vaccine hesitancy—a systematic review. Vaccine. 2015;33(34):4180–90.

Johnston K, O'Reilly CL, Scholz B, Mitchell I. The experiences of pharmacists during the global COVID-19 pandemic: a thematic analysis using the jobs demands-resources framework. Res Social Adm Pharm. 2022;18(9):3649–55.

Jones EAK, Mitra AK, Bhuiyan AR. Impact of COVID-19 on mental health in adolescents: a systematic review. Int J Environ Res Public Health. 2021;18(5):2470.

Kampf G, Scheithauer S, Lemmen S, Saliou P, Suchomel M. COVID-19-associated shortage of alcohol-based hand rubs, face masks, medical gloves, and gowns: proposal for a risk-adapted approach to ensure patient and healthcare worker safety. J Hosp Infect. 2020;105(3):424–7.

Kasperkiewicz M, Strong R, Mead K, Yale M, Zillikens D, Woodley DT, Recke A. COVID-19 vaccine acceptance and hesitancy in patients with immunobullous diseases: a cross-sectional study of the international pemphigus and pemphigoid foundation. Br J Dermatol. 2022;186(4):737–9.

Khan YH, Rasheed M, Mallhi TH, Salman M, Alzarea AI, Alanazi AS, Alotaibi NH, Khan SUD, Alatawi AD, Butt MH, Alzarea SI, Alharbi KS, Alharthi SS, Algarni MA, Alahmari AK, Almalki ZS, Iqbal MS. Barriers and facilitators of childhood COVID-19 vaccination among parents: a systematic review. Front Pediatr. 2022;10(November):1–19.

Knebel C, Ertl M, Lenze U, Suren C, Dinkel A, Hirschmann MT, von Eisenhart-Rothe R, Pohlig F. COVID-19-related cancellation of elective orthopaedic surgery caused increased pain and psychosocial distress levels. Knee Surg Sports Traumatol Arthrosc. 2021;29(8):2379–85.

Knight H, Jia R, Ayling K, Bradbury K, Baker K, Chalder T, Morling JR, Durrant L, Avery T, Ball JK, Barker C, Bennett R, McKeever T, Vedhara K. Understanding and addressing vaccine hesitancy in the context of COVID-19: development of a digital intervention. Public Health. 2021;201:98–107.

Koh SWC, Liow Y, Loh VWK, Liew SJ, Chan Y-H, Young D. COVID-19 vaccine acceptance and hesitancy among primary healthcare workers in Singapore. BMC Primary Care. 2022;23(1):81.

Kricorian K, Civen R, Equils O. COVID-19 vaccine hesitancy: misinformation and perceptions of vaccine safety. Hum Vaccin Immunother. 2022;18(1):1950504.

Kuang Y, Shen M, Wang Q, Xiao Y, Lv C, Luo Y, Zhu W, Chen X. Association of outdoor activity restriction and income loss with patient-reported outcomes of psoriasis during the COVID-19 pandemic: a web-based survey. J Am Acad Dermatol. 2020;83(2):670–2.

Lai J, Ma S, Wang Y, Cai Z, Hu J, Wei N, Wu J, Du H, Chen T, Li R, Tan H, Kang L, Yao L, Huang M, Wang H, Wang G, Liu Z, Hu S. Factors associated with mental health outcomes among health care workers exposed to coronavirus disease 2019. JAMA Netw Open. 2020;3(3):e203976.

Larson HJ, Jarrett C, Eckersberger E, Smith DMD, Paterson P. Understanding vaccine hesitancy around vaccines and vaccination from a global perspective: a systematic review of published literature, 2007–2012. Vaccine. 2014;32(19):2150–9.

Larson HJ, Gakidou E, Murray CJL. The vaccine-hesitant moment. N Engl J Med. 2022;387(1):58–65.

Lee SK, Sun J, Jang S, Connelly S. Misinformation of COVID-19 vaccines and vaccine hesitancy. Sci Rep. 2022;12(1):13681.

Li HOY, Pastukhova E, Brandts-Longtin O, Tan MG, Kirchhof MG. YouTube as a source of misinformation on COVID-19 vaccination: a systematic analysis. BMJ Glob Health. 2022;7(3):1–6.

Lockyer B, Islam S, Rahman A, Dickerson J, Pickett K, Sheldon T, Wright J, McEachan R, Sheard L. Understanding COVID-19 misinformation and vaccine hesitancy in context: findings from a qualitative study involving citizens in Bradford, UK. Health Expect. 2021;24(4):1158–67.

Loh CH, Chong Tam SY, Oh CC. Teledermatology in the COVID-19 pandemic: a systematic review. JAAD Int. 2021;5:54–64.

Lou NM, Montreuil T, Feldman LS, Fried GM, Lavoie-Tremblay M, Bhanji F, Kennedy H, Kaneva P, Harley JM. Nurses' and physicians' distress, burnout, and coping strategies during COVID-19: stress and impact on perceived performance and intentions to quit. J Contin Educ Health Prof. 2022;42(1):E44–52.

Luchetti M, Lee JH, Aschwanden D, Sesker A, Strickhouser JE, Terracciano A, Sutin AR. The trajectory of loneliness in response to COVID-19. Am Psychol. 2020;75(7):897–908.

Lund J, Sadler P, McLarty E. The effect of COVID-19 on surgical training. Surgery (Oxford). 2021;39(12):829–33.

Lv S, Wang L, Zou X, Wang Z, Qu B, Lin W, Yang D. A case of acute Telogen effluvium after SARS-CoV-2 infection. Clin Cosmet Investig Dermatol. 2021;14:385–7.

MacDonald NE. Vaccine hesitancy: definition, scope and determinants. Vaccine. 2015;33(34):4161–4.

Magid M, Reichenberg JS. An evidence-based approach to starting a Psychodermatology clinic. JAMA Dermatol. 2020;156(6):617.

Mahil SK, Dand N, Mason KJ, Yiu ZZN, Tsakok T, Meynell F, Coker B, McAteer H, Moorhead L, Mackenzie T, Rossi MT, Rivera R, Mahe E, Carugno A, Magnano M, Rech G, Balogh EA, Feldman SR, De La Cruz C, Choon SE, Naldi L, Lambert J, Spuls P, Jullien D, Bachelez H, McMahon DE, Freeman EE, Gisondi P, Puig L, Warren RB, Di Meglio P, Langan SM, Capon F, Griffiths CEM, Barker JN, Smith CH, Shah A, Barea A, Romero-Maté A, Singapore A, Paolino A, Mwale A, Morales Callaghan AM, Martinez A, DeCrescenzo A, Pink AE, Jones A, Sergeant A, Essex A, Bewley A, Makrygeorgou A, van Huizen A, Pérez-Suárez B, Farida B, Claréus BW, Prims CT, Davis C, Quinlan C, Maybury C, Cesar GA, Barclay C, Greco C, Brassard D, Cummings D, Kolli D, Descamps V, Genao DR, Carras E, Hawryluk E, Martínez-García E, Klujszo E, Dwyer E, Toni E, Sonkoly E, Loayza E, Daudén E, Valenzuela F, Popov G, King G, Celine G, Aparicio G, Johnston GA, Cardozo GA, Pearson I, Yanguas I, Weisman J, Carolan JE, Hughes J, Ortiz-Salvador JM, Carrascosa JM, Schwartz JJ, Jackson K, Kerisit KG, Wu K, Asfour L, de Graaf L, Lesort C, Meuleman L, Eidsmo L, Skov L, Gribben L, Rustin M, Velasco M, Panchal M, Lakhan M, Franco MD, Svensson ML, Vandaele M, Marovt M, Zargari O, De Caso P, Varela P, Jenkin P, Phan C, Hampton P, Goldsmith P, Bak R, Speeckaert R, Romiti R, Woolf R, Mercado-Seda R, Khatun R, Ceovic R, Taberner R, Cohen RW, Stefanescu S, Kirk S, Reeken S, Ayob S, Pérez-Barrio S, Piaserico S, Hoey S, Torres T, Talme T, Desai TV, van Geest AJ, King V, Di Lernia V, Koreja Z, Hasab VZ. Factors associated with adverse COVID-19 outcomes in patients with psoriasis—insights from a global registry–based study. J Allergy Clin Immunol. 2021a;147(1):60–71.

Mahil SK, Yates M, Langan SM, Yiu ZZN, Tsakok T, Dand N, Mason KJ, McAteer H, Meynell F, Coker B, Vincent A, Urmston D, Vesty A, Kelly J, Lancelot C, Moorhead L, Bachelez H, Bruce IN, Capon F, Contreras CR, Cope AP, De La Cruz C, Di Meglio P, Gisondi P, Hyrich K, Jullien D, Lambert J, Marzo-Ortega H, McInnes I, Naldi L, Norton S, Puig L, Sengupta R, Spuls P, Torres T, Warren RB, Waweru H, Weinman J, Griffiths CEM, Barker JN, Brown MA, Galloway JB, Smith CH. Risk-mitigating behaviours in people with inflammatory skin and joint disease during the COVID-19 pandemic differ by treatment type: a cross-sectional patient survey*. Br J Dermatol. 2021b;185(1):80–90.

Mahil SK, Yates M, Yiu ZZN, Langan SM, Tsakok T, Dand N, Mason KJ, McAteer H, Meynell F, Coker B, Vincent A, Urmston D, Vesty A, Kelly J, Lancelot C, Moorhead L, Bachelez H, Capon F, Contreras CR, De La Cruz C, Di Meglio P, Gisondi P, Jullien D, Lambert J, Naldi L, Norton S, Puig L, Spuls P, Torres T, Warren RB, Waweru H, Weinman J, Brown MA, Galloway JB, Griffiths CM, Barker JN, Smith CH. Describing the burden of the COVID-19 pandemic in people with psoriasis: findings from a global cross-sectional study. J Eur Acad Dermatol Venereol. 2021c;35(10):e636–40.

Majid U, Ahmad M, Zain S, Akande A, Ikhlaq F. COVID-19 vaccine hesitancy and acceptance: a comprehensive scoping review of global literature. Health Promot Int. 2022;37(3):daac078.

Manchia M, Gathier AW, Yapici-Eser H, Schmidt MV, de Quervain D, van Amelsvoort T, Bisson JI, Cryan JF, Howes OD, Pinto L, van der Wee NJ, Domschke K, Branchi I, Vinkers CH. The impact of the prolonged COVID-19 pandemic on stress resilience and mental health: a critical review across waves. Eur Neuropsychopharmacol. 2022;55(January):22–83.

Mangini CSM, de Vasconcelos RCF, Rodriguez EVR, de Oliveira IRL. Social isolation: main dermatosis and the impact of stress during the COVID-19 pandemic. Einstein (Sao Paulo). 2022;20(2):eAO6320.

Marahatta S, Singh A, Pyakurel P. Self-cosmetic care during the COVID-19 pandemic and its psychological impacts: facts behind the closed doors. J Cosmet Dermatol. 2021;20(10):3093–7.

Marasca C, Ruggiero A, Napolitano M, Fabbrocini G, Megna M. May COVID-19 outbreaks lead to a worsening of skin chronic inflammatory conditions? Med Hypotheses. 2020;143(January):109853.

Marasca C, De Rosa A, Fabbrocini G, Cantelli M, Patrì A, Vastarella M, Gallo L, di Vico F, Poggi S, Ruggiero A. Psychological teleconsultations in patients suffering from chronic skin diseases during the COVID-19 era: a service to improve patients' quality of life. J Dermatol Treat. 2022;33(3):1736–7.

McMahon DE, Gallman AE, Hruza GJ, Rosenbach M, Lipoff JB, Desai SR, French LE, Lim H, Cyster JG, Fox LP, Fassett MS, Freeman EE. Long COVID in the skin: a registry analysis of COVID-19 dermatological duration. Lancet Infect Dis. 2021;21(3):313–4.

Mieczkowska K, Deutsch A, Borok J, Guzman AK, Fruchter R, Patel P, Wind O, McLellan BN, Mann RE, Halverstam CP. Telogen effluvium: a sequela of COVID-19. Int J Dermatol. 2021;60(1):122–4.

Misery L, Fluhr J-W, Beylot-Barry M, Jouan N, Hamann P, Consoli S-G, Schollhammer M, Charleux D, Bewley A, Rathod D. Psychological and professional impact of COVID-19 lockdown on French dermatologists: data from a large survey. Ann Dermatol Venereol. 2021;148(2):101–5.

Montero-Vilchez T, Cuenca-Barrales C, Martinez-Lopez A, Molina-Leyva A, Arias-Santiago S. Skin adverse events related to personal protective equipment: a systematic review and meta-analysis. J Eur Acad Dermatol Venereol. 2021;35(10):1994–2006.

Moreno R, Díez J-L, Diarte J-A, Macaya F, de la Torrre Hernández J-M, Rodríguez-Leor O, Trillo R, Alonso-Briales J, Amat-Santos I, Romaguera R, Díaz J-F, Vaquerizo B, Ojeda S, Cruz-González I, Morena-Salas D, Pérez de Prado A, Sarnago F, Portero P, Gutierrez-Barrios A, Alfonso F, Bosch E, Pinar E, Ruiz-Arroyo J-R, Ruiz-Quevedo V, Jiménez-Mazuecos J, Lozano F, Rumoroso J-R, Novo E, Irazusta FJ, García Del Blanco B, Moreu J, Ballesteros-Pradas SM, Frutos A, Villa M, Alegría-Barrero E, Lázaro R, Paredes E. Consequences of canceling elective invasive cardiac procedures during Covid-19 outbreak. Catheter Cardiovasc Interv. 2021;97(5):927–37.

Mościcka P, Chróst N, Terlikowski R, Przylipiak M, Wołosik K, Przylipiak A. Hygienic and cosmetic care habits in polish women during COVID-19 pandemic. J Cosmet Dermatol. 2020;19(8):1840–5.

Murrell DF, Arora G, Rudnicka L, Kassir M, Lotti T, Goldust M. A dermatologist's perspective of the COVID-19 outbreak. Dermatol Ther. 2020;33(4):e13538.

Nagaraj MB, Weis HB, Weis JJ, Cook GS, Bailey LW, Shoultz TH, Farr DE, AbdelFattah KR, Dultz LA. The impact of COVID-19 on surgical education. J Surg Res. 2021;267:366–73.

Narang T, Bhandari A, Mehta H, Narang K, Handa S, Dogra S. Effect of lockdown due to COVID-19 on health and lifestyle of psoriasis patients: a web-based survey. Indian Dermatol Online J. 2022;13(5):625.

Nasseh J, Podevin C, Ternynck C, Zephir H, Letarouilly JG, Flipo RM, Nachury M, Chenivesse C, Hachulla E, Launay D, Staumont-Salle D, Dezoteux F. Self-reported impact of the early 2020 COVID-19 crisis on the healthcare pathway during and after lockdown in patients with chronic immune-mediated inflammatory diseases: a practical survey. J Patient Exp. 2022;9:19–22.

Navin MC, Oberleitner LM-S, Lucia VC, Ozdych M, Afonso N, Kennedy RH, Keil H, Wu L, Mathew TA. COVID-19 vaccine hesitancy among health-care personnel who generally accept vaccines. J Community Health. 2022;47(3):519–29.

Nazlı ŞB, Yığman F, Sevindik M, Deniz Özturan D. Psychological factors affecting COVID-19 vaccine hesitancy. Irish J Med Sci (1971). 2022;191(1):71–80.

Nicola M, Alsafi Z, Sohrabi C, Kerwan A, Al-Jabir A, Iosifidis C, Agha M, Agha R. The socio-economic implications of the coronavirus pandemic (COVID-19): a review. Int J Surg. 2020;78:185–93.

Niesert A-C, Oppel EM, Nellessen T, Frey S, Clanner-Engelshofen BM, Wollenberg A, French LE, Reinholz M. "Face mask dermatitis" due to compulsory facial masks during the SARS-CoV-2 pandemic: data from 550 health care and non-health care workers in Germany. Eur J Dermatol. 2021;31(2):199–204.

Nowak SA, Gidengil CA, Parker AM, Matthews LJ. Association among trust in health care providers, friends, and family, and vaccine hesitancy. Vaccine. 2021;39(40):5737–40.

Patel A, Jafferany M. Multidisciplinary and holistic models of care for patients with dermatologic disease and psychosocial comorbidity. JAMA Dermatol. 2020;156(6):686.

Pathoulas JT, Olson SJ, Idnani A, Farah RS, Hordinsky MK, Widge AS. Cross-sectional survey examining skin picking and hair pulling disorders during the COVID-19 pandemic. J Am Acad Dermatol. 2021;84(3):771–3.

Pendlebury GA, Oro P, Haynes W, Merideth D, Bartling S, Bongiorno MA. The impact of COVID-19 pandemic on dermatological conditions: a novel, comprehensive review. Dermatopathology. 2022;9(3):212–43.

Pires C. Global predictors of COVID-19 vaccine hesitancy: a systematic review. Vaccine. 2022;10(8):1349.

Pirro F, Caldarola G, Chiricozzi A, Tambone S, Mariani M, Calabrese L, D'Urso DF, De Simone C, Peris K. The impact of COVID-19 pandemic in a cohort of Italian psoriatic patients treated with biological therapies. J Dermatol Treat. 2022;33(2):1079–83.

Prabani KIP, Weerasekara I, Damayanthi HDWT, Yasmin F, Najeeb H, Moeed A, Naeem U, Asghar MS, Chughtai NU, Yousaf Z, Seboka BT, Ullah I, Lin CY, Pakpour AH, Sallam M, Mohebi S, Parham M, Sharifirad G, Gharlipour Z, Kafadar AH, Tekeli GG, Jones KA, Stephan B, Dening T, Pires C, Hussain B, Latif A, Timmons S, Nkhoma K, Nellums LB. COVID-19 vaccine hesitancy in the United States: a systematic review. Vaccine. 2022;9(January):1–15.

Prochwicz K, Antosz-Rekucka R, Kałużna-Wielobób A, Sznajder D, Kłosowska J. Negative affectivity moderates the relationship between attentional control and focused skin picking. Int J Environ Res Public Health. 2022;19(11):6636.

Ramphul K. "Zoom dysmorphia": the rise of a new issue amidst the pandemic. Acta Biomed. 2021;92(6):e2021348.

Rensch G, Barton V, Ragland P. Disruption of the medical supply chain by the COVID-19 pandemic adversely affecting dermatologic surgery. Dermatol Surg. 2022;48(4):477–8.

Richardson VL, Garcia-Albea VR, Bort NL, Mayne SL, Nolen ME, Bobonich MA. Reflections of COVID-19 on dermatology practice. J Dermatol Nurses Assoc. 2021;13(1):49–53.

Ricketts EJ, Peris TS, Grant JE, Valle S, Cavic E, Lerner JE, Lochner C, Stein DJ, Dougherty DD, O'Neill J, Woods DW, Keuthen NJ, Piacentini J. Clinical characteristics of youth with trichotillomania (hair-pulling disorder) and excoriation (skin-picking) disorder. Child Psychiatry Hum Dev. 2022.

Roberts JE, Smith AM, Wilkerson AH, Chandra A, Patel V, Quadri SSA, Mann JR, Brodell RT, Nahar VK. "Psychodermatology" knowledge, attitudes, and practice among health care professionals. Arch Dermatol Res. 2020;312(8):545–58.

Roberts V, Chan J, Davies J, Angus J. The benefits of an integrated liaison psychiatry and dermatology service for complex dermatology patients—a case series. Skin Health Dis. 2022;2:e159.

Rodríguez BO, Sánchez TL. The psychosocial impact of COVID-19 on health care workers. Int Braz J Urol. 2020;46(Suppl 1):195–200.

Romer D, Jamieson KH. Conspiracy theories as barriers to controlling the spread of COVID-19 in the U.S. Soc Sci Med. 2020;263:113356.

Saladino V, Algeri D, Auriemma V. The psychological and social impact of Covid-19: new perspectives of well-being. Front Psychol. 2020;11:577684.

Sharquie KE, Jabbar RI. COVID-19 infection is a major cause of acute telogen effluvium. Irish J Med Sci (1971). 2022;191(4):1677–81.

Shen M, Xiao Y, Yuan Y, Chen X, Li J. Perceived stress links income loss and urticaria activity during the coronavirus disease 2019 pandemic. Ann Allergy Asthma Immunol. 2021;126(1):89–90.

Soutou B, Tomb R. The multifaceted engagement of the dermatologist in the Covid-19 pandemic. SN Comprehens Clin Med. 2020;2(9):1388–92.

Stamu-O'Brien C, Carniciu S, Halvorsen E, Jafferany M. Psychological aspects of COVID-19. J Cosmet Dermatol. 2020;19(9):2169–73.

Stamu-O'Brien C, Jafferany M, Carniciu S, Abdelmaksoud A. Psychodermatology of acne: psychological aspects and effects of acne vulgaris. J Cosmet Dermatol. 2021;20(4):1080–3.

Steinhoff M, Suárez A, Feramisco J, Koo J. Psychoneuroimmunology of psychological stress and atopic dermatitis: pathophysiologic and therapeutic updates. Acta Dermato Venereologica. 2012;92(1):7–15.

Stickley A, Koyanagi A. Loneliness, common mental disorders and suicidal behavior: findings from a general population survey. J Affect Disord. 2016;197:81–7.

Storey D. COVID-19 vaccine hesitancy. Glob Health Sci Pract. 2022;10(1):e2200043.

Strategic Advisory Group of Experts. Meeting of the Strategic Advisory Group of Experts on Immunization, November 2011—conclusions and recommendations. Wkly Epidemiol Rec. 2012;87(1):1–16.

Tammaro A, Parisella FR, Adebanjo GAR. Cutaneous long COVID. J Cosmet Dermatol. 2021;20(8):2378–9.

Torales J, Díaz NR, Barrios I, Navarro R, García O, O'Higgins M, Castaldelli-Maia JM, Ventriglio A, Jafferany M. Psychodermatology of skin picking (excoriation disorder): a comprehensive review. Dermatol Ther. 2020;33(4):e13661.

Trott M, Johnstone J, Pardhan S, Barnett Y, Smith L. Changes in body dysmorphic disorder, eating disorder, and exercise addiction symptomology during the COVID-19 pandemic: a longitudinal study of 319 health club users. Psychiatry Res. 2021;298:113831.

van Kessel SAM, Olde Hartman TC, Lucassen PLBJ, van Jaarsveld CHM. Post-acute and long-COVID-19 symptoms in patients with mild diseases: a systematic review. Fam Pract. 2022;39(1):159–67.

Wilson SL, Wiysonge C. Social media and vaccine hesitancy. BMJ Glob Health. 2020;5(10):e004206.

Wong C, Tay W, Hap X, Chia F. Love in the time of coronavirus: training and service during COVID-19. Singapore Med J. 2020;51(1):1–1.

Xiao X, Wong RM. Vaccine hesitancy and perceived behavioral control: a meta-analysis. Vaccine. 2020;38(33):5131–8.

Xie Z, Yang Y, Zhang H. Mask-induced contact dermatitis in handling COVID-19 outbreak. Contact Dermatitis. 2020;83(2):166–7.

Xiong J, Lipsitz O, Nasri F, Lui LMW, Gill H, Phan L, Chen-Li D, Iacobucci M, Ho R, Majeed A, McIntyre RS. Impact of COVID-19 pandemic on mental health in the general population: a systematic review. J Affect Disord. 2020;277(July):55–64.

Yu J, Chen JK, Mowad CM, Reeder M, Hylwa S, Chisolm S, Dunnick CA, Goldminz AM, Jacob SE, Wu PA, Zippin J, Atwater AR. Occupational dermatitis to facial personal protective equipment in health care workers: a systematic review. J Am Acad Dermatol. 2021;84(2):486–94.

Zimmerman T, Shiroma K, Fleischmann KR, Xie B, Jia C, Verma N, Lee MK. Misinformation and COVID-19 vaccine hesitancy. Vaccine. 2022;41:136.

Oral COVID-19 Antiviral Agents in Dermatology Outpatient Treatment

14

Kathleen Shu-En Quah, Xiaoling Huang, Laurent Renia, and Hazel H. Oon

Introduction

In December 2019, the first cases of COVID-19 were reported, with an ensuing rapid spread to many countries across the world. On 11 March 2020, the World Health Organization (WHO) declared the COVID-19 outbreak a pandemic. Since then, there were more than two million deaths reported in the European region. Tremendous efforts have been focussed on developing vaccines and medications for the prevention and treatment of COVID-19 to minimise complications from this infection (WHO 2022).

Two oral antiviral medications, nirmatrelvir-ritonavir (NMV/r, Paxlovid™) and molnupiravir (Lagevrio™), have been developed and used in the treatment of patients with mild COVID-19 at risk of developing severe disease resulting in hospitalisation or mortality (U.S. Food and Drug Administration 2022a, b). Unfortunately, the use of these COVID-19 therapies is complicated by clinically significant drug-drug interactions (DDIs) with ritonavir and many commonly prescribed medications, including dermatologic medications. Dermatologists should be familiar with DDIs involving NMV/r, molnupiravir and dermatologic medications to support safe and prompt initiation of COVID-19 treatment while keeping the underlying dermatologic condition controlled. A systematic review, together with a manual search of the various drug interaction checkers, was conducted in July 2022 to collate DDIs between dermatologic medications, NMV/r and molnupiravir (Quah et al. 2022). However, with the rapid approval of new medications, as well as more information on drug interactions, it is imperative to continue to update the DDIs to keep abreast of changes for optimal patient care.

This chapter will summarise the DDIs between NMV/r, molnupiravir and dermatologic medications, with a focus on the potential adverse events and suggested management of co-medications that interact with NMV/r and molnupiravir.

K. S.-E. Quah
Yong Loo Lin School of Medicine, National University of Singapore, Singapore, Singapore
e-mail: kathleenquahse@u.nus.edu

X. Huang
Pharmacy Department, National Skin Centre, Singapore, Singapore
e-mail: xlhuang@nsc.com.sg

L. Renia
Lee Kong Chian School of Medicine, Nanyang Technological University, Singapore, Singapore

A*STAR Infectious Diseases Labs, Singapore, Singapore
e-mail: lcsrenia@ntu.edu.sg

H. H. Oon (✉)
National Skin Centre, Singapore, Singapore
e-mail: hazeloon@nsc.com.sg

© The Author(s), under exclusive license to Springer Nature Switzerland AG 2023
H. H. Oon, C. L. Goh (eds.), *COVID-19 in Dermatology*, Updates in Clinical Dermatology,
https://doi.org/10.1007/978-3-031-45586-5_14

Methods

A search using the Liverpool COVID-19 Drug Interaction Checker, Micromedex, Lexicomp and the National Institutes of Health COVID-19 Treatment Guidelines from inception to 28 December 2022 was conducted to identify DDI between dermatologic medications, NMV/r and molnupiravir (University of Liverpool 2022; Micromedex Solutions 2022; UpToDate 2022; National Institutes of Health 2023a). The Liverpool COVID-19 Drug Interaction Checker is the leading database for DDI with COVID-19 therapies (University of Liverpool 2022). Micromedex and Lexicomp were selected as the drug interaction checkers due to their accuracy, completeness and ease of use (Micromedex Solutions 2022; UpToDate 2022; Patel and Beckett 2016; Kheshti et al. 2016). Furthermore, these sources are updated with information on new drugs, pharmacovigilance and pharmaceutical publications. More than one drug interaction resources has been used due to the inconsistency in recommendations provided among the various drug interaction resources (Monteith and Glenn 2021).

For drugs that do not have information in all four drug interaction resources, the drug monograph was referred to determine whether the drug is an inhibitor, inducer or substrate of the CYP3A4, CYP2D6, CYP2B6, CYP2C19, CYP2C9, CYP1A2 and P-glycoprotein (P-gp) to predict potential drug interactions with NMV/r or molnupiravir. The prescribing information of the interacting drugs were then reviewed for the need for drug discontinuation, dosage reduction or continued use with close monitoring.

Results and Discussion

Therapeutic Management of Nonhospitalised Adults with COVID-19

All patients with COVID-19 should be offered symptomatic management, including rest, adequate fluid intake, antipyretics, analgesia and antitussives. Access to a healthcare provider, with access by telehealth where possible, and advice for in-person consultation and emergency services should be given (National Institutes of Health 2023b).

For adults with mild-to-moderate COVID-19 at high risk of progression to severe disease, not requiring hospitalisation and supplemental oxygen, NMV/r is currently recommended by the NIH COVID-19 Treatment Guidelines Panel as the first-line (recommendation rating AIIa) and most efficacious oral COVID-19 therapy available (National Institutes of Health 2023b). In the EPIC-HR trial, NMV/r administered within 5 days of symptom onset was demonstrated to reduce the risk of hospitalisation or mortality at day 28 by 88.9% compared to placebo, greater than that reported for remdesivir in the PINETREE trial (87% relative reduction) and molnupiravir (30% relative reduction) in the MOVe-OUT study (Jayk Bernal et al. 2022; Gottlieb et al. 2022). However, NMV/r may not be suitable for all patients due to its potential for significant DDIs with co-administered medications.

Remdesivir intravenous infusion over a 3-day period and started within 7 days of symptom onset is a second-line preferred agent (recommendation rating BIIa) (National Institutes of Health 2023b). Remdesivir is a nucleotide prodrug of an adenosine analogue which binds to viral RNA polymerase and inhibits viral replication by terminating RNA transcription prematurely. It retains in vitro neutralisation activity against the Omicron variant and its subvariants (Food and Drug Administration 2022). If remdesivir is unsuitable or infusion access is unavailable or logistically challenging, molnupiravir is an alternative agent (recommendation rating CIIa) (National Institutes of Health 2023b).

Nirmatrelvir-Ritonavir (NMV/r)

Nirmatrelvir is a SARS-CoV-2-3CL protease inhibitor involved in the prevention of viral replication in COVID-19 and other coronavirus infections. This is co-administered with ritonavir, which is a pharmacoenhancer and strong CYP450 3A4 enzyme inhibitor, to inhibit the metabolism of nirmatrelvir, a CYP3A4 substrate, and maintain its plasma concentrations at therapeutic levels (Paxlovid 2021).

Drug-Drug Interactions

The DDIs of NMV/r mainly include other CYP3A4 substrates, due to ritonavir-mediated CYP3A4 inhibition, maximal within 48 h from the first dose of NMV/r, resulting in increased drug plasma concentration and risk of concentration-dependent toxicity (Katzenmaier et al. 2011). Concomitant administration of NMV/r with CYP3A4 inhibitors increases the plasma concentration of NMV/r and the risk of adverse effects from NMV/r. In contrast, CYP3A4 inducers reduce the plasma concentration of NMV/r, causing significant decline in therapeutic effect with potential for development of viral resistance.

Ritonavir is an irreversible CYP3A4 inhibitor; hence, these DDIs persist even after its discontinuation as time is required for the resolution of CYP3A4 inhibition through the synthesis of new CYP3A4 enzymes. This is dependent on multiple factors including the patient's age, with a longer time to resolution occurring in older patients. Significant resolution of CYP3A4 inhibition by 80% occurs after 48 h and 72 h from the last dose of NMV/r, in adults aged 20 to 50 years old and above 60 years old, respectively (Stader et al. 2020). Hence, a 3-day rule may be used to guide the management of DDI with NMV/r; medications that interact with NMV/r may be safely restarted or returned to their original dose 3 days following the last dose of NMV/r in most individuals.

As the treatment course of NMV/r for COVID-19 is only a duration of 5 days, chronic dermatologic medications with drug interactions should be withdrawn or dose adjusted, as clinically appropriate, for a short duration of 8 days to allow safe treatment with NMV/r. Since NMV/r is currently the most effective oral antiviral therapy against COVID-19, DDI should be managed where feasible to allow its use (National Institutes of Health 2023c).

Commonly used dermatologic drugs that have significant drug interactions with NMV/r are described below, along with the potential side effects and recommendations on management. The principles of management of these DDIs are further summarised in Table 14.1 for ease of reference.

Antibiotics

Macrolides have been used to treat acne, rosacea and other staphylococcal skin infections. During co-administration with NMV/r, the CYP3A4-mediated metabolism of clarithromycin and erythromycin is inhibited by ritonavir, with the elevated plasma concentration of these macrolides increasing the risk of side effects such as hepatotoxicity and QT interval prolongation (Erythro-Base 2014; Biaxin 2017). For erythromycin, recommendations include to stop use or replace with other antibiotics with lesser interaction with NMV/r during the course of NMV/r and for 3 days after the last dose of NMV/r; examples include replacing with tetracycline class antibiotics for acne and rosacea and penicillin or cephalosporin class antibiotics for staphylococcal skin infections, barring any drug allergies. Clarithromycin, which is less dependent on CYP3A4 metabolism than erythromycin, may be continued with careful monitoring for adverse effects, with dose reduction only required in patients with renal impairment (KDIGO Stage ≥ 3, with creatinine clearance (CrCl) ≤ 60 mL/min). Clarithromycin prescribing information suggests dose reduction by 50% and 75% in patients with CrCl 30–60 mL/min and <30 mL/min, respectively (Biaxin 2017).

However, replacement with another antibiotic is recommended for use of clarithromycin in non-tuberculous mycobacterial infections. Although the co-administration of clarithromycin and ritonavir in NMV/r increases the plasma concentration of clarithromycin, there is a decrease in the plasma concentration of the active metabolite 14-OH-clarithromycin. The efficacy of clarithromycin therapy may be compromised, and thus, considerations should be made for replacement with other antibiotics as appropriate (Biaxin 2017).

Table 14.1 Summary of drug interactions between dermatologic medications and nirmatrelvir-ritonavir (NMV/r)[a]

Dermatologic medications	Common indications	Effect of NMV/r/on plasma drug concentration	Potential adverse effects	Recommended management
Antibiotics				
Clarithromycin	Acne Rosacea Staphylococcal skin infections Non-tuberculous mycobacterium infections	↑ Clarithromycin but ↓ clarithromycin active metabolites (Dependent on CYP3A4 metabolism)	Hepatotoxicity QT interval prolongation	Consider alternative antibiotics for mycobacterial infections since efficacy may be compromised. (Micromedex, Lexicomp) Carefully monitor for adverse effects, particularly in patients with renal impairment No dose adjustment is necessary in patients with normal renal function. Avoid clarithromycin doses higher than 1000 mg/day Dose reduction by 50% and 75% in patients with CrCl 30–60 mL/min and <30 mL/min, respectively (Biaxin 2017) (Lexicomp Risk Rating D, Micromedex Severity Major)
Clindamycin	Hidradenitis suppurativa Staphylococcal skin infections	↑ Clindamycin (Dependent on CYP3A4 metabolism)	Gastrointestinal symptoms Nephrotoxicity	Carefully monitor for adverse effects (Lexicomp Risk Rating C; Micromedex however states no drug interactions)
Clofazimine	Leprosy	↑ Clofazimine (Dependent on CYP3A4 metabolism)	QT interval prolongation	Carefully monitor for adverse effects, including ECG monitoring. (Micromedex Severity Major) Lexicomp and Liverpool COVID-19 Drug Interaction Checker indicate no drug interactions expected
Erythromycin	Acne Rosacea Staphylococcal skin infections	↑ Erythromycin (Dependent on CYP3A4 metabolism)	Gastrointestinal symptoms Hepatotoxicity QT interval prolongation	Stop or replace with another antibiotic that has lesser interaction with NMV/r during and for 3 days after the last dose of NMV/r (NIH). Alternatively, carefully monitor for adverse effects, including ECG monitoring, and consider dose reduction (Lexicomp Risk Rating D, Micromedex Severity Major)
Rifampicin	Hidradenitis suppurativa Staphylococcal skin infections Non-tuberculous mycobacterium infections	↓ NMV/r (rifampicin is a CYP3A4 inducer)	Reduced therapeutic effects of NMV/r Risk of loss of virological response	Concomitant use of rifampicin is contraindicated Consider alternative COVID-19 treatment or anti-mycobacterial therapy (e.g. rifabutin) or alternative treatment for hidradenitis suppurativa (Lexicomp Risk Rating X, Micromedex Severity Contraindicated)

Metronidazole	Rosacea Bacterial vaginosis Trichomoniasis	–	QT interval prolongation (metronidazole and ritonavir both cause QT interval prolongation)	Carefully monitor for adverse effects, including ECG monitoring, or consider avoiding the concomitant administration of metronidazole and NMV/r in susceptible patients (Micromedex Severity Major) Lexicomp and Liverpool COVID-19 Drug Interaction Checker indicate no significant drug interactions expected
Tinidazole	Bacterial vaginosis Trichomoniasis	↑ Tinidazole (Dependent on CYP3A4 metabolism)	Clinical consequences unknown	No dose adjustment or additional monitoring necessary (Lexicomp Risk Rating B)
Anti-fungal agents				
Fluconazole	Dermatophyte infections Pityriasis versicolor Candidiasis	↑ NMV/r (fluconazole is a CYP3A4 inhibitor)	Gastrointestinal symptoms Transaminitis QT interval prolongation	Carefully monitor for adverse effects, including ECG monitoring (Lexicomp Risk Rating B, Micromedex Severity Contraindicated) Liverpool COVID-19 Drug Interaction Checker indicates no drug interactions expected
Itraconazole	Dermatophyte infections Onychomycosis Pityriasis versicolor	↑ Itraconazole (Dependent on CYP3A4 metabolism) ↑ NMV/r (itraconazole is an CYP3A4 inhibitor)	Gastrointestinal symptoms Transaminitis QT interval prolongation	Avoid high doses (>200 mg/day) of itraconazole, and carefully monitor for adverse effects (Sporanox 2001) (Lexicomp Risk Rating D, Micromedex Severity Moderate)
Ketoconazole	Dermatophyte infections Pityriasis versicolor	↑ Ketoconazole (Dependent on CYP3A4 metabolism) ↑ NMV/r (ketoconazole is an CYP3A4 inhibitor)	Gastrointestinal symptoms Transaminitis QT interval prolongation	Avoid high doses (>200 mg/day) of ketoconazole, and carefully monitor for adverse effects (Nizoral 2014) (Lexicomp Risk Rating C, Micromedex Severity Major)
Anti-parasitic agents				
Albendazole	Parasitic worm infections	↓ Albendazole (ritonavir is an inducer of hepatic metabolism of albendazole)		Monitor for poorer clinical response to albendazole therapy. (Lexicomp Risk Rating C)
Ivermectin	Scabies	↑ Ivermectin (Dependent on CYP3A4 metabolism and P-glycoprotein efflux)	Neurotoxicity	Potential interaction (Liverpool COVID-19 Drug Interaction Checker) Lexicomp indicates no drug interactions expected Carefully monitor for adverse effects, including signs and symptoms of neurotoxicity

(continued)

Table 14.1 (continued)

Dermatologic medications	Common indications	Effect of NMV/r/on plasma drug concentration	Potential adverse effects	Recommended management
Antihistamines				
Bilastine	Angioedema and other allergic dermatological reactions Atopic dermatitis Urticaria Pruritus	↑ Bilastine (Dependent on P-glycoprotein efflux)	QT interval prolongation	Discontinue bilastine during NMV/r treatment, especially in patients with moderate-to-severe renal impairment, and resume bilastine 3 days after the last dose of NMV/r (Lexicomp Risk Rating X)
Hydroxyzine		↑ Hydroxyzine (Dependent on CYP3A4 metabolism)	QT interval prolongation Torsade de Pointes	Potential interaction (Liverpool COVID-19 Drug Interaction Checker) Pre-emptive dose adjustment not required but may be considered; continue and monitor for adverse effects (NIH). May consider close ECG monitoring for QT interval prolongation. (Lexicomp Risk Rating B, Micromedex Severity Major)
Rupatadine fumarate		↑ Rupatadine fumarate (Dependent on CYP3A4 metabolism)	QT interval prolongation Torsade de Pointes	Concomitant use of rupatadine with NMV/r is contraindicated (Rupall 2017) Discontinue rupatadine during NMV/r treatment, and resume rupatadine 3 days after the last dose of NMV/r (Lexicomp Risk Rating X)
Cetirizine Fexofenadine Levocetirizine		↑ Cetirizine ↑ Fexofenadine ↑ Levocetirizine (Dependent on P-glycoprotein efflux and CYP3A4 metabolism)	Greater central antihistamine effects (reduced alertness, longer reaction times) (Lexicomp)	No dose adjustment or additional monitoring necessary (Lexicomp Risk Rating B)

Systemic glucocorticoids

Dexamethasone	Vitiligo	↑ Dexamethasone (Dependent on CYP3A4 metabolism)	Systemic glucocorticoid effects (hyperglycaemia, Cushing's syndrome, adrenal suppression) Prednisolone has a lower likelihood for adverse effects than the other systemic glucocorticoids discussed herein, when taken concomitantly with NMV/r	Dexamethasone dose<16 mg daily is not expected to have significant interaction For high doses at >16 mg daily, the dose of dexamethasone should be reduced by 50%; resume the usual dose 3 days after completing NMV/r (Liverpool COVID-19 Drug Interaction Checker) Adjust dexamethasone dose, and monitor for adverse effects (NIH) (Lexicomp Risk Rating C, Micromedex Severity Major)
Hydrocortisone	Angioedema Anaphylaxis	↑ Hydrocortisone (Dependent on CYP3A4 metabolism)		Carefully monitor for adverse effects (Lexicomp Risk Rating C) The Micromedex Drug Reference and Liverpool COVID-19 Drug Interaction Checker indicate no interactions expected
Methylprednisolone	Pemphigus	↑ Methylprednisolone (Dependent on CYP3A4 metabolism)		Carefully monitor for adverse effects (Lexicomp Risk Rating C, Micromedex Severity Major) Liverpool COVID-19 Drug Interaction Checker indicates no interactions expected
Prednisolone	Allergic contact dermatitis Atopic dermatitis Bullous pemphigoid Pemphigus Urticaria Vitiligo	↑ Prednisolone (Dependent on CYP3A4 metabolism)		No dose adjustment or additional monitoring necessary (Lexicomp Risk Rating B) The Micromedex Drug Reference and Liverpool COVID-19 Drug Interaction Checker indicate no interactions expected
Prednisone	Allergic contact dermatitis Angioedema Urticaria	↑ Prednisone (Dependent on CYP3A4 metabolism)		Not expected to have clinically relevant interaction (NIH) Carefully monitor for adverse effects. (Lexicomp Risk Rating B, Micromedex Severity Major) Liverpool COVID-19 Drug Interaction Checker indicates no interactions expected

(continued)

Table 14.1 (continued)

Dermatologic medications	Common indications	Effect of NMV/r/on plasma drug concentration	Potential adverse effects	Recommended management
Immunomodulators				
Ciclosporin	Atopic dermatitis Psoriasis	↑ Ciclosporin (Dependent on CYP3A4 metabolism)	Renal impairment Hypertension	Discontinue ciclosporin during treatment, and resume 3 days after the last dose of NMV/r If unable to stop ciclosporin, consider alternative COVID-19 treatment. (Liverpool COVID-19 Drug Interaction Checker) (Lexicomp Risk Rating D, Micromedex Severity Major)
Cyclophosphamide	Autoimmune diseases Dermatomyositis Mycosis fungoides	↑ Cyclophosphamide (Dependent on CYP3A4 and CYP2B6 metabolism)	Oral mucositis Neutropaenia Infection	Carefully monitor for adverse effects (Lexicomp Risk Rating C, Micromedex Severity Major)
Tofacitinib	Psoriatic arthritis	↑ Tofacitinib (Dependent on CYP3A4 metabolism)	Transaminitis Neutropenia Infection	If possible, pause tofacitinib, and resume the original dose 3 days after the completion of NMV/r treatment. Alternatively, reduce the total daily dose by half on NMV/r, and resume the original dose 3 days after the completion of NMV/r treatment (Liverpool COVID-19 Drug Interaction Checker) Avoid tofacitinib XR, and replace with immediate-release tofacitinib (Xeljanz 2018) Carefully monitor for adverse effects (Lexicomp Risk Rating D, Micromedex Severity Moderate)
Upadacitinib	Atopic dermatitis Psoriatic arthritis	↑ Upadacitinib (Dependent on CYP3A4 metabolism)	Infection Thrombosis	Carefully monitor for adverse effects at upadacitinib 15 mg daily dosing (Rinvoq 2022). Avoid higher doses (30 mg/day) of upadacitinib during NMV/r treatment and 3 days following the completion of NMV/r treatment Carefully monitor for adverse effects (Lexicomp Risk Rating D, Micromedex Severity Major)

Anti-acne agents				
Combined oral contraceptives *Oestradiol* Ethinyloestradiol	Acne Prevention of pregnancy	↓ Ethinyloestradiol (Probable CYP2C9 and CYP1A2 metabolism)	Irregular bleeding Venous thrombosis Dyslipidaemia Hyperkalaemia (drospirenone) Hepatotoxicity (cyproterone) Hot flashes (cyproterone)	Carefully monitor for adverse effects Reduction in contraceptive efficacy is unlikely to be clinically significant given the short course of NMV/r. However, patients on oestrogen-containing hormonal contraception are advised to consider additional non-hormonal method of contraception during and up to one menstrual cycle after completing the course of NMV/r (Paxlovid 2021) (Lexicomp Risk Rating D for ethinyloestradiol and all progestogens except for cyproterone, Lexicomp Risk Rating C for cyproterone)
Progestogen (progestin) Chlormadinone acetate Dienogest Levonorgestrel Norethindrone Norgestimate Norgestrel Drospirenone Cyproterone acetate		↑ Chlormadinone acetate ↑ Dienogest ↑ Levonorgestrel ↑ Norethindrone ↑ Norgestimate ↑ Norgestrel ↑ Drospirenone ↑ Cyproterone acetate (Dependent on CYP3A4 metabolism)		
Isotretinoin	Acne	↑ Isotretinoin (Dependent on CYP3A4 and CYP2C8 metabolism)	Hepatotoxicity Hypertriglyceridemia Myopathy Mucocutaneous effects Visual disturbance Mood disorders	Potential interaction (Liverpool COVID-19 Drug Interaction Checker) Consider stopping isotretinoin during treatment and resuming 3 days after the last dose of NMV/r. If co-administration is necessary, monitor closely for isotretinoin toxicity The Micromedex Drug Reference and Lexicomp Drug Interaction Checker indicate no interactions expected
Hair agents				
Dutasteride	Androgenetic alopecia	↑ Dutasteride (Dependent on CYP3A4 metabolism)	Erectile dysfunction Decreased libido	Carefully monitor for adverse effects, and consider dose reduction if adverse effects are observed (Lexicomp Risk Rating C)

(continued)

Table 14.1 (continued)

Dermatologic medications	Common indications	Effect of NMV/r/on plasma drug concentration	Potential adverse effects	Recommended management
Other commonly encountered drugs in dermatology patients				
Colchicine	Leukocytoclastic vasculitis Neutrophilic dermatoses Sweet's syndrome Urticarial vasculitis	↑ Colchicine (Dependent on CYP3A4 metabolism) Risk of serious toxicity	Acute colchicine toxicity (gastrointestinal symptoms, seizures, bone marrow suppression, multi-organ failure)	Concomitant use of colchicine with NMV/r is contraindicated, especially in patients with renal or hepatic impairment (Paxlovid 2021) Discontinue colchicine during NMV/r treatment if possible A colchicine dose adjustment is required in patients who are taking or have taken NMV/r within the last 14 days. Recommendations on dose adjustment for dermatologic indications are not available but can be inferred from dose adjustment for other indications For the treatment of a gout flare-up during NMV/r treatment, the adjusted dose of colchicine is 0.6 mg once and then 0.3 mg 1 h later (repeated no earlier than every 3 days) For the prevention of gout flare, if the original dose is 0.6 mg two times daily, the adjusted dose is 0.3 mg once daily If the original dose is 0.6 mg once daily, the adjusted dose is 0.3 mg every other day In patients with familial Mediterranean fever with concomitant use of NMV/r, the maximum daily dose of colchicine is 0.6 mg (may be given as 0.3 mg twice daily) (Colcrys 2012). (Lexicomp Risk Rating X, Micromedex Severity Contraindicated)

HMG-CoA reductase inhibitors Atorvastatin Rosuvastatin	Dyslipidaemia e.g. in acne patients taking isotretinoin or psoriasis patients taking acitretin	↑ Atorvastatin (Atorvastatin is less dependent on CYP3A4 metabolism than simvastatin or lovastatin) ↑ Rosuvastatin (Ritonavir causes the inhibition of drug transporters)	Myopathy Rhabdomyolysis Transaminitis	Consider stopping atorvastatin during treatment and resuming 3 days after the last dose of NMV/r. If concomitant intake of atorvastatin and NMV/r is required, atorvastatin dose should be reduced to 10 mg daily, and resume the usual dose 3 days after the completion of NMV/r. (Liverpool COVID-19 Drug Interaction Checker) Consider withholding rosuvastatin during NMV/r treatment. There is no need to withhold rosuvastatin either before or after the completion of the NMV/r therapy (Lexicomp). If concurrent intake of rosuvastatin and NMV/r is required, maximum rosuvastatin dose should be 10 mg daily. (Liverpool COVID-19 Drug Interaction Checker) Carefully monitor for adverse effects (Micromedex Severity Major, Lexicomp Risk Rating D for Atorvastatin and Rosuvastatin)
Simvastatin Lovastatin		↑ Simvastatin ↑ Lovastatin (Dependent on CYP3A4 metabolism)		Concurrent use of simvastatin or lovastatin with NMV/r is contraindicated (Paxlovid 2021) Stop use at least 12 h prior to the first dose of NMV/r, and resume 5 days after the last dose (Lexicomp Risk Rating X, Micromedex Severity Contraindicated)

[a]Consult the Liverpool COVID-19 Drug Interactions website, Micromedex, Lexicomp and the National Institutes of Health COVID-19 Treatment Guidelines for updated drugs (University of Liverpool 2022; Micromedex Solutions 2022; UpToDate 2022; National Institutes of Health 2023a; Paxlovid 2021). If a drug is not listed here, co-administration cannot be automatically assumed to be safe

Rifampicin, an anti-tuberculosis agent, may be used in patients with hidradenitis suppurativa as well as in staphylococcal and non-tuberculous mycobacterial infections (Rifampin 2019). Rifampicin is a potent CYP3A4 inducer; thus, concomitant administration with NMV/r would cause decreased plasma concentrations of nirmatrelvir and ritonavir, which are both CYP3A4 substrates, with a significant decline in the therapeutic effect of NMV/r, poor treatment outcomes as well as potential for the development of viral resistance to NMV/r (U.S. Food and Drug Administration 2021a). As the induction effect of rifampicin on CYP3A4 persists for a prolonged duration after discontinuation, it is not sufficient to stop rifampicin use prior to starting NMV/r therapy (Paxlovid 2021). Hence, for patients on rifampicin, the use of alternative COVID-19 treatment, such as molnupiravir, is recommended.

Clindamycin and clofazimine are also dependent on CYP3A4 metabolism; hence, careful monitoring for adverse effects is recommended as well. According to Micromedex, the concomitant use of metronidazole and NMV/r may lead to a higher risk of QT interval prolongation ad arrhythmias as both drugs can prolong QT interval. ECG monitoring during the co-administration or avoidance of this combination are recommended for susceptible patients. The Liverpool COVID-19 Drug Interaction Checker and Lexicomp, however, did not consider this interaction as clinically significant. NMV/r may increase the serum concentration of tinidazole to a limited extent. No dosage adjustment or additional monitoring is required during the concomitant administration of tinidazole and NMV/r.

A list of commonly used antibiotics in dermatologic conditions with no significant interactions with NMV/r and which may be safely continued during the treatment course of NMV/r without dose adjustments or additional monitoring is included in Table 14.2.

Anti-Fungal Agents

The systemic azoles, fluconazole, itraconazole and ketoconazole, are prescribed in the treatment of resistant or extensive dermatophyte infections,

Table 14.2 Preferred systemic dermatologic medications during nirmatrelvir-ritonavir (NMV/r) treatment[a]

Antibiotics	Immunomodulators
Azithromycin	Abrocitinib
Cephalosporins	Acitretin
Dapsone	Apremilast
Isoniazid	Azathioprine
Penicillins	Baricitinib
Pyrazinamide	Dimethyl fumarate
Sulfonamides	Methotrexate
Tetracyclines	Mycophenolate mofetil
Anti-fungals	Sulfasalazine
Griseofulvin	**Anti-acne agents**
Nystatin	Spironolactone
Terbinafine	**Hair agents**
Antivirals	Finasteride
Aciclovir	Minoxidil
Valaciclovir	**Miscellaneous: statins**
Antihistamines	Fluvastatin
Buclizine	Pravastatin
Chlorpheniramine	
Desloratadine	
Diphenhydramine	
Loratadine	
Biologics	
Adalimumab	
Anakinra	
Brodalumab	
Certolizumab	
Dupilumab	
Etanercept	
Guselkumab	
Infliximab	
Ixekizumab	
Omalizumab	
Risankizumab	
Rituximab	
Secukinumab	
Spesolimab	
Tildrakizumab	
Ustekinumab	

[a]Consult the Liverpool COVID-19 Drug Interactions website, Micromedex, Lexicomp and the National Institutes of Health COVID-19 Treatment Guidelines for updated drugs (University of Liverpool 2022; Micromedex Solutions 2022; UpToDate 2022; National Institutes of Health 2023a)

pityriasis versicolor and other cutaneous fungal infections. All of these three azoles have significant DDIs with NMV/r, as they are CYP3A4 inhibitors and would result in elevated plasma concentrations of NMV/r, with increased risk of NMV/r adverse effects. In addition, itraconazole and ketoconazole are also substrates of CYP3A4; hence, ritonavir-mediated CYP3A4 inhibition would result in increased plasma concentrations of these two azoles and greater risk of adverse effects including gastrointestinal side effects, transaminitis as well as QT interval prolongation caused by ketoconazole.

For fluconazole, recommendations include careful ECG monitoring, as both fluconazole and ritonavir are known to prolong the QT interval with risk of an additive effect in concomitant use (Diflucan 2022). Recommendations for itraconazole and ketoconazole are for the use of a reduced dose, at a daily dose not exceeding 200 mg, in addition to monitoring for side effects (Sporanox 2001; Nizoral 2014).

Anti-Parasitic Agents

The anti-helminthic agent albendazole is used in the systemic treatment of parasitic worm infections such as cutaneous larva migrans. In co-administration with ritonavir, induction of hepatic metabolism of albendazole occurs, resulting in decreased plasma concentration (Corti et al. 2009). As a result, monitoring for reduced clinical response to albendazole therapy is suggested in co-administration during NMV/r treatment.

Ivermectin is used off-label for the treatment of scabies. As it is a substrate of CYP3A4 and P-gp, NMV/r which is a strong CYP3A4 and P-gp inhibitor may increase the concentration of ivermectin in the brain, leading to a higher risk of neurotoxicity. Careful monitoring of adverse effects including neurotoxicity is recommended in patients taking both ivermectin and NMV/r.

Antiviral Agents

Aciclovir and valaciclovir are commonly used agents in the treatment of viral skin infections such as herpes simplex, herpes zoster (shingles) and varicella zoster (chickenpox). Valaciclovir is a prodrug that is rapidly hydrolysed to aciclovir, following which both subsequently undergo renal excretion. No clinically significant DDIs are expected between these antiviral agents and NMV/r; hence, no dosage adjustment or additional monitoring is currently recommended.

Antihistamines

Antihistamines are one of the most commonly prescribed drugs in dermatology, ranging from use in pruritic skin dermatoses to allergic cutaneous reactions such as urticaria and angioedema. Clinically significant drug interactions exist between ritonavir and several antihistamines, including the first-generation antihistamine, hydroxyzine, and second-generation antihistamines, bilastine and rupatadine.

Hydroxyzine, dependent on hepatic CYP3A4 metabolism, when co-administered with the CYP3A4 inhibitor ritonavir, will result in higher hydroxyzine plasma concentrations and increased risk of adverse effects, including QT interval prolongation (Hydroxyzine 2018). Recommendations offered range from monitoring for adverse effects, dose reduction and close ECG monitoring for a prolonged QT interval.

Bilastine and rupatadine have significant DDIs with NMV/r as they are dependent on P-gp-mediated efflux and CYP3A4 metabolism, respectively, both of which are inhibited by ritonavir. This leads to an increase in plasma concentrations of the antihistamines and the risk of side effects such as QT interval prolongation. It is recommended to discontinue these antihistamines during the NMV/r treatment course and for an additional 3 days after the last dose.

Other second-generation antihistamines such as cetirizine, fexofenadine and levocetirizine are also dependent on P-gp-mediated efflux and CYP3A4 metabolism. Drug interaction with ritonavir may lead to increased central antihistamine effects including drowsiness and prolonged reaction times, with minimal risk of severe adverse effects such as QT interval prolongation. No dosage adjustment or additional monitoring is currently suggested.

Desloratadine, loratadine, chlorpheniramine, diphenhydramine and buclizine are the preferred choices of antihistamine during NMV/r treatment, for which no clinically significant interactions are expected, and are summarised in Table 14.2.

Systemic Glucocorticoids

Short courses of oral glucocorticoids are used to treat severe acute exacerbations of atopic dermatitis. Many frequently used glucocorticoids, such as dexamethasone, methylprednisolone and hydrocortisone, are dependent on CYP3A4-mediated metabolism. As such, co-administration with NMV/r may increase systemic glucocorticoid exposure and risk of adverse effects such as hyperglycaemia (Prednisolone 2022). The risk of glucocorticoid-induced adrenal suppression and Cushing's syndrome is likely low in patients treated with a 5-day duration of NMV/r. Low-dose dexamethasone at ≤16 mg daily is not expected to have significant interaction, but for high doses at >16 mg daily, the dose of dexamethasone should be reduced by 50% and the usual dose resumed 3 days after completing NMV/r (University of Liverpool 2022).

Prednisolone has a lower likelihood of adverse events compared with other systemic glucocorticoids discussed herein, and when given concurrently with NMV/r, hence, it may be considered as an alternative if clinically appropriate.

Biologics

Even though NMV/r interacts with some conjugated monoclonal antibodies, it does not to date interact with dermatological biologics. Dermatological biologics, if clinically indicated to continue during the COVID-19 infection, may be safely continued during treatment with NMV/r without the need for dose adjustment or additional clinical monitoring (Table 14.2).

Systemic Immunomodulators

Ciclosporin is a calcineurin inhibitor that is used in the treatment of severe, resistant atopic dermatitis and psoriasis. Ciclosporin is primarily metabolised by hepatic and intestinal CYP3A4 enzymes; hence, ritonavir-mediated CYP3A4 inhibition during concomitant administration will greatly increase its plasma concentration, with a significantly increased risk of ciclosporin toxicity, including systemic hypertension, nephrotoxicity and hepatotoxicity (Neoral 2009). It is recommended to discontinue ciclosporin during NMV/r treatment and resume it 3 days after the last dose in view of increased risk of ciclosporin toxicity during concomitant administration with NMV/r.

Cyclophosphamide is an alkylating agent used in chemotherapy for cutaneous T-cell lymphomas and in the treatment of severe, refractory autoimmune skin conditions (Kim and Chan 2017). It is administered as a prodrug and requires activation by hepatic CYP450 enzymes, including CYP2B6 and CYP3A4. As ritonavir is a CYP2B6 inducer, concomitant use of cyclophosphamide with NMV/r results in an increased risk for toxic effects such as oral mucositis and neutropaenia, for which patients should be carefully monitored (Cyclophosphamide 2013).

Janus kinase (JAK) inhibitors are a relatively new treatment for autoimmune diseases such as psoriatic arthritis, for which tofacitinib and upadacitinib have both been approved for use, with the latter recently approved by FDA for use in atopic dermatitis as well (Xeljanz 2018; Rinvoq 2022). Metabolism of both tofacitinib and upadacitinib is mediated primarily by hepatic CYP3A4; hence, co-administration with NMV/r will result in an elevated plasma concentration of the active drugs via ritonavir-mediated CYP3A4 inhibition. If possible, tofacitinib should be paused during NMV/r treatment and for 3 days after the completion of treatment (University of Liverpool 2022). Alternatively, reduce the total daily dose of tofacitinib by half while on NMV/r, and resume the original dose 3 days after treatment. The immediate-release formulation is recommended (Xeljanz 2018). For upadacitinib, a maximum daily dose of 15 mg is recommended (Rinvoq 2022). Dose reductions for both tofacitinib and upadacitinib should be carried out throughout the course of NMV/r treatment and for another 3 days from the completion of the last dose. In addition, the patients should be monitored for adverse effects.

Systemic immunomodulators that may be co-administered safely with NMV/r without clinically significant DDIs include abrocitinib, acitretin, apremilast, azathioprine, baricitinib, dimethyl fumarate, methotrexate, mycophenolate mofetil and sulfasalazine, as listed in Table 14.2.

Anti-Acne Agents

Oral contraceptives with anti-androgenic properties are used in the treatment of acne, hirsutism and polycystic ovarian syndrome (PCOS) with underlying hyperandrogenism and adult female acne. Combined oral contraceptive pills (COCPs) contain the synthetic oestrogen ethinyloestradiol in formulations with various progestins. In co-administration with ritonavir, plasma concentration of ethinyloestradiol has shown to be reduced, most likely via ritonavir-mediated CYP2C9 and CYP1A2 induction. Progesterone, however, is primarily metabolised by CYP3A4 with resultant elevated plasma concentrations due to DDI with ritonavir, increasing the risk of side effects such as irregular menstrual bleeding and venous thrombosis. Additional side effects with certain progestins include the risk of hyperkalaemia with drospirenone and hepatotoxicity and hot flashes with cyproterone acetate. Recommendations for the co-administration of progestin-only pills or COCPs with NMV/r include careful monitoring for adverse effects. In addition, patients taking COCPs should be advised to consider non-hormonal contraceptives for prevention of pregnancy during and up to one menstrual cycle after completing the course of NMV/r, although it is unlikely that a reduction in contraceptive efficacy from reduced plasma concentration of ethinyloestradiol during the short course of NMV/r will be clinically significant (Paxlovid 2021).

With the inhibition of CYP2C8 and CYP3A4 by NMV/r, isotretinoin concentrations may increase when co-administered with NMV/r. Consider stopping isotretinoin during treatment and resuming 3 days after the last dose of NMV/r. If co-administration is necessary, monitor closely for isotretinoin toxicity.

Hair Agents

5-Alpha-reductase inhibitors, such as dutasteride and finasteride, have shown to be effective in the treatment of male androgenetic alopecia through the inhibition of dihydrotestosterone production. Dutasteride is dependent on CYP3A4 metabolism; drug interaction with ritonavir, a CYP3A4 inhibitor, will result in an elevated plasma concentration of dutasteride and increased risk of side effects including erectile dysfunction and decreased libido. Close monitoring for these adverse effects is suggested for dutasteride if used concomitantly with NMV/r (Avodart 2013). A dose reduction of dutasteride may be considered if adverse effects are observed. Finasteride can be co-administered with NMV/r without the need for additional monitoring.

Minoxidil, also used in the treatment of androgenetic alopecia, is not expected to have DDI with NMV/r, and systemic treatment may be safely continued without changes in dosage or additional monitoring.

Other Commonly Encountered Drugs in Dermatology Patients

The longitudinal care of patients with chronic skin conditions includes the management of their comorbid conditions. Several non-dermatologic medications commonly encountered and used by dermatologists with significant drug-drug interactions with NMV/r are highlighted below.

Colchicine is an anti-gout agent that is also used in the treatment of dermatologic conditions, e.g. leukocytoclastic and urticarial vasculitis and neutrophilic dermatoses, including Sweet's syndrome. Colchicine is primarily dependent on hepatic CYP3A4 metabolism. During co-administration with the potent CYP3A4 inhibitor ritonavir, colchicine plasma concentrations will be greatly increased, with risk of potentially life-threatening acute colchicine toxicity, presenting with severe gastrointestinal symptoms, bone marrow suppression, seizures and multi-organ failure (Davis et al. 2013). As such, the use of colchicine during NMV/r treatment is contraindicated, especially in patients with renal or hepatic impairment. For patients who are currently or have recently been treated with NMV/r within the last 14 days and requiring colchicine therapy, the use of an alternative agent is recommended, or else colchicine should be given at a reduced dose as is summarised in Table 14.1.

Dyslipidaemia is a common comorbidity in all fields of medicine. In dermatology, this is especially prevalent in patients with conditions which have been linked to metabolic syndrome, such as psoriasis and hidradenitis suppurativa, and in those receiving medications such as retinoids (e.g. isotretinoin, acitretin) and ciclosporin, with side effects that predispose patients to dyslipidaemia (Shenoy et al. 2015). Of the HMG-CoA reductase inhibitors, lovastatin, simvastatin and to a lesser degree atorvastatin are primarily dependent on CYP3A4 metabolism. Hence, the co-administration of these statins with CYP3A4 inhibitor ritonavir may increase the risk of statin-induced myopathy and rhabdomyolysis. Lovastatin and simvastatin should be discontinued at least 12 h before the first dose of NMV/r, during treatment and for the next 5 days after the last dose (Kiser et al. 2008). For atorvastatin, it is recommended to temporarily discontinue or reduce dose to 10 mg daily with resumption of the usual dose 3 days after completing NMV/r treatment. Rosuvastatin has been demonstrated in previous studies to have an elevated plasma concentration when co-administered with ritonavir, possibly due to the inhibition of drug transporters by ritonavir (Kiser et al. 2008). As such, recommendations for rosuvastatin include to discontinue temporarily or reduce dose to 10 mg daily during NMV/r treatment. Only the HMG-CoA reductase inhibitors pravastatin and fluvastatin are not expected to have clinically significant interactions with NMV/r and may be continued during NMV/r therapy.

Molnupiravir (U.S. Food and Drug Administration 2021b)

Molnupiravir is a prodrug, which is subsequently converted to the active metabolite β-D-N^4-hydroxycytidine (NHC), phosphorylated and incorporated by viral RNA polymerase into viral RNA, causing SARS-CoV-2 viral replication to be inhibited (Extance 2022). As of December 2022, molnupiravir is still under the Emergency Use Authorisation by FDA and currently not approved for use in the European Union yet (European Medicines Agency 2021; FDA 2021). Further studies are needed to explore any potential long-term mutagenic effects of molnupiravir to the host (Rahmah et al. 2022).

Although no drug-drug interactions involving molnupiravir have been identified yet, in vitro studies show that molnupiravir and its metabolite NHC are not substrates, inducers or inhibitors of major drug metabolising CYP450 enzymes. They are also not substrates of P-glycoprotein or breast cancer resistance protein (BCRP) efflux transporters, which are important mediators of intestinal absorption and subsequent excretion of drugs (U.S. Food and Drug Administration 2021b). Hence, for patients clinically indicated for oral COVID-19 antiviral therapy but with contraindications to NMV/r therapy, molnupiravir may be a viable alternative for clinicians to consider. Molnupiravir is not recommended for use during pregnancy. Women should not breastfeed during therapy and for 4 days after the last dose of molnupiravir. Women of reproductive potential should abstain or use reliable contraception during therapy and for 4 days after the last dose of molnupiravir. Sexually active men should avoid conception during therapy and for 3 months after the last dose (National Institutes of Health 2022).

Limitations

Despite the efforts to produce a comprehensive and in-depth review on drug interactions between dermatologic medications and the current two oral COVID-19 medications, drugs that are still pending approval by EMA and FDA are not included due to limited information. At the time of literature search, some of the drugs in this chapter were not listed on the Liverpool COVID-19 Drug Interaction Checker and cannot be assumed to be safe when taken with NMV/r, although attempts were made to corroborate with the individual drug monographs. The information in this chapter is based on a literature search ending on 28 December 2022. The recommendations and practices may differ with time and between regions.

Conclusion

Clinically significant drug-drug interactions exist between NMV/r and numerous dermatologic medications, primarily due to CYP3A4 inhibition caused by ritonavir. Chronic dermatologic medications with drug interactions should be withdrawn or dose adjusted as appropriate for the duration of 8 days to enable safe treatment with NMV/r. For patients taking medications with complicated drug interactions with NMV/r that are not suitable for temporary discontinuation or dose reduction, molnupiravir may be considered as an alternative oral COVID-19 therapy.

Disclaimer This document is intended for use by experienced clinicians and pharmacists. The information in this chapter is not meant to replace professional clinical judgment in individual situations. The risk/benefit profile for the individual patient should be considered when starting, stopping or altering medications. Patients should be closely monitored for therapeutic benefit and adverse events. The authors and their respective institutions are not responsible for inaccuracies in information or claims of injuries.

Funding This study is supported by the Singapore National Medical Research Council Centre Grant II Seed funding and National Skin Centre Medical Department Fund.

References

Avodart (dutasteride) [package insert]. Mississauga, ON: GlaxoSmithKline; 2013.

Biaxin (clarithromycin) [package insert]. North Chicago, IL: AbbVie; 2017.

Colcrys (colchicine) [package insert]. Deerfield, IL: Takeda Pharmaceuticals America; 2012.

Corti N, Heck A, Rentsch K, Zingg W, Jetter A, Stieger B, et al. Effect of ritonavir on the pharmacokinetics of the benzimidazoles albendazole and mebendazole: an interaction study in healthy volunteers. Eur J Clin Pharmacol. 2009;65(10):999–1006.

Cyclophosphamide [package insert]. Deerfield, IL: Baxter Healthcare; 2013.

Davis MW, Wason S, Digiacinto JL. Colchicine-antimicrobial drug interactions: what pharmacists need to know in treating gout. Consult Pharm. 2013;28(3):176–83.

Diflucan (fluconazole) [Package insert on the internet]. New York, NY: Roerig Div Pfizer; 2022. https://labeling.pfizer.com/showlabeling.aspx?id=575.

Erythro-Base (erythromycin) [package insert]. Vaughan, ON: AA Pharma; 2014.

European Medicines Agency. COVID-19 treatments. 2021. https://www.ema.europa.eu/en/human-regulatory/overview/public-health-threats/coronavirus-disease-covid-19/treatments-vaccines/covid-19-treatments. Accessed 25 Dec 2022.

Extance A. Covid-19: what is the evidence for the antiviral molnupiravir? BMJ. 2022;377:o926.

FDA. Coronavirus (COVID-19) update: FDA authorizes additional oral antiviral for treatment of COVID-19 in certain adults. 2021. https://www.fda.gov/news-events/press-announcements/coronavirus-covid-19-update-fda-authorizes-additional-oral-antiviral-treatment-covid-19-certain. Accessed 25 Dec 2022.

Food and Drug Administration. Remdesivir (Veklury) [package insert]. 2022. https://www.accessdata.fda.gov/drugsatfda_docs/label/2022/214787Orig1s015lbl.pdf.

Gottlieb RL, Vaca CE, Paredes R, et al. Early remdesivir to prevent progression to severe COVID-19 in outpatients. N Engl J Med. 2022;386(4):305–15. https://www.ncbi.nlm.nih.gov/pubmed/34937145.

Hydroxyzine (hydroxyzine) [package insert]. Vaughan, ON: AA Pharma; 2018.

Jayk Bernal A, Gomes da Silva MM, Musungaie DB, et al. Molnupiravir for oral treatment of COVID-19 in non-hospitalized patients. N Engl J Med. 2022;386(6):509–20. https://www.ncbi.nlm.nih.gov/pubmed/34914868.

Katzenmaier S, Markert C, Riedel KD, Burhenne J, Haefeli WE, Mikus G. Determining the time course of CYP3A inhibition by potent reversible and irreversible CYP3A inhibitors using a limited sampling strategy. Clin Pharmacol Ther. 2011;90(5):666–73.

Kheshti R, Aalipour M, Namazi S. A comparison of five common drug-drug interaction software programs regarding accuracy and comprehensiveness. J Res Pharm Pract. 2016;5(4):257–63.

Kim J, Chan JJ. Cyclophosphamide in dermatology. Australas J Dermatol. 2017;58(1):5–17.

Kiser JJ, Gerber JG, Predhomme JA, Wolfe P, Flynn DM, Hoody DW. Drug/drug interaction between lopinavir/ritonavir and rosuvastatin in healthy volunteers. J Acquir Immune Defic Syndr. 2008;47(5):570–8.

Micromedex Solutions. Micromedex Drug Interactions. 2022. https://www.micromedexsolutions.com/micromedex2/librarian/CS/7CF77C/ND_PR/evidencexpert/ND_P/evidencexpert/DUPLICATIONSHIELDSYNC/D9DBBD/ND_PG/evidencexpert/ND_B/evidencexpert/ND_AppProduct/evidencexpert/ND_T/evidencexpert/PFActionId/evidencexpert.FindDrugInteractions?navitem=topInteractions&isToolPage=true. Accessed 28 Dec 2022.

Monteith S, Glenn T. Comparison of potential psychiatric drug interactions in six drug interaction database programs: a replication study after 2 years of updates. Hum Psychopharmacol Clin Exp. 2021;36(6):e2802.

National Institutes of Health. Molnupiravir. 2022. https://www.covid19treatmentguidelines.nih.gov/therapies/antivirals-including-antibody-products/molnupiravir/. Accessed 1 Jan 2023.

National Institutes of Health. Drug-drug interactions between Ritonavir-Boosted Nirmatrelvir (Paxlovid) and concomitant medications. 2023a. https://www.covid19treatmentguidelines.nih.gov/therapies/antivirals-including-antibody-products/ritonavir-boosted-nirmatrelvir%2D%2Dpaxlovid-/paxlovid-drug-drug-interactions/. Accessed 1 Jan 2023.

National Institutes of Health. COVID-19 treatment guidelines panel. Coronavirus disease 2019 (COVID-19) treatment guidelines. 2023b. https://www.covid19treatmentguidelines.nih.gov/. Accessed 1 Jan 2023.

National Institutes of Health. Ritonavir-Boosted Nirmatrelvir (Paxlovid). 2023c. https://www.covid19treatmentguidelines.nih.gov/therapies/antiviral-therapy/ritonavir-boosted-nirmatrelvir%2D%2Dpaxlovid-/.

Neoral (cyclosporine) [package insert]. East Hanover, NJ: Novartis Pharmaceuticals; 2009.

Nizoral (ketoconazole) [package insert]. Titusville, NJ: Janssen Pharmaceuticals; 2014.

Patel RI, Beckett RD. Evaluation of resources for analyzing drug interactions. J Med Libr Assoc. 2016;104(4):290–5.

Paxlovid (nirmatrelvir and ritonavir) [package insert on the internet]. New York, NY: Pfizer Laboratories Div Pfizer; 2021. https://labeling.pfizer.com/ShowLabeling.aspx?id=16474.

Prednisolone (systemic): drug information [Internet]. Accessed 28 Dec 2022.

Quah KSE, Huang X, Renia L, Oon HH. Drug interactions between common dermatological medications and the oral anti-COVID-19 agents nirmatrelvir-ritonavir and molnupiravir. Ann Acad Med Singapore. 2022;51(12):774–86.

Rahmah L, Abarikwu SO, Arero AG, Jibril AT, Fal A, Flisiak R, et al. Oral antiviral treatments for COVID-19: opportunities and challenges. Pharmacol Rep. 2022;74:1–24.

Rifampin (rifampicin): Drug information. [Internet]; 2019.

Rinvoq (upadacitinib) [package insert]. North Chicago, IL: AbbVie; 2022.

Rupall (rupatadine) [package insert]. Verdun, QC: Pediapharm; 2017.

Shenoy C, Shenoy MM, Rao GK. Dyslipidemia in dermatological disorders. N Am J Med Sci. 2015;7(10):421–8.

Sporanox (itraconazole) [package insert]. Titusville, NJ: Janssen Pharmaceuticals; 2001.

Stader F, Khoo S, Stoeckle M, Back D, Hirsch HH, Battegay M, et al. Stopping lopinavir/ritonavir in COVID-19 patients: duration of the drug interacting effect. J Antimicrob Chemother. 2020;75(10):3084–6.

U.S. Food and Drug Administration. Fact sheet for healthcare providers: emergency use authorisation for Paxlovid. 2021a. https://www.fda.gov/media/155050/download.

U.S. Food and Drug Administration. Fact sheet for healthcare providers: emergency use authorisation for Lagevrio (molnupiravir) capsules. 2021b. https://www.fda.gov/media/155054/download.

U.S. Food and Drug Administration. Coronavirus (COVID-19) update: FDA authorizes first oral antiviral for treatment of COVID-19. 2022a. https://www.fda.gov/news-events/press-announcements/coronavirus-covid-19-update-fda-authorizes-first-oral-antiviral-treatment-covid-19. Accessed 28 Dec 2022.

U.S. Food and Drug Administration. Coronavirus (COVID-19) update: FDA authorizes additional oral antiviral for treatment of COVID-19 in Certain Adults. 2022b. https://www.fda.gov/news-events/press-announcements/coronavirus-covid-19-update-fda-authorizes-additional-oral-antiviral-treatment-covid-19-certain. Accessed 28 Dec 2022.

University of Liverpool. Liverpool COVID-19 drug interaction. 2022. https://www.covid19-druginteractions.org/checker. Accessed 28 Dec 2022.

UpToDate. Lexicomp drug interactions. 2022. https://www.uptodate.com/drug-interactions/?source=responsive_home#di-druglist. Accessed 28 Dec 2022.

WHO. Coronavirus disease (COVID-19) pandemic [Internet]. https://www.who.int/europe/emergencies/situations/covid-19. Accessed 23 Dec 2022.

Xeljanz (tofacitinib) [package insert]. New York, NY: Pfizer; 2018.

The Economic Impact of COVID-19 on Dermatology

15

Valencia Long, Ellie Choi, and Phillip Phan

Introduction

In this chapter, we explore the economic impact of COVID-19 on the practice of dermatology. To understand this issue, we first review the impact of COVID-19 on the macro economy and its healthcare system. This "embeddedness" approach is a theoretical framework employed by economic sociologists to model how shocks are propagated through a system that consists of many sub-systems (Granovetter 1985). Figure 15.1 illustrates the framework of the chapter, which we organize into five sections. We begin with the impact of COVID-19 on the global economy and the consumption of healthcare, followed by a discussion of government responses and its economic effects. We then discuss the effects on dermatology providers and finances and the role of technology. We conclude with a discussion on the way forward.

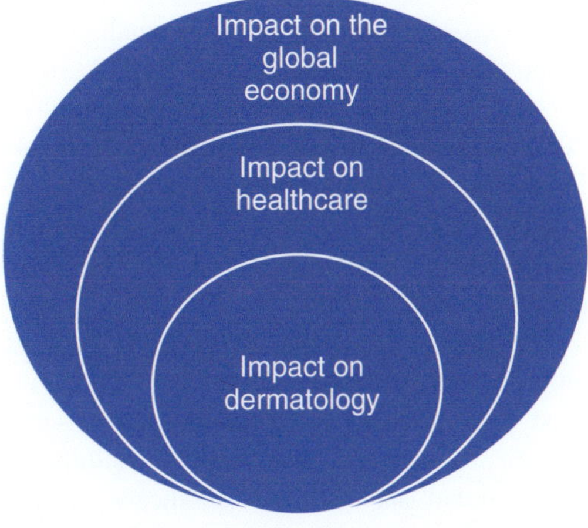

Fig. 15.1 The discussion framework for this chapter

COVID-19 and Its Impact on the Global Economy

By most accounts, COVID-19 is a once-in-a-century global health disaster that quickly became an economic disaster. Some of the economic fallout is due to the natural contraction in consumption as a consequence of the early uncertainty around a disease that few understood, even experts. Other fallout can be attributed to infection control policies such as lockdowns and social distancing aimed at limiting viral transmission and managing hospital capacity.

The onset of the COVID-19 pandemic was accompanied by a large-scale global economic

V. Long · E. Choi
Division of Dermatology, National University Health System, Singapore, Singapore

P. Phan (✉)
Department of Medicine and Carey Business School, Johns Hopkins University and Medicine, Baltimore, MD, USA
e-mail: pphan@jhu.edu

© The Author(s), under exclusive license to Springer Nature Switzerland AG 2023
H. H. Oon, C. L. Goh (eds.), *COVID-19 in Dermatology*, Updates in Clinical Dermatology,
https://doi.org/10.1007/978-3-031-45586-5_15

downturn due to the widespread movement restrictions and lockdowns, manpower and supply chain disruptions, and reduced consumption. China was the first country to be impacted and saw a gross domestic product (GDP) contraction of 6.8% in Q1 2020 (China Economic Quarterly 2020; Cheng 2022). Other economies followed, with the US economy shrinking at an annual rate of 32.9% in Q2 2020 (U.S. Bureau of Economic Analysis 2020) and the UK at 20.4% (Smith 2023). China saw a 2.2% real GDP growth in 2020 compared to 6% in 2019, a contraction of 4 percentage points year on year. The US GDP shrank to 3.4% and the UK by −9.3%, and Singapore, one of the most robust small country economies in the world, recorded a GDP growth at −4.1% in 2020 (World Economic Outlook 2022). According to the International Monetary Fund World Economic Outlook Update, the estimated cumulative output loss since the start of the pandemic through 2024 is US$13.8 trillion (Al Mutair et al. 2022).

Despite the slowdown of economic output, global health spending saw massive increases to cope with the costs of infection control, social welfare, testing, and, later, vaccine rollouts. In 2020, global spending on healthcare reached US$9 trillion, or 10.8% of global GDP. Increased health spending compounded existing health system challenges by exacerbating inequalities in health and health coverage as countries scrambled to reprioritize and reallocate health budgets. Global spending was skewed toward high-income countries, such as the USA spending US$300 billion to pre-purchase vaccines. Despite accounting for 15% of the world's population, high-income countries accounted for 80% of the total health spending in 2020, with the USA making up 44% of all spending in 2020.

Government Response to COVID-19 and Its Effects

Compared to previous pandemics, COVID-19 was distinguished by the intrusiveness of government interventions, manifested in lockdowns, curfews, mask and vaccine mandates, and mandatory business and school closures. While these occurred to varying degrees across the world, with China adopting the most restrictive, the impacts were similar in direction.

Expenditure on Healthcare

Globally, governments responded with varying degrees and combinations of travel quarantines, lockdowns, social distancing, and vaccinations (Richards et al. 2022). These measures were met with varying degrees of efficacy and costs, depending on the degree to which existing healthcare systems could be quickly restructured, managed, and financed. Governments were faced with providing financial support and creating adaptive and responsive milieus for frontline healthcare providers.

Governments utilized various methods to cope with their COVID-19 responses. These included the compensation of healthcare providers for pandemic-related income loss using general taxes and national health insurance funds. For example, South Korea utilized the National Health Insurance (NHI) fund to create a health insurance advance payment system to compensate medical institutions for revenue losses and additional costs during COVID-19 movement restrictions (Yun et al. 2022). In addition, the Korean government attempted to reflect the actual demand for COVID-19 medical services through co-payment support.

In the USA, government pandemic-related spending fell into four buckets. The first was income protection to support the forced closures of public places (restaurants and bars, entertainment venues and concert halls, theme parks, etc.). The second was business protection to stave off bankruptcy and support faster reopening. The third was payments to healthcare providers for surge capacity and suspension of elective procedures and ambulatory care. The fourth was payments to pharmaceutical companies for vaccines, personal protection equipment (PPE), test kits, and the infrastructure for widespread testing. These expenditures, which occurred in two tranches between 2020 and 2021, amounted to

US$4.5 trillion (The Federal Response 2022), which boosted household demand for goods and services and led to a 40-year-high inflation.

In other parts of the world, governments responded aggressively by modifying their provider-payment mechanisms or creating new payment schemes altogether (Waitzberg et al. 2022; McClellan et al. 2021).

Expenditure on Material

The early days saw a rapid increase in demand for PPE, spiking shortages worldwide. In a retrospective review of market prices for PPE during the first pandemic surge in Chicago, Lora et al. found that disposable gown cost per unit (CPU) peaked at US$12 during the first week of March, 13.7 times higher than pre-pandemic prices; the average gown CPU was 7.5 times higher. N95 respirators peaked at a CPU of US$12, eight times higher than pre-pandemic prices. Face mask CPU peaked at US$0.55, 11 times higher than the regular price. Gloves averaged 2.5 times higher than the pre-pandemic CPU (Mena Lora et al. 2021). By Oct 2021, data from Premier Inc., a healthcare improvement company working with 4400 US hospitals and health systems and more than 250,000 providers and organizations, reported that US hospitals spent more than US$3 billion on PPE (Premier Data 2021). The shortages and costs can be attributed, as with other goods, to the integrated supply chains beginning in China, which went into repeated factory closures during the period (Gereffi 2020).

Expenditure on ICU and Chronic Care

Globally, no country was spared from the massive increase in critical care expenditures. A Singapore tertiary acute care hospital serving 1900 beds reported pandemic-related expenditure in 2020 to be US$45.39 million, a significant increase from prior years (Cai et al. 2022). The largest categories of expenses were surge facilities and patient care supplies. Outpatient visits dropped by 30% and elective surgeries by 50% in

the aftermath of the "circuit breaker" (lockdown), putting more pressure on hospital finances.

The economic strain from long COVID cannot be underestimated. A US study (DeMartino et al. 2022) compared healthcare resource use (HRU) for patients with and without COVID-19 diagnoses over 6 months and found that total healthcare costs were significantly higher among patients with COVID-19 than controls (mean differences: US$3706 for commercial insurance; US$10,595 for Medicare; both p < 0.001). Though the incremental HRU and cost burden of COVID-19 decreased over time, patients with COVID-19 continued to have significantly higher total costs through the fifth month of recovery. During follow-up, patients with COVID-19 had significantly higher rates of complications than controls (commercial insurance, 52.8% vs. 29.0% with any; Medicare, 74.5% vs. 47.9% with any; both $p < 0.001$), continuing to suffer from such symptoms as cough, dyspnea, and fatigue.

Expenditure on COVID-19 Vaccinations

COVID-19 vaccines were considered a key tool for fighting the pandemic. Analysts projected the cost of lockdowns to far outweigh the expected costs of vaccinations globally (Hafner et al. 2022). That said, by March 2022, the USA spent an additional US$22.5 billion for securing oral antiviral treatments, monoclonal antibodies, pre-exposure prophylaxis, operating critical testing initiatives, and follow-on vaccine research. By December 2022, the US federal government spent $25.3 billion on vaccinations or about 1.2 billion doses of Pfizer and Moderna COVID-19 vaccines, with an average purchase price of $20.69 per dose (Kates et al. 2022).

Impact on Non-COVID-Related Healthcare

At the peak of the pandemic (May–July 2020), essential health services faced disruptions, defined by WHO as a change of 5–50% in service provision or use, because of infection control policies. According to the WHO, the 5 most disrupted services (from a list of 25) were rehabilitation services (91% of surveyed countries), dental services (91%), non-communicable disease (NCD) diagnosis and treatment, family planning and contraception, and outreach services for immunizations (European Observatory on Health S, Policies, World Health Organization 2020). Of these, the disruptions to dental and rehabilitation services were the direct result of infection control policies that limited or suspended outpatient and elective inpatient services and community-based care.

The disruption of essential services included NCD management (69%), family planning and contraception (68%), treatment for mental health disorders (61%), antenatal care (56%), and cancer diagnosis and treatment (55%). While the WHO did not assess dermatological service delivery during the pandemic peak, we expect similar outcomes since dermatological disease falls under the NCD and cancer diagnosis categories that were surveyed.

There were marked differences across income groups in terms of NCD service provision. While 50% of low-income countries reported disruptions to services for cardiovascular (CVD) emergencies, only 17% of high-income countries reported any disruptions. Likewise, 58% of low-income countries reported disruptions to cancer treatment services compared to 26% of high-income countries. Based on these patterns, it is likely that dermatological services were also less disrupted in high-income than low-income countries.

The Disproportionate Impact of COVID-19 on Health Outcomes

The impact on health outcomes across the world is disproportionate and has been more adverse in lower-income and/or minority groups. Ethnic minorities and lower-educated and low-wage workers were more often in jobs less amenable to remote work. These workers were at higher risk of acquiring infections and/or job and income losses (OECD 2022; Kaye et al. 2021). The OECD reported that employment rates across 28 OECD countries dropped by 3.3% for migrants compared to 2.3% for natives in Q2 2020. Migrants were slower to recover employment with the discrepancy persisting into 2021 (OECD 2022). During Q2 2020 in the USA, blacks and Hispanics experienced a 10% decrease in employment compared to 7.3% for whites.

Impact of COVID-19 Vaccinations on the Global Economy

To date, there is limited data on the economic effects of vaccinations. Sandmann et al. examined the potential health and economic value of COVID-19 vaccinations in the UK and found that introducing vaccinations led to incremental monetary gains from a healthcare perspective (Sandmann et al. 2021). The finding of improved economic activity from vaccinations was corroborated by Deb et al. (Deb et al. 2022) and Agarwal and Gopinath, who found that vaccinating 40% of the world's population by 2021 cost about $50 billion, while benefits reached $9 trillion in economic gains, mostly from the reopening of economies and resumption of trade (Ogundari 2022).

Vaccines had second-order economic effects through spillovers, especially in systemically important economies such as the USA. Deb et al. found that a neighboring country's COVID-19 cases can have a significant effect on a country's own pandemic course, amplifying its own caseload despite vaccinations or containment measures (Deb et al. 2023). Although foreign COVID-19 cases could dampen a country's local economic activity, foreign COVID-19 vaccinations had a similar opposite effect because of global trade linkages. Deb et al. (2022) stress the economic importance of vaccinating a large share of the global population. Evidence from Deb et al. (2023) show that an outbreak of communicable disease among trading partners severely impacted their domestic economies. This suggests the importance of ensuring a global distribution of vaccines, especially by sharing vaccine oversupply from advanced economies with developing, underserved economies (Deb et al. 2022).

Impact of School Closures on the Global Economy

As a direct result of public infection control policies to restrict movement, many governments ordered the closing of schools. Waitzberg et al. (2022) identified two related long-run economic costs of school closures. Students whose schooling were interrupted by the pandemic faced long-term losses in income. National economies with less skilled labor forces faced lower economic growth, attenuating societal welfare. Specifically, Christakis et al. (2020) found that school closures at the end of the 2019–2020 school year were associated with 13.8 million years of life lost with OECD estimates of the costs of learning losses to be a 3% decline in lifetime earnings. A loss of a third of a year of learning resulted in a long-term economic impact of US$14 trillion (Hanushek and Woessmann 2020). The spillover on overall economic productivity is likely even higher as companies are not able to fill positions that require higher skills and thus suffer lost productivity (Psacharopoulos et al. 2021).

The notion that lost years of schooling are "not so bad if it affects everyone" is based on the erroneous assumption of fixed national economic pie and that education serves to distribute the pie. Rather, Hanushek argues that "overall economic growth effects show that higher skills of one person do not come at the expense of the economic opportunities of others." The overall economic costs of lost learning are not less if they affect all pupils equally (Hanushek and Woessmann 2020). As the economic pie shrinks, everyone is affected because lower education level attenuates national productivity, elevates financial burdens on social security systems, and reduces tax revenues for social needs (Hanushek and Woessmann 2020).

Impact of COVID-19 on Dermatology and Dermatologists

The Medscape Physician Compensation Report, an annual survey of physicians in the USA, reported a fall in annual income reported by dermatologists from US$411,000 pre-pandemic in 2019 to US$394,000 in 2020 during the peak of the pandemic. Indeed, this was reflected by the drop in average weekly dermatology patient visits, which dramatically decreased from 149.7 visits (95% CI, 139.6–159.9 visits) from mid-February 2020 to 28.2 visits (95% CI, 23.7–32.7 visits) by mid-April 2020. Weekly visits recovered to 96.5 (95% CI, 93.0–100.0 visits) by mid-May 2020 ($p < 0.0001$), accompanied by the recovery of annual income to US$428,000 by 2021. The reasons cited for loss of income in 2020 were job loss, fewer hours, and fewer patients. Non-COVID-related factors were also cited.

Impact on STI Screening and Transmission

Early COVID-19 pandemic advisories from the US Centers for Disease Control and Prevention (CDC) provided the basis for the care of sexually transmitted infections (STI). Apart from redeploying STI specialists to perform contact tracing during the pandemic and recommending deferment of routine screening visits until after the initial emergency response, the CDC also advised practitioners to consider telemedicine-based triage, syndromic management, identification of additional at-risk individuals, and referral to other clinics and pharmacies.

Changes in sexual health screening had negative outcomes on sexually transmitted infections' (STIs') prevention and control and were comparable to delays that were witnessed in cancer diagnosis and treatment (Cancino et al. 2020). Much like the early stages of cancer, STIs such as chlamydia and gonorrhea are often asymptomatic in about 80% of female cases and require age-

and sexual behavior-based screening (Pinto et al. 2021). The long-term sequelae of STIs are often unrecognized and include a higher risk of HIV infection, pelvic inflammatory disease, infertility, ectopic pregnancy, and other adverse outcomes during pregnancy.

During the COVID-19 pandemic, the shift in testing methods toward symptomatic patients compromised the identification of asymptomatic cases, particularly with chlamydia in male and female individuals. A preventive health study by Pinto et al. revealed that chlamydia and gonorrhea testing reached a nadir in early April 2020, with decreases (relative to baseline) of 59% in female patients and 63% in male patients (Pinto et al. 2021). Declines in testing were strongly associated with increases in weekly positivity rates for chlamydia ($R^2 = 0.96$) and gonorrhea ($R^2 = 0.85$). This resulted in an expected missed 27,659 (26.4%) chlamydia and 5577 (16.5%) gonorrhea cases, from March 2020 through June 2020. Other studies by Bonett et al. corroborate this finding (Bonett et al. 2021).

The implications of delayed or missed testing are critical and bear consideration for physicians in addressing the expected post-pandemic STI epidemic. It is unclear whether STI incidence declined due to COVID-19 mitigation/physical distancing methods or if only diagnosis rates and observed case load had decreased. Continued at-risk sexual behaviors with reduced emphasis on STI testing could imply an emergence of cases and disease complications over the next few years. Disparities within global marginalized communities that are disproportionately impacted and underserved continue to be most affected by STIs and require access to testing and treatment options.

Anticipating the downstream effects in the STI landscape, practitioners should capitalize on primary care and/or point-of-service care in pharmacy/health clinic settings that could provide additional pitstops for testing and treatment. Riding on existing telehealth infrastructure can see STI testing alongside home-based COVID-19 testing. Studies have shown that self-collection methods were feasible and preferred by patients (Spielberg et al. 2014).

Impact on Oncologic Dermatology

Within the healthcare industry, the sharp rise in COVID-19 infections led to a surge in demand for medical services, including the need for inpatient and ICU beds, and logistics services for testing and the distribution of personal protective equipment such as masks. Healthcare systems countered this demand for COVID-19 care by diverting/displacing resources from elective services, non-essential services, and routine ambulatory services. The impact of these decisions is unlikely to be apparent for some time, but early indications suggest that the decline of routine cancer screening is likely to show up in higher rates of late-stage cancer and mortality (Cancino et al. 2020). The more direct effects of suspension in outpatient visits also show up in the increased mortality of cancer patients due to disruptions in treatment (Han et al. 2022). In fast-moving cancers such as melanoma, there are reports that newly discovered melanomas were thicker during the pandemic period in comparison to the pre-pandemic era. This was attributed to missed routine appointments (Weston et al. 2021). Based on projections, the net economic burden due to increased late-stage melanomas with annualized average costs (including medical and prescription drug costs) would have risen from US$6.3 billion to US$7.1 billion (Mariotto et al. 2020).

Impact on Aesthetic Dermatology

As physical distancing constraints heightened, services deemed not to be an essential good faced an inevitable decline. Non-urgent dermatological surgical procedures were postponed or cancelled due to the fear of infection transmission (due to close physical contact between physician and patient), leading to fewer performed cosmetic procedures, particularly at the beginning of the COVID-19 pandemic. At the same time, social distancing measures necessitated more video calls, creating increased dissatisfaction in personal appearances. Pikoos et al. (2021) described this phenomenon to be the "Zoom effect."

Other authors including Chen et al. (2021) and Rice et al. (2020) described a type of "Zoom dysmorphia," postulating that body dysmorphia disorder could be triggered by prolonged staring and self-reflection of individuals' digitally projected image, as aspects of the technological interface and front-facing cameras in video conferencing can distort facial proportions, causing or worsening the perception of problems in one's own appearance. This illusion may exacerbate the appearance of facial dark spots and create unnecessary concern for users (Rice et al. 2021).

The focus on neck-up appearances was reflected in a survey of 134 dermatologists conducted by Rice et al.; patients were reported to be most concerned with regions from the neck up, most notably the forehead/glabella, eyes, neck, and hair. Specific concerns identified in this physician survey were upper-face wrinkles, circles/bags under the eyes, dark spots, and neck sagging. In comparison, concerns neck down were comparatively less reported.

In a cross-sectional survey of 295 respondents by Chen et al. (2021), the authors recognized that increased video calling utilization was associated with increased acceptance of aesthetic surgery. Long hours of inactivity from heightened social distancing measures also likely increased the demand for services such as liposuction.

During the COVID-19 pandemic, rapid uptake of vaccines had also been associated with the occurrence of vaccine-related adverse events in body areas where aesthetic procedures were performed. Reports of body areas that previously experienced tissue filler injections saw post-COVID vaccination complications of swelling, erythema, and tenderness in the injected sites (Aryanian et al. 2022; Michon 2021; Osmond and Kenny 2021). Acute onset of breast implant seroma after the COVID vaccine was attributed to the post-vaccination immune response (Kayser et al. 2021). Finally, though rare, botulinum toxin was reported to interact with COVID vaccines (Guo et al. 2021). Skin/soft tissue reactions are attributed to result from vaccine adjuvants, which led to autoimmune/inflammatory syndromes induced by adjuvants (ASIA) (Shoenfeld and Agmon-Levin 2011). Other postulated mechanisms included interaction between the skin ACE-2 receptors and the vaccine's spike protein (Munavalli et al. 2022).

The literature reports that vaccine-induced reactions in previously cosmetically manipulated areas can be immediate or delayed, with onset ranging from hours to 10 days after the first or second doses of the vaccines (Kalantari et al. 2022). However, latency of up to after 1 year post-procedure has also been observed (Rauso et al. 2021). Aesthetic dermatologists therefore counselled patients to space the intervals between aesthetic procedures and COVID vaccines. Although there is no current consensus on the time span for safety, a lag of 3–4 weeks seemed reasonable, with practitioners advising a longer lag for individuals with established sensitivity to fillers, those with pre-existing autoimmune disorders, or those on immunosuppressive drugs (Aryanian et al. 2022). Pre-treatments with corticosteroid and antihistamines have also been described in the literature (Aryanian et al. 2022).

Impact of Technology

The discussion of COVID-19 impact on aesthetic dermatology relates to our discussion on the impact of the pandemic on and of technology generally. The COVID-19 pandemic demonstrated that teledermatology was a valid and effective mode of treating common chronic skin conditions such as atopic dermatitis, acne, and psoriasis, on top of a myriad of other conditions that were amenable for teledermatologic care. Systematic reviews reflected that apart from AD, acne, and psoriasis, a wide range of oncodermatology cases, hair disorders, infantile hemangiomas, infective dermatoses (such as tinea and intertrigo), photodermatitis, pityriasis rosea, and pyogenic granulomas were all amenable to teledermatology (Loh et al. 2021). Conditions considered by physicians to be more challenging to manage over teledermatology included those with underlying privacy concerns such as hidradenitis suppurativa (Ruggiero et al. 2023).

Increased Use of Teledermatology

The COVID-19 pandemic saw a rapid rise in teledermatology utilization. Prior to the pandemic, teledermatology tended to be utilized for inpatient consultations, with comparatively reduced uptake in private practices due to uncertainties with reimbursement policies. In the USA, the pandemic led to increased flexibility regarding telehealth requirements implemented under the Coronavirus Aid, Relief, and Economic Security Act (Singh et al. 2022). As the Centers for Medicare and Medicaid Services eased restrictions on what constituted a "telehealth" visit, more states enacted parity laws, which reimbursed telehealth as a regular office visit (compared to 16 states which did so pre-pandemic), leading to increased private uptake of teledermatology.

The Cost-Effectiveness of Teledermatology

A medical treatment is generally considered to be cost-effective based on the following conditions: if it provides an added health benefit at an equal or lower cost than the opposing treatment, if it provides an added health benefit that is worth an additional cost, or if it provides a lesser health benefit but comes with cost savings that are more valuable than the health benefit lost.

In pre-pandemic times, analyses of the US Department of Veterans Affairs' store-and-forward program demonstrated that compared with conventional referrals, teledermatology incurred comparably lower costs to the health system and society (Wang et al. 2020). Studies also reported that in nursing home settings, store-and-forward teledermatology was a cost-effective alternative to in-person consults (Brinker et al. 2018; López-Liria et al. 2022).

In the early days of teledermatology, Eminović et al. (2010) applied cost minimization analysis, to compare teledermatology and conventional process costs per dermatology care episode. Adopting a health systems/societal perspective, total mean costs of investment, general practitio-

ner, dermatologists, out-of-pocket expenses, and employer costs were calculated. The authors conclude that teledermatology, when applied to all dermatology referrals, had a probability of 0.11 of being cost-effective to society. Interestingly, they recommended that cost savings by teledermatology could be achieved if the distance to a dermatologist is larger ($\geq$75 km) or when more in-person consultations ($\geq$37%) can be avoided. This foreshadowed the usefulness of teledermatology during the pandemic, when social distancing was mandated, and when the provision of dermatological care to less served rural areas became even more challenging.

When the mean costs of managing newly referred dermatology patients within a teledermatology triage system were compared with the conventional dermatology care model, at Zuckerberg San Francisco General Hospital and Trauma Center (ZSFG) in California, it was found that the triage system was associated with statistically significant cost savings of US$140.12 per patient over a 6-month period (June through December 2017), compared with conventional care. The mean cost per patient within the teledermatology triage model was US$559.84, and the estimated mean cost per patient within the conventional care model was US$699.96. This study reflected annual savings of US$441,378 for an estimated annual dermatology referral volume of 3150 patients. Further sensitivity analysis done in the study reported that teledermatology consultations would need to be more than four times more costly for the teledermatology triage and conventional care models to become cost neutral (Zakaria et al. 2021).

From a chronic dermatological care perspective, Parsi et al. (2012) demonstrated in a real-world study that the costs of follow-up psoriasis care done online cost 1.7 times less than in-person visits (US$315 vs. US$576). Zakaria et al. (2021) reported, via decision tree modelling, that implementing teledermatology triage systems for managing newly referred dermatology patients within a managed care setting in the USA can generate significant cost savings (in terms of personnel costs associated with primary care provider visits, dermatology clinic visits, and technological costs) for individuals.

For patients requiring chronic wound management, Le Goff-Pronost et al. (2018) affirmed the ability of teledermatology to produce cost savings in their pragmatic real-world study. The authors found that telemedicine costs were found to be €4583 less costly per patient compared with standard practice over 9 months, with shorter healing times for patients who adopted telemedicine as opposed to those who had traditional follow-ups. Other studies by Vidal-Alaball et al. (2018) and Whited et al. (2003) corroborated similar findings of cost savings to individuals suffering from a spectrum of dermatological disorders.

In terms of reduction of in-person consultations, López-Villegas et al. (2022) demonstrated that teledermatology saved more than 50% of visits with respect to face-to-face consultations within the public healthcare system. These findings were corroborated by Vidal-Alaball et al. (2018), Yang et al. (2019), and Zarca et al. (2018). In the post-pandemic era, a systematic review by López-Liria et al. (2022) compared the cost-effectiveness of two follow-up methods (face-to-face and telemedicine) used in dermatology over the last 10 years (pre- and post-pandemic), demonstrating that teledermatology consistently provided substantial savings in relation to in-person consultations.

Despite an abundance of literature documenting the merits of teledermatology, there are existing barriers to uptake. These include the lack of reliable systems for reimbursement. A large survey carried by the American Academy of Dermatology (AAD) in 2021 of 5000 participants revealed that reimbursement concerns formed the majority (69.8%) of all reported barriers (Kennedy et al. 2021). Although the pandemic has likely improved the flexibility of reimbursement for telephonic consults, reimbursement policies for store-and-forward services would similarly likely benefit from review. The comparatively low reimbursement rates for store-and-forward teledermatology consults may undervalue the time and expertise of the practicing dermatologists (Long and Chandran 2022).

Cultural and socioeconomic circumstances influence the successful uptake of teledermatology. A single-center US study demonstrated via multivariate analyses that independent factors associated with lower rates of telemedicine use were patients identifying as black/African American and having a non-English preferred language (Duan et al. 2022). In that study, patients on public insurance were also found to have significantly lower odds of telemedicine use despite widely expanded telehealth coverage by US health insurance plans. Low-income households may experience gaps in access to technology and internet connectivity that are requisites for teledermatology visits. Differential digital literacy and connectedness among cultural and socioeconomic groups create inequity in teledermatology uptake and care delivery.

Physicians need to be sensitive and remain current on patient communication preferences (Long and Chandran 2022). In a mixed-methods study of 942 participants, there was decreased willingness to use teledermatology with the easing of COVID-19 movement restrictions, and 48.5% reported a poorer experience with teledermatology compared to in-person consultations (Choi et al. 2022). Lastly, perhaps not all dermatological conditions would be met by equal enthusiasm among patients and providers when managed using teledermatology. This is particularly so if patients have skin involvement in sensitive body areas. Studies have shown that there is relative reluctance of dermatologists to use teledermatology for conditions such as hidradenitis suppurativa with mixed levels of willingness from patients (Ruggiero et al. 2023; Long et al. 2023; Okeke et al. 2022). Significant challenges cited include the need for photography of hard-to-reach or sensitive areas, difficulties in accurate assessment of disease severity, and inability to palpate lesions (Long et al. 2023).

As the world continues with COVID-19 fading into the background, healthcare delivery and needs will continue to change. While teledermatology was regarded as a "necessity" in pandemic lockdowns, the lifting of restrictions now affords individuals the option of keeping teledermatology consults, switching to face-to-face consults, or a hybrid. As previous studies in adult and pediatric teledermatology have shown, store-and-forward and live interactive teledermatology could be diagnostically comparable, while hybrid models may further help ameliorate physician-patient diagnostic and logistical difficulties (Long and Chandran 2022). Offering individuals hybrid models of care could increase acceptability of teledermatology and maintain uptake over time.

Lessons Learned and the Way Forward

In this final section, we explore the way forward by reflecting on the lessons learned, not only for the next pandemic but for the practice of dermatology. In the previous section, we discussed the impact of the pandemic on the accelerated adoption of teledermatology, which is economically the most significant impact of COVID-19 on the discipline and its providers. We also suggested that providers and healthcare facilities should not take for granted the embrace of the technology since early evidence suggests a pullback from the enthusiasm that fueled its rise. Instead, we believe that such technology and related technologies such as remote monitoring and remote testing need to be tuned to the specific presenting complaint and stage of consult. Initial consults that require visual characterization of the condition is not likely to shift to teledermatology in any meaningful way, absent the restrictions imposed by social distancing mandates. Having said this, we would be remiss when discussing the way forward without first acknowledging the impact and implications of countries relaxing their COVID-19 infection control policies, including the extreme case of China.

China's Rapid Reopening and Beyond

Rapid reopening, consisting of the sudden stoppage of testing, and social distancing and isolation measures, combined with mass infections (800 M+ by some estimates) and the risk of new variants arising from a differentially vaccinated population, threaten to reignite COVID-19 in antigenically naïve populations through the sudden reopening of international travel and takedown of quarantine requirements. Reopening of factories and return to work may see the rise in GDP and easing of supply chain problems experienced during the zero-COVID period. In this situation, the impact on dermatology services and practice is likely to be greatest on elective cosmetic procedures. However, 3 years of lockdowns may have created hesitancy among the population, which may need time to regain the confidence for discretionary consumption of healthcare to pre-pandemic levels.

While the rest of the world worried about the "great resignation," the mass dropout of workers from the labor force, China will likely experience the reverse. Workers who lost their jobs would likely hope to return to work as soon as possible. The millions of health workers employed to staff the hundreds of thousands of testing facilities, now finding themselves jobless, will need placement in other industries. A voracious appetite for jobs would likely buttress the country's factory output and supply chains.

The economic implications of China's sudden reopening extend globally. The Hong Kong and Shanghai Banking Corporation (HSBC) believes that, as a major player in the global economy, China's GDP by the first quarter of 2024 may be 10% higher than it would have been in the first 3 months of 2023. This would roughly translate to China accounting for two-thirds of global growth in that period (The Economist 2023).

Export markets serving China's pent-up demand would likely be boosted. These include traditional exporters like Chile, and Brazil, that fill China's appetite for commodities. With outbound travel lifted, tourism is anticipated to spike across the world. Thailand, a popular destination, could enjoy a three-percentage-point boost to growth as China fully reopens (The Economist 2023). Reopening would aid Hong Kong in the export and tourism markets, which may see a boost to GDP by almost 8% (The Economist 2023).

Over time, China's recovery may also lead to other undesirable side effects. In other big economies, the binding constraint on economic expansion is monetary policy, as central banks raise interest rates to suppress inflation. With reopening, China's demand for commodities and metals may raise global demand and increase price pressures, with central banks around the world adopting tighter monetary policy to offset the inflationary threat. In such a scenario, the impact of China's reopening on the rest of the world might show up not in higher growth but in higher inflation or interest rates. In November 2022, Goldman Sachs reckoned the price of copper would increase to US$9000 per ton within 12 months and has by January 2023 speculated that the equivalent price would reach US$11,000 (The Economist 2023; Mining.com 2023).

Lessons from Singapore's Model of Pandemic Management

Singapore has been lauded to be one of the most effective nations in combating the pandemic and curbing disease spread. This was made possible through governmental strategies in the following areas. Firstly, liberal testing was performed on the population, with implementation of contact tracing to arrest the chain of transmission. Public Health Preparedness Clinics (PHPCs) were activated across the country to dispense medications, administer vaccinations, and provide subsidized treatments. They served as intermediaries between the community and hospitals, to improve efficiency in healthcare delivering and alleviating stress on hospitals (Liao et al. 2022). Together with infection control, Singapore was among the first countries to adopt mRNA vaccines on 30 December 2020, which it pushed to the population through mandates and incentives.

Beginning with healthcare workers who were considered most at risk, the vaccination campaign swiftly reached senior citizens and vulnerable populations and eventually included the young adult population and children. Within a year, by 29 December 2021, 87% of the population had been fully vaccinated, defined as receiving two shots of the mRNA vaccine at the time (Liao et al. 2022). Due to high vaccination rates, vaccination-

differentiated mobility measures could be introduced in early 2021, where vaccinated individuals enjoyed high degrees of freedom for daily activities, while unvaccinated individuals continued to experience mobility restrictions.

Transparency from the Singapore government regarding the COVID-19 situation fostered public willingness to cooperate and adhere to infection control policies. This was facilitated over press releases, situation reports, and the Gov.sg WhatsApp channel which disseminated important daily public updates (Kuguyo et al. 2020). Such measures came with a cost, such as the government had to reallocate 10 years of planned infrastructure improvement, such as water security, expenditures toward COVID-19 response. The long-term impact of delayed or reprioritized infrastructure spending is unknown but is an area of concern for policymakers.

Building Resiliency for Healthcare and Dermatology

The COVID-19 pandemic exposed the weaknesses of health systems' preparedness and responses across the world, compelling countries to rapidly adjust their public health measures. The World Health Organization (WHO) Regional Office for Europe issued some key takeaway points including the following. Health security could be improved by prioritizing known capacity gaps. The pandemic highlighted the strengths of many aspects of the 2005 International Health Regulations (IHR) and existing frameworks such as the Cartagena Protocol on Biosafety and the Fair and Equitable Sharing of Benefits Arising from their Utilization to the Convention on Biological Diversity (Europe WHOROf 2021).

In the context of COVID-19, severe and widespread as it may have been, it is also important to draw from lessons learned from previous infectious disease outbreaks (e.g., Ebola, SARS, MERS-CoV, and Zika). Governments should address the gaps identified in the IHR (2005) and existing frameworks so that they can mount a robust response in future pandemics (Kluge et al. 2018). In particular, the WHO reminded policymakers that the IHR (2005) core capacities need to be fortified by capabilities and competencies at all levels of government, by healthcare providers, and by communities, noting that early pandemic responses were slower than the spread of the virus (Europe WHOROf 2021). For example, the prepositioning of PPE, testing capacity, and public health communications need to be taken seriously while balancing the costs of doing so against national budgetary priorities.

The WHO lists some strategies for emergency preparedness and readiness going forward in their 71st virtual session in 2021 (Europe WHOROf 2021). For dermatologists, key learning points include the need to be ready for medical countermeasures. The WHO suggests that systems should ensure "Unhindered access to diagnostics and care for all, including the marginalized and vulnerable." During the pandemic, underserved groups were most affected by the limited access to diagnostics (such as in STI management), which represents an important area of focus for dermatologists. The experience from COVID-19 suggests that teledermatology is an area with immense potential and may serve to reduce disparities in healthcare access in many underserved and marginalized communities (Maddukuri et al. 2021). Effort should be invested in streamlining the expansion of teledermatology services, improving implementation, such that the service could be more equitable among all communities. An explicit consideration of the economics of teledermatology, and telemedicine in general, with a focus on cost-effectiveness and the role that government can play in enhancing the technology infrastructure to support wide deployment cannot be understated. The good news is that, as we have shown in this chapter, prior studies have pointed the way to building the appropriate economic models to support the implementation policies.

References

Al Mutair A, Layqah L, Alhassan B, Alkhalifah S, Almossabeh M, AlSaleh T, et al. Estimated cost of treating hospitalized COVID-19 patients in Saudi Arabia. Sci Rep. 2022;12(1):21487.

Aryanian Z, Ehsani A, Razavi Z, Hamzelou S, Mohseni Afshar Z, Hatami P. The COVID-19 pandemic and its impact on esthetic dermatology. J Cosmet Dermatol. 2022;21(12):6557–61.

Bonett S, Petsis D, Dowshen N, Bauermeister J, Wood SM. The impact of the COVID-19 pandemic on sexually transmitted infection/human immunodeficiency virus testing among adolescents in a large pediatric primary care network. Sex Transm Dis. 2021;48(7):e91–e3.

Brinker TJ, Hekler A, von Kalle C, Schadendorf D, Esser S, Berking C, et al. Teledermatology: comparison of store-and-forward versus live interactive video conferencing. J Med Internet Res. 2018;20(10):e11871.

Cai Y, Kwek S, Tang SSL, Saffari SE, Lum E, Yoon S, et al. Impact of the COVID-19 pandemic on a tertiary care public hospital in Singapore: resources and economic costs. J Hosp Infect. 2022;121:1–8.

Cancino RS, Su Z, Mesa R, Tomlinson GE, Wang J. The impact of COVID-19 on cancer screening: challenges and opportunities. JMIR Cancer. 2020;6(2):e21697.

Chen J, Chow A, Fadavi D, Long C, Sun AH, Cooney CM, et al. The zoom boom: how video calling impacts attitudes towards aesthetic surgery in the COVID-19 era. Aesthet Surg J. 2021;41(12):NP2086.

Cheng E. China sets GDP target of 'around 5.5%' for 2022. CNBC; 2022. https://www.cnbc.com/2022/03/05/china-on-deck-to-reveal-its-2022-gdp-target.html.

China Economic Quarterly Q1 2020—PwC CN. https://www.pwccn.com/en/research-and-insights/china-economic-quarterly-q1-2020.html.

Choi ECE, Heng LW, Tan SY, Phan P, Chandran NS. Factors influencing use and perceptions of teledermatology: a mixed-methods study of 942 participants. JAAD Int. 2022;6:97–103.

Christakis DA, Van Cleve W, Zimmerman FJ. Estimation of US Children's educational attainment and years of life lost associated with primary school closures during the coronavirus disease 2019 pandemic. JAMA Netw Open. 2020;3(11):e2028786.

Deb P, Furceri D, Jimenez D, Kothari S, Ostry JD, Tawk N. The effects of COVID-19 vaccines on economic activity. Swiss J Econ Stat. 2022;158(1):3. https://doi.org/10.1186/s41937-021-00082-0

Deb P, Furceri D, Jimenez D, Kothari S, Ostry JD, Tawk N. Determinants of COVID-19 vaccine rollouts and their effects on health outcomes. Appl Health Econ Health Policy. 2023;21:71–89.

DeMartino JK, Swallow E, Goldschmidt D, Yang K, Viola M, Radtke T, et al. Direct health care costs associated with COVID-19 in the United States. J Manag Care Spec Pharm. 2022;28(9):936–47.

Duan GY, Ruiz De Luzuriaga AM, Schroedl LM, Rosenblatt AE. Disparities in telemedicine use during the COVID-19 pandemic among pediatric dermatology patients. Pediatr Dermatol. 2022;39(4):520–7.

Eminović N, Dijkgraaf MG, Berghout RM, Prins AH, Bindels PJE, de Keizer NF. A cost minimisation analysis in teledermatology: model-based approach. BMC Health Serv Res. 2010;10(1):251.

Europe WHOROf. Response to the COVID-19 pandemic: lessons learned to date from the WHO European region. 2021.

European Observatory on Health S, Policies, World Health Organization. Regional Office for E. Managing health systems on a seesaw: balancing the delivery of essential health services whilst responding to COVID-19. Eur Secur. 2020;26(2):63–7.

Gereffi G. What does the COVID-19 pandemic teach us about global value chains? The case of medical supplies. J Int Bus Policy. 2020;3(3):287–301.

Granovetter M. Economic action and social structure: the problem of embeddedness. Am J Sociol. 1985;91(3):481–510.

Guo X, Li T, Wang Y, Jin X. Sub-acute hypersensitive reaction to botulinum toxin type a following Covid-19 vaccination: case report and literature review. Medicine (Baltimore). 2021;100(49):e27787.

Hafner M, Yerushalmi E, Fays C, Dufresne E, Van Stolk C. COVID-19 and the cost of vaccine nationalism. Rand Health Q. 2022;9(4):1.

Han S, Zhuang Q, Chiang J, Tan SH, Chua GWY, Xie C, et al. Impact of cancer diagnoses on the outcomes of patients with COVID-19: a systematic review and meta-analysis. BMJ Open. 2022;12(2):e044661.

Hanushek EA, Woessmann L. The economic impacts of learning losses. Paris: OECD; 2020.

Kalantari Y, Aryanian Z, Mirahmadi SM, Alilou S, Hatami P, Goodarzi A. A systematic review on COVID-19 vaccination and cosmetic filler reactions: a focus on case studies and original articles. J Cosmet Dermatol. 2022;21(7).

Kates J, Cox C, Michaud J. How much could COVID-19 vaccines cost the U.S. after commercialization? 2022. https://www.kff.org/coronavirus-covid-19/issue-brief/how-much-could-covid-19-vaccines-cost-the-u-s-after-commercialization/.

Kaye AD, Okeagu CN, Pham AD, Silva RA, Hurley JJ, Arron BL, et al. Economic impact of COVID-19 pandemic on healthcare facilities and systems: international perspectives. Best Pract Res Clin Anaesthesiol. 2021;35(3):293–306.

Kayser F, Fourneau H, Mazy OC, Mazy S. Breast implant seroma: a SARS-CoV-2 mRNA vaccine side effect. J Clin Ultrasound. 2021;49(9):984–6.

Kennedy J, Arey S, Hopkins Z, Tejasvi T, Farah R, Secrest AM, et al. Dermatologist perceptions of Teledermatology implementation and future use after COVID-19: demographics, barriers, and insights. JAMA Dermatol. 2021;157(5):595–7.

Kluge H, Martín-Moreno JM, Emiroglu N, Rodier G, Kelley E, Vujnovic M, et al. Strengthening global health security by embedding the international health regulations requirements into national health systems. BMJ Glob Health. 2018;3(Suppl 1): e000656.

Kuguyo O, Kengne AP, Dandara C. Singapore COVID-19 pandemic response as a successful model framework for low-resource health care settings in Africa? OMICS. 2020;24(8):470–8.

Le Goff-Pronost M, Mourgeon B, Blanchère JP, Teot L, Benateau H, Dompmartin A. Real-world clinical evaluation and costs of telemedicine for chronic wound management. Int J Technol Assess Health Care. 2018;34(6):567–75.

Liao Z, Menon D, Zhang L, Lim Y-J, Li W, Li X, et al. Management of the COVID-19 pandemic in Singapore from 2020 to 2021: a revisit. Reports. 2022;5(3):35.

Loh CH, Chong Tam SY, Oh CC. Teledermatology in the COVID-19 pandemic: a systematic review. JAAD Int. 2021;5:54–64.

Long V, Chandran NS. A glance at the practice of pediatric Teledermatology pre- and post-COVID-19: narrative review. JMIR Dermatol. 2022;5(2):e34228.

Long V, Choi EC-E, Chen Z, Kamil MAA, Rajagopalan M, McMeniman E, et al. Dermatologists' perceptions of the use of teledermatology in managing hidradenitis Suppurativa: survey study. JMIR Dermatol. 2023;6:e43910.

López-Liria R, Valverde-Martínez M, López-Villegas A, Bautista-Mesa RJ, Vega-Ramírez FA, Peiró S, et al. Teledermatology versus face-to-face dermatology: an analysis of cost-effectiveness from eight studies from Europe and the United States. Int J Environ Res Public Health. 2022;19(5):2534.

Lopez-Villegas A, Bautista-Mesa RJ, Acosta-Robles P, Hidalgo-Serrano D, Aguirre-Ortega FJ, Castellano-Ortega MA, et al. Analysis of healthcare costs incurred in regional hospitals in Andalusia (Spain) during the COVID-19 pandemic. Int J Environ Res Public Health. 2022;19(23).

Maddukuri S, Patel J, Lipoff JB. Teledermatology addressing disparities in health care access: a review. Curr Dermatol Rep. 2021;10(2):40–7.

Mariotto AB, Enewold L, Zhao J, Zeruto CA, Yabroff KR. Medical care costs associated with cancer survivorship in the United States. Cancer Epidemiol Biomarkers Prev. 2020;29(7):1304–12.

McClellan M, Rajkumar R, Couch M, Holder D, Pham M, Long P, et al. Health care payers COVID-19 impact assessment: lessons learned and compelling needs. In: NAM Perspectives. Discussion Paper. Washington, DC: National Academy of Medicine; 2021.

Mena Lora A, Ali M, Spencer S, Takhsh E, Krill C, Bleasdale S. Cost of personal protective equipment during the first wave of COVID-19. Antimicrob Stewardship Healthc Epidemiol. 2021;1(S1):s49.

Michon A. Hyaluronic acid soft tissue filler delayed inflammatory reaction following COVID-19 vaccination - a case report. J Cosmet Dermatol. 2021;20(9):2684–90.

Mining.com. Copper rises while Goldman predicts prices reaching $11,000 in a year. 2023. https://www.mining.com/copper-rises-while-goldman-predicts-prices-reaching-11000-in-a-year/.

Munavalli GG, Guthridge R, Knutsen-Larson S, Brodsky A, Matthew E, Landau M. COVID-19/SARS-CoV-2 virus spike protein-related delayed inflammatory reaction to hyaluronic acid dermal fillers: a challenging clinical conundrum in diagnosis and treatment. Arch Dermatol Res. 2022;314(1):1–15.

OECD. The unequal impact of COVID-19: a spotlight on frontline workers, migrants and racial/ethnic minorities. 2022. https://www.oecd.org/coronavirus/policy-responses/the-unequal-impact-of-covid-19-a-spotlight-on-frontline-workers-migrants-and-racial-ethnic-minorities-f36e931e/.

Ogundari K. The COVID-19 vaccine rollout and labor market recovery in the U.S: a note. SN Bus Econ. 2022;2(7):75.

Okeke CAV, Shipman WD, Perry JD, Kerns ML, Okoye GA, Byrd AS. Treating hidradenitis suppurativa during the COVID-19 pandemic: teledermatology exams of sensitive body areas. J Dermatolog Treat. 2022;33(2):1163–4.

Osmond A, Kenny B. Reaction to dermal filler following COVID-19 vaccination. J Cosmet Dermatol. 2021;20(12):3751–2.

Parsi K, Chambers CJ, Armstrong AW. Cost-effectiveness analysis of a patient-centered care model for management of psoriasis. J Am Acad Dermatol. 2012;66(4):563–70.

Pikoos TD, Buzwell S, Sharp G, Rossell SL. The zoom effect: exploring the impact of video calling on appearance dissatisfaction and interest in aesthetic treatment during the COVID-19 pandemic. Aesthet Surg J. 2021;41(12):NP2066.

Pinto CN, Niles JK, Kaufman HW, Marlowe EM, Alagia DP, Chi G, et al. Impact of the COVID-19 pandemic on chlamydia and gonorrhea screening in the U.S. Am J Prev Med. 2021;61(3):386–93.

Premier Data: The State of PPE Supply One Year into COVID-19. 2021. https://www.premierinc.com/newsroom/blog/premier-data-the-state-of-ppe-supply-one-year-in-to-covid-19.

Psacharopoulos G, Collis V, Patrinos HA, Vegas E. The COVID-19 cost of school closures in earnings and income across the world. Comp Educ Rev. 2021;65(2):271–87.

Rauso R, Lo Giudice G, Zerbinati N, Nicoletti GF, Fragola R, Tartaro G. Adverse events following COVID-19 vaccine in patients previously injected with facial filler: scoping review and case report. Appl Sci. 2021;11(22):10888.

Rice SM, Graber E, Kourosh AS. A pandemic of dysmorphia: "zooming" into the perception of our appearance. Fac Plast Surg Aesthet Med. 2020;22(6):401–2.

Rice SM, Siegel JA, Libby T, Graber E, Kourosh AS. Zooming into cosmetic procedures during the COVID-19 pandemic: the provider's perspective. Int J Womens Dermatol. 2021;7(2):213–6.

Richards F, Kodjamanova P, Chen X, Li N, Atanasov P, Bennetts L, et al. Economic burden of COVID-19: a systematic review. Clinicoecon Outcomes Res. 2022;14:293–307.

Ruggiero A, Marasca C, Fabbrocini G, Villani A, Martora F. Teledermatology in the management of hidradenitis suppurativa: should we improve this service? J Cosmet Dermatol. 2023;22:677.

Sandmann FG, Davies NG, Vassall A, Edmunds WJ, Jit M. The potential health and economic value of SARS-CoV-2 vaccination alongside physical distancing in the UK: a transmission model-based future scenario analysis and economic evaluation. Lancet Infect Dis. 2021;21(7):962–74.

Shoenfeld Y, Agmon-Levin N. 'ASIA'—autoimmune/inflammatory syndrome induced by adjuvants. J Autoimmun. 2011;36(1):4–8.

Singh J, Albertson A, Sillerud B. Telemedicine during COVID-19 crisis and in post-pandemic/post-vaccine world-historical overview, current utilization, and innovative practices to increase utilization. Healthcare (Basel). 2022;10(6):1041.

Smith E. UK enters recession after GDP plunged by a record 20.4% in the second quarter. 2023. https://www.cnbc.com/2020/08/12/uk-gdp-plunged-by-a-record-20point4percent-in-the-second-quarter.html.

Spielberg F, Levy V, Lensing S, Chattopadhyay I, Venkatasubramanian L, Acevedo N, et al. Fully integrated e-services for prevention, diagnosis, and treatment of sexually transmitted infections: results of a 4-county study in California. Am J Public Health. 2014;104(12):2313–20.

The Economist. What the great reopening means for China—and the world. 2023. https://www.economist.com/finance-and-economics/2023/01/02/what-the-great-reopening-means-for-china-and-the-world.

The Federal Response to COVID-19: USAspending.gov; 2022. https://www.usaspending.gov/disaster/covid-19?publicLaw=all.

U.S. Bureau of Economic Analysis (BEA). Gross Domestic Product, 2nd Quarter 2020 (Advance Estimate) and Annual Update. https://www.bea.gov/news/2020/gross-domestic-product-2nd-quarter-2020-advance-estimate-and-annual-update.

Vidal-Alaball J, Garcia Domingo JL, Garcia Cuyàs F, Mendioroz Peña J, Flores Mateo G, Deniel Rosanas J, et al. A cost savings analysis of asynchronous teledermatology compared to face-to-face dermatology in Catalonia. BMC Health Serv Res. 2018;18(1):650.

Waitzberg R, Gerkens S, Dimova A, Bryndová L, Vrangbæk K, Jervelund SS, et al. Balancing financial incentives during COVID-19: a comparison of provider payment adjustments across 20 countries. Health Policy. 2022;126(5):398–407.

Wang RH, Barbieri JS, Nguyen HP, Stavert R, Forman HP, Bolognia JL, et al. Clinical effectiveness and cost-effectiveness of teledermatology: where are we now, and what are the barriers to adoption? J Am Acad Dermatol. 2020;83(1):299–307.

Weston GK, Jeong HS, Mu EW, Polsky D, Meehan SA. Impact of COVID-19 on melanoma diagnosis. Melanoma Res. 2021;31(3):280–1.

Whited JD, Datta S, Hall RP, Foy ME, Marbrey LE, Grambow SC, et al. An economic analysis of a store and forward teledermatology consult system. Telemed J E Health. 2003;9(4):351–60.

World Economic Outlook. Real GDP growth. 2022. https://www.imf.org/external/datamapper/NGDP_RPCH@WEO.

Yang X, Barbieri JS, Kovarik CL. Cost analysis of a store-and-forward teledermatology consult system in Philadelphia. J Am Acad Dermatol. 2019;81(3):758–64.

Yun E, Ko HJ, Ahn B, Lee H, Jang WM, Lee JY. Expanding medical surge capacity to counteract COVID-19: South Korea's medical fee adjustment through the National Health Insurance System. Risk Manag Healthc Policy. 2022;15:2031–42.

Zakaria A, Miclau TA, Maurer T, Leslie KS, Amerson E. Cost minimization analysis of a Teledermatology triage system in a managed care setting. JAMA Dermatol. 2021;157(1):52–8.

Zarca K, Charrier N, Mahé E, Guibal F, Carton B, Moreau F, et al. Tele-expertise for diagnosis of skin lesions is cost-effective in a prison setting: a retrospective cohort study of 450 patients. PloS One. 2018;13(9):e0204545.

Index

© The Editor(s) (if applicable) and The Author(s), under exclusive license to Springer Nature
Switzerland AG 2023
H. H. Oon, C. L. Goh (eds.), *COVID-19 in Dermatology*, Updates in Clinical Dermatology,
https://doi.org/10.1007/978-3-031-45586-5

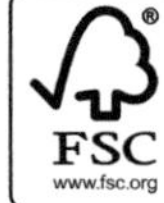

MIX
Papier aus verantwortungsvollen Quellen
Paper from responsible sources
FSC® C105338

If you have any concerns about our products,
you can contact us on
ProductSafety@springernature.com

In case Publisher is established outside the EU,
the EU authorized representative is:
Springer Nature Customer Service Center GmbH
Europaplatz 3, 69115 Heidelberg, Germany

Printed by Libri Plureos GmbH
in Hamburg, Germany